Career Planning for Nurses

DATE DUE

About the
ONLINE COMPANION™

Delmar Publishers offers a series of Online Companions™. Through the Delmar site on the World Wide Web, the Online Companions™ let readers access online companions that update the information in the books.

The *Nurse's Guide to Career Planning* Online Companion™ provides links to various up-to-date resources on the internet, including discussion groups, résumé and career tips and resources, and much more.

To access the site simply point your browser to:

http://www.delmar.com

Online Services

Delmar Online
To access a wide variety of Delmar products and services on the World Wide Web, point your browser to:
      http://www.delmar.com
      or email: info@delmar.com

thomson.com
To access International Thomson Publishing's home site for information on more than 34 publishers and 20,000 products, point your browser to:
      http://www.thomson.com
      or email: findit@kiosk.thomson.com

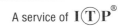

A service of I(T)P®

Career Planning for Nurses

Bette Case, PhD, RN, C

Delmar Publishers

I(T)P™ An International Thomson Publishing Company

Albany • Bonn • Boston • Cincinnati • Detroit • London • Madrid • Melbourne
Mexico City • New York • Pacific Grove • Paris • San Francisco • Singapore • Tokyo
Toronto • Washington

NOTICE TO THE READER

Delmar Staff
  Publisher: William Brottmiller
  Assistant Editor: Hilary A. Everson-Schrauf
  Project Editor: Judith Boyd Nelson
  Production Coordinator: Barbara A. Bullock
  Art/Design Coordinator: Carol D. Keohane

COPYRIGHT © 1997
By Delmar Publishers
a division of International Thomson Publishing Inc.

The ITP logo is a trademark under license.

Printed in the United States of America

For information, contact:

Delmar Publishers
3 Columbia Circle, Box 15015
Albany, New York 12212-5015

International Thomson Publishing Europe
Berkshire House 168-173
High Holborn
London, WC1V7AA
England

Thomas Nelson Australia
102 Dodds Street
South Melbourne, 3205
Victoria, Australia

Nelson Canada
1120 Birchmont Road
Scarborough, Ontario
Canada M1K 5G4

International Thomson Editores
Campos Eliseos 385, Piso 7
Col Polanco
11560 Mexico D F Mexico

International Thomson Publishing GmbH
Königswinterer Strasse 418
53227 Bonn
Germany

International Thomson Publishing Asia
221 Henderson Road
#05-10 Henderson Building
Singapore 0315

International Thomson Publishing—Japan
Hirakawacho Kyowa Building, 3F
2-2-1 Hirakawacho
Chiyoda-ku, Tokyo 102
Japan

1 2 3 4 5 6 7 8 9 10 XXX 02 01 00 99 98 97 96

Library of Congress Cataloging-in-Publication Data
Career planning for nurses/ [edited by] Bette Case.
    p. cm.
  Includes bibliographical references and index.
  ISBN 0-8273-7165-9
  1. Nursing—Vocational guidance.   I. Case, Bette.
  [DNLM: 1. Career Mobility.   2. Nursing.   3. Vocational Guidance.
WY 16 C2709 1997]
RT82.C285 1997
610.73' 06' 9—dc20
DNLM/DLC
for Library of Congress
                                                                96-21218
                                                                    CIP

Table of Contents

Preface   ix

Contributors   x

Acknowledgements   xii

Introduction   xvii

Chapter 1   **Where Are You Taking Your Career?**   1
Introduction 1 • Economic, Societal, and Industrial Trends 4 • Seizing Career Opportunities 9 • Public Perception of Nurses 16 • Strategies That Work Best 17 • Summary 27 • References 27 • Appendix 1.1 The National Student Nurses' Association, Inc. 29

Chapter 2   **Changing Your Direction**   35
Introduction 35 • What is a Career? 37 • The Career Path 38 • Myths About Nursing Careers 39 • Knowing Your Wants and Needs 41 • Motivators 44 • Sources of Help 45 • Hindrances 51 • Ways to Succeed 52 • Summary 56 • References 57

Chapter 3   **Managing Your Career**   59
Introduction 59 • Assessing the Market 60 • Locating Information 61 • Networking 61 • Self-Assessment 62 • Profiting from Your Résumé 66 • Interviewing 69 • Finding Greater Satisfaction in Your Current Position 73 • An Ongoing Plan for Self-Management 75 • Summary 76 • References 76 • Appendix 3.1 Career Mapping Exercise 77 • Appendix 3.2 Sample Basic Résumé 80 • Appendix 3.3 Sample Résumé for Advanced Skills 82 • Appendix 3.4 Sample Cover Letter 85

Chapter 4   **Creating Your Own Job: Using Nonlinear Strategies to Reach Your Career Goals**   87
Introduction 87 • Linear Career Paths 89 • Nonlinear Career Paths 90 • Your Current Place on the Linear-Nonlinear Continuum 92 • Before Practicing Nonlinear Thinking 98 • Techniques for Practicing Nonlinear Thinking 100 • Exercise 4.1: What Can You Do With a . . . ? 100 • Exercise 4.2: List That Career! 100 • Exercise 4.3: What's Your Angle? 101 • Exercise 4.4: Putting It Together 101 • Keeping the Creative Juices Flowing 102 • Some Final Words 103 • Summary 103 • References 103

Chapter 5   Nursing Informatics   **105**
Introduction 105 • Nurse As Communicator 106 • Nurse As Programmer 110 • The Nurse As Vendor Representative 112 • Other Opportunities in Informatics 114 • Educational Preparation 115 • Nursing on the Internet 116 • Resources for Further Information 117 • Summary 117 • References 117

Chapter 6   The RN in Redesigned Organizations   **119**
Introduction 119 • Implications of Redesign for the RN 120 • Characteristics and Skills Needed in Redesigned Organizations 126 • The Restructuring Controversy 129 • Resources for Further Information 130 • Summary 131 • References 132

Chapter 7   Nurse Case Management   **133**
Introduction 133 • Managed Care 133 • The Opportunities for Nurses 135 • The Process 135 • Nurse Case Management Models 135 • Attributes of the Nurse Case Manager 153 • Finding or Marketing Case Management Work 156 • Resources for Further Information 157 • Summary 159 • References 159

Chapter 8   The Nurse Practitioner, Nurse Anesthetist, and Nurse Midwife   **161**
Introduction 161 • Nurse Practitioners 162 • The Nurse Anesthetist 166 • The Nurse Midwife 169 • Contributions to Health Care 172 • Issues 172 • Resources for Further Information 175 • Summary 175 • References 176

Chapter 9   The Clinical Nurse Specialist   **179**
Introduction 179 • An Overview of the Specialty 180 • CNS Roles 181 • Characteristics of the CNS 190 • CNS Practice Models 192 • Learning More About a CNS Career 196 • CNS As a Career Choice 197 • Summary 199 • References 200

Chapter 10   The Nurse-Manager-to-Executive Track   **203**
Introduction 203 • Changes in Management Competencies 204 • Self-Assessment for the Management Track 209 • Seven Tips for a Successful Management Career 212 • Summary 217 • References 217

Chapter 11   Home Health Care   **219**
Introduction 219 • The Growth of Home Health Care 220 • Differences Between Hospital and Home Care Nursing 222 • Roles and Variations in Home Health Nursing 226 • The Nursing Process in Home Care 231 • Qualifications 232 • Resources for Further Information 233 • Summary 233 • References 233

Chapter 12 **Occupational Health Nursing, Employee Health, Nursing and Case Management in the Workplace** 235

Introduction 235 • Tracing the Subspecialties 236 • Professional and Certification Associations 236 • Historical Interrelationships Among OHN, EHN, and CM 239 • OHN and EHN 242 • CM in the Workplace 253 • Future Opportunities in OHN, EHN, and CM 256 • Summary 257 • References 257

Chapter 13 **Entrepreneurial Nursing** 259

Introduction 259 • Defining Entrepreneurial Nursing 260 • Being an Entrepreneur 263 • Getting Started As an Entrepreneur 268 • Entrepreneurial Interaction and Collaboration 281 • Special Concerns in Entrepreneurial Practice 286 • Resources for Further Information 287 • Summary 287 • References 287

Chapter 14 **Legal Roles** 289

Introduction 289 • The Nurse Legal Consultant 290 • The Nurse Risk Manager 292 • The Nurse Attorney 295 • Summary 298 • References 298

Chapter 15 **Nursing Opportunities in the Public Sector: Military and Public Service** 299

Introduction 299 • Military Nursing 300 • PHS 302 • Federal Civic Service System 304 • Basic Requirements 306 • Colleagues 308 • Geographic Variations and Opportunities 310 • Educational Opportunities 312 • Other Benefits 313 • Resources for Further Information 315 • Summary 316

Chapter 16 **Educator Roles** 317

Introduction 317 • The Educator Role Today 318 • Trends in Society, Health Care, and Education 318 • The Educational Process 320 • Adult Learning Principles 323 • Attributes and Qualifications of the Effective Educator 324 • Differences Among Educator Roles 326 • Sampling Educator Roles 335 • Summary 336 • References 337

Chapter 17 **Taking Off with Your Career** 339

Introduction 339 • Ways Nurses Are Working in the 1990s 340 • New Words, New Ways of Thinking 342 • Strategies for Success 343 • If You're a New Graduate 346 • If Your Job Has Been Eliminated 347 • If You've Been Out of Nursing for a While 347 • More Paths to Explore 348 • Summary 351 • References 351

Index 353

DEDICATION

For the first nurse I knew, my mother, Marion S. Barnes, R.N. and for the memory of my father, Earle E. Barnes, Jr., M.D., with whom she practiced.

PREFACE

If you are considering a career in nursing, preparing for a career in nursing, or practicing nursing, *Career Planning for Nurses* was written for you. The contributors and I reflected on our own experiences as well as spoke to nurse colleagues who practice many different dimensions of nursing in many different parts of the country and the world. We deeply appreciate the contributions of those colleagues whom we recognize in the **Acknowledgments**. We also recognize many others who have enriched our professional lives and aided us in formulating the information, thoughts, and advice that we share in this book. The book represents the experiences and careers of over one hundred nurses.

The book places nursing career planning in the context of trends in society, industry and healthcare. We describe changes in nursing roles that effect all nurses—even those who do not choose to seek new opportunities. We also project and predict future developments in various dimensions of nursing practice.

You will discover helpful insights for career planning as you complete the self-tests, evaluation tools and exercises, and read the vignettes. You will also find strategies for marketing yourself and for coping with and thriving in the changing healthcare environment.

The chapters focus on many different types of nursing career options. They include information about work environment, relationships with other health professionals, educational requirements and personal dispositions that fit well in various career paths. Sources of further information accompany each chapter.

The contributing authors and I present this book with a great deal of pride in our profession and with confidence in the value and future evolution of nursing in our healthcare system and in our society. We hope the book will help you find a personally fulfilling path to participating in the future of our profession.

Bette Case, PhD, RN, C
Chicago, Illinois
1996

Contributors

Beth A. Bongard, MA
Prinicipal
Bongard-Ross, Organizational
    Development
Olympia Fields, Illinois

Nancy Brent, JD, MS, RN
Health Law and Legal Representation
Chicago, Illinois

Bette Case, PhD, RN, C
Independent Consultant
Chicago, Illinois

Judith A. Combs, RN, BSN
Nurse Case Manager, Child and Family
    Services
Carondelet Health Services
Tucson, Arizona

Joyce P. Crutchfield, PhD, RN, CNP
Associate Professor
University of Nebraska Medical Center
    College
Lincoln, Nebraska

Kay Davis, EdD, RN
Past President, National Nurses in
    Business Association
Owner, Director
NES
Marina del Rey, California

Jean B. Doerge, RN, MS
Assistant to Vice President of Care
    Continuum
Carondelet Health Services
Tucson, Arizona

Benne Druckenmiller, RN, BSN
New Canaan, Connecticut
formerly Clinical Supervisor, Home
    Care/Hospice Department
Holy Cross Hospital
Silver Spring, Maryland

Elizabeth J. Falter, RN, BS, MS, CNAA
President, Falter & Associates
Croton-on-Hudson, New York

Ann Gunnett, MSN, RN
Assistant Professor
Department of Acute and
    Long-Term Care
University of Maryland at Baltimore
Baltimore, Maryland

Margaret Hadley, RN, MSN
Assistant Director, Home Care/Hospice
    Department
Holy Cross Hospital
Silver Spring, Maryland

Sandra A. Holmes, MSN, RN, Captain,
    Nurse Corps, US Navy (Ret.)
Staff Development Consultant
Escondido, California

Audrey L. Klopp, PhD, RN, CS, ET,
    NHA
Director of Nursing
Plymouth Place
LaGrange Park, Illinois

Vicky A. Mahn, RN, MS, CCRN
System Associate for Quality and
    Clinical Case Management
Carondelet Health Care Corporation
Tucson, Arizona

Diane J. Mancino, EdD, RN, CAE
Executive Director
National Student Nurses'
    Association, Inc.
New York, New York

Dennis Ondrejka, RN, MS, COHN
Manager of Employee Health and
    Infection Control
National Jewish Hospital
Denver, Colorado

Rose Pfefferbaum, PhD, RN
Director of Gerontology
Phoenix College
Phoenix, Arizona

Joan E. Stempel, RN, MS, CCM
Community Nurse Case Manager
Development and Evaluation
  Coordinator
Carondelet Hospice Services
Tucson, Arizona

Karen Van Wie, RN, BSN
Child-Family Nurse Case Management
Carondelet Health Services
Tucson, Arizona

Bonnie Wilson, PhD, RN
Assistant Director, Nursing
Chandler Regional Hospital
Chandler, Arizona

ACKNOWLEDGMENTS

I deeply appreciate the work of the contributing authors who thoughtfully shared their expertise. I am grateful to Alice Stein for giving me the opportunity to develop the project and to my colleagues who critiqued the manuscript: Lori Angarone, Kay Bensing, Lisa Bové, Beverly Chickerella, Carrol Gold, Loretta Seigley, and Paula Tinghitella. I am also grateful to Hilary Schrauf, Assistant Editor for Delmar Publishers for her support, encouragement, assistance, and competence, and to Rosemary Camilleri for helping me learn to write. I thank my daughter, Barbara, and my family and friends for inspiring and encouraging me. Finally, I thank Bob DiLeonardi for the many ways in which he helped me to complete this project.

Bette Case, PhD, RN, C
Chicago, IL
1996

CHAPTER 2

The authors gratefully acknowledge the following nurses for telling their career stories.

Veronica Bender, MA, RN
Manager of CQI Services
Senior Consultant, Metricor
Louisville, Kentucky

Katherine Brown-Saltzman
Clinical Nurse Specialist, Pain
    Management and Bereavement
UCLA Medical Center
Los Angeles, California

Mary Cramer-Simpson, MSN, RN, C
Director, Customer Service Department
The Ohio State University Medical
    Center
Columbus, Ohio

Michele Deck, BSN, MEd, ACCE-R,
    RN
President, G.A.M.E.S.
Metairie, Louisiana

Linda Goldberg, EdD, RN
Assistant Provost, Kutztown University
    of Pennsylvania, Kutztown,
    Pennsylvania, presentation at
    Dimensions in Academic Leadership,
    sponsored by The Medical College of
    Pennsylvania-Hahnemann University, Orlando, Florida, January 9,
    1995.

Jan Henderson
Regional Director, Health Care
    Compensation Consulting, Ernst &
    Young
Chicago, Illinois

Stephen Horner, BSN, RN
Information Services, Columbia HCA
Nashville, Tennessee

Gayle McMurry, BSN, MS, RN, JD
Attorney, independent practice
Chicago, Illinois

Linda Moskowitz, RN, JD
Support Center Leader for
    Transition/Continuity of Care
University of Chicago Hospitals
Chicago, Illinois

Lisa Murphy, RN, MS
Customer Resource Manager, Stericycle
Chicago, Illinois

Jennifer Schwarz
Organizational Development Consultant
Buffalo Grove, Illinois

Sandra Shelley, DNSc, RN, CNAA,
    CHE
Founder and President, Sandra Shelley
    & Associates
Western Springs, Illinois

Charlotte Whitaker, MS, RN
Associate Administrator, Patient Care
    Services
Valley Hospital Medical Center
Las Vegas, Nevada

Elaine Yarling
Manager, Employment and Labor
    Relations
Mount Sinai Hospital and Medical
    Center
Chicago, Illinois

Jeff Zurlinden, MS, RN
Director, Chicago Clinical Programs for
    Research on AIDS
Chicago, Illinois

CHAPTER 9

The author wishes to sincerely thank the following nurses for sharing small parts of their complex roles as clinical nurse specialists. Their contributions helped to more clearly illustrate the diversity inherent in this role.

Susan Galanes, RN, MS, CCRN
Clinical Nurse Specialist, Pulmonary
    Nursing
Suburban Lung Associates
Winfield, Illinois

Carol Gawron, RN, MSN, CETN
Clinical Nurse Specialist
Private Practice
Downers Grove, Illinois

Ann Henrick, PhD, RN, FAAN
Clinical Nurse Specialist, Cardiac
    Research
Edward Hines, Jr. VA Hospital
Maywood, Illinois

Mary McCarthy, MSN, CS, CETN
Clinical Nurse Specialist/Enterostomal
    Therapy
Michael Reese Hospital & Medical
    Center
Chicago, Illinois

Christa Schroeder, RN, MSN
Clinical Nurse Specialist, Oncology &
    Bone Marrow Transplantation
Michael Reese Hospital & Medical
    Center
Chicago, Illinois

CHAPTER 13

The Buckman Company, Inc.
1000 Burnett Avenue, Suite 250
Concord, California 94520
510-356-2640

Critical Care Associates, Inc.
484 Bloomfield Avenue
Montclair, New Jersey 07042
201-746-5990

Gail Wick & Associates
5420 New Wellington Close
Atlanta, Georgia 30327
404-252-9341

The National Nurses in Business
 Association
56 McArthur Avenue
Staten Island, New York 10312
800-331-6534
fax: 718-317-0858

CHAPTER 16

The author respectfully acknowledges the following leaders in education, who shared their experiences, insights, and predictions.

Roberta Abruzzese, EdD, RN, FAAN
Consultant in Continuing Education
 and Staff Development
Garden City, New York

Grif Alspach, EdD, MSN, RN, FAAN
Consultant, Nursing Staff Development
 and Competency-Based Education
Annapolis, Maryland

Marilyn Bunt, PhD, RN
Dean and Professor
Lewis University College of Nursing
Romeoville, Illinois

Sandra Byers, PhD, RN, CNAA
Vice President, Corporate Health Affairs
 Peer Review Systems
Westerville, Ohio

Patsy Colwell, BSN, MN, RN
Orthopedic Clinical Case Manager
Good Samaritan Regional Medical Center
Pheonix, Arizona

Dorothy J. del Bueno, EdD, RN
Partner, Performance Management
 Associates
Professor, University of Pennsylvania
Philadelphia, Pennsylvania

Gloria Donnelly, PhD, RN, FAAN
Dean and Professor, College of Nursing
Allegheny University
Philadelphia, Pennsylvania

Elizabeth Falter, MS, RN, CNAA
Falter & Associates
Croton-on-Hudson, New York

Venner M. Farley, EdD, RN
President, Innovative Nursing
 Consultants
Orange, California

Kathleen J. Fischer, MA, RN, C, CNAA
Director of Educational Services for
 Nursing
University of Michigan Hospitals
Ann Arbor, Michigan

Meg Gulanick, PhD, RN
Assistant Professor, The Marcella
 Niehoff School of Nursing
Loyola University of Chicago
Chicago, Illinois

Suzanne Hall-Johnson, MN, RN
Director, Hall Johnson
 Communications
Lakewood, Colorado

Rosalyn Jazwiec, EdD, RN
Director of Education and Training
Kaiser Foundation Hospital
Fontana, California

Mitzi Jobes, RN, MS
Systems Director, Clinical Education
Samaritan Health Systems
Pheonix, Arizona

Karen Kelly, PhD, RN, C, CNAA
Director of Practice and Research
Association of Women's Health,
    Obstetric and Neonatal Nurses
    (AWHONN)
Washington, DC

Kathleen C. Kelly, PhD, RN
Assistant Professor and Director of the
    Office of Continuing Nursing
    Education
The University of Iowa College of
    Nursing
Iowa City, Iowa

Susan Kennerly, PhD, RN
Associate Dean, Academic Affairs,
    College of Nursing and Health
University of Cincinnati
Cincinnati, Ohio

Alice Kuramoto, PhD, RN, FAAN
Professor, University of Wisconsin-
    Milwaukee School of Nursing
Milwaukee, Wisconsin

Dianne Leonard, EdD, RN, CNAA
Director, Nursing Education,
    Greensboro AHEC
Visiting Associate Professor, University
    of North Carolina Greensboro
Greensboro, North Carolina

Elizabeth Miller, BSN, RN
Program Director, Cardiac
    Rehabilitation
Good Samaritan Regional Medical
    Center
Pheonix, Arizona

Vi Moran, MS, RN
Owner and Consultant, Vi-Moran
    Associates
Madison, Wisconsin

Alma Mueller, EdM, BSN, RN
Program Director and Professor of
    Nursing
Front Range Community College
Westminster, Colorado

Jody Pelusi, RN, RT, MS, ONC, FNP
Clinical Nurse Specialist, Oncology and
    Cancer Program Coordinator
Maryville Samaritan Medical Center
Pheonix, Arizona

Belinda Puetz, PhD, RN
Editor, *Journal of Nursing Staff
    Development*
Administrator, National Nursing Staff
    Development Organization
President, Puetz and Associates
Pensacola, Florida

Michele Knoll Puzas, RN, C, MHPE
Pediatric Nurse Specialist and Chair,
    Patient Education Committee
Michael Reese Hospital and Medical
    Center
Chicago, Illinois
Editorial Advisory Board, *Patient
    Education Management*

Nancy Ridenour, PhD, RN, C, FNC
Associate Dean, Graduate Programs
Texas Tech University Health Sciences
    Center
School of Nursing
Lubbock, Texas

Lori Rodriquez, RN, C, MA, MSN
Director of Education
Camino Healthcare System
Mountain View, California

Christa Schroeder, MSN, RN
Clinical Nurse Specialist, Oncology
Michael Reese Hospital and Medical
    Center
Chicago, Illinois

Mary Simpson, MSN, RN, C
Director, Customer Service Department
The Ohio State University Hospital
Columbus, Ohio

Alice Stein, MA, RN
Associate Dean, College of Nursing
    Allegheny University
Philadelphia, Pennsylvania

Christine Tanner, PhD, RN, FAAN
Editor, *Journal of Nursing Education*
Professor of Community Healthcare
    Systems
Oregon Health Sciences University,
    School of Nursing
Portland, Oregon

Dori Taylor-Sullivan, PhD, RN, CNA
Assistant Vice President for Organiza-
    tion and Staff Development
University of Connecticut Health
    Center
Farmington, Connecticut

Madeline Wake, PhD, RN, FAAN
Dean, Marquette University College of
    Nursing
Milwaukee, Wisconsin

Janice Ward, MSN, RN, C
Director, Central Staff Development
Indiana University Medical Center
Indianapolis, Indiana

Kathy Weiland
Director, Health Education
Humana Health Care Plans
Chicago, Illinois

Francine Wolgin, MSN, RN, CNA
President, National Nursing Staff
    Development Organization
Director, Operations Support and
    Practice Development
St. Joseph Mercy Hospital
Ann Arbor, Michigan

INTRODUCTION

When Bette Case first brought this project to me, my initial reaction was, "That is the best idea I've heard in a year!" In a time when so much emphasis is being placed on downsizing, rightsizing, and layoffs, it is easy to focus on what is becoming scarcer in nursing. To do so, however, completely misses the unique nature of our time. Today, the opportunities available to nurses are expanding so quickly that they defy categorization. The question, properly phrased, should not be, "What jobs are available?" but, rather, "What is it that I want to do?"

When I graduated from nursing school in 19__, the options available were to work in a hospital or a doctor's office, or to teach. Opportunities for advancement were limited to the immediate supervision of other nurses. Today, the preponderance of positions may still lie within hospital walls, but the ratio is shifting daily to include more and more varied positions outside of traditional delivery sites. Within the hospital, nurses with advanced degrees are practicing subspecialties. Discharge planners are managing utilization of resources and are overseeing the continuity of patient care. Management positions are no longer limited to unit supervision, but now reach the senior vice president level. Outside the hospital, nurses are leveraging physicians in a huge number of settings. They are working in home care, treating patients on the patients' own schedules, and they are acting as consultants in numerous fields including (but not limited to) insurance, law, and hospital reengineering. The range of options is dazzling.

Every nurse is a witness to the changes sweeping health care today, and every nurse will be affected by these changes. The trick is to take advantage of change. To do so, however, we may need help—help in seeing what others have done so that we can see how far the boundaries have been pushed; help in refining visions of what we would like to do; and help in identifying the skills we can bring to bear in making our visions our realities. Readers will find that *Career Planning for Nurses* provides this help.

Connie Curran, EdD, RN, FAAN
President, CurranCare
North Riverside, Illinois

Chapter One

Where Are You Taking Your Career?

Bette Case

INTRODUCTION

Marion, president of the school of nursing alumni, approached the podium to introduce the banquet speaker. The speaker's topic for the annual reunion banquet had attracted the best turnout in years. The topic, "Thriving in Your Career," interested many alumni in various phases of their respective careers. Looking out at the audience, Marion reflected on the personal experiences that stimulated so many of her fellow alumni to attend.

Many new graduates looked eagerly toward the podium, each awaiting that hot tip that would lead to a desirable nursing position in a downsized job market. Paul, one of the new graduates, had earned a bachelor's degree in psychology before entering nursing school. He entered nursing school to improve his job and career prospects, but not yet found a position he wants in a hospital. He's trying to decide whether to take a job in an extended care facility in the city or apply for one of the positions being advertised at some of the nearby community hospitals.

Felicia has worked in an oncology unit since graduating five years ago. She recently enrolled in a certification program in therapeutic touch. The notion of intervening in energy fields intrigues her. She has read reports of increased pain relief and sense of well-being among oncology patients exposed to therapeutic touch. She's even been thinking about opening her own practice in therapeutic touch after earning her certificate. When she shared her thoughts with fellow alumni over dinner, however, some of their responses shocked her. Though some supported the idea of nurses applying alternative therapies, Sally dismissed the whole approach as "New Age bunk."

Sally admits to feeling burned out after working in critical care for ten years. The hospital where she works is opening a subacute unit, and she's seriously considering applying for a staff position. She knows her critical care skills will serve her well in subacute care, but she wonders how she'll react to caring for more patients and long-term patients.

Millie has managed a busy nursing unit for six years. During recent downsizing, her unit merged with another, and administration eliminated her job. Millie's boss has offered her a staff nurse position in a new outpatient clinic. She wonders whether she should go back to school to prepare for a nurse practitioner role. She enjoyed management and wants to explore opportunities to apply her management skills, maybe even outside of nursing.

Leah served as a staff nurse on a surgical unit for five years, but that was fifteen years ago. In the fifteen years since, she raised three children, managed a household, and participated actively in her community. She feels ready to reenter nursing now but wonders whether she has any relevant skills. After all, presurgical and postsurgical care have changed dramatically since she practiced as a staff nurse. She thinks she might do well in home health because she's so connected to her community, but she feels intimidated by the high technology and high degree of independence. She hasn't been able to find a refresher course, although a few years ago she received advertising of such courses from many of the local hospitals.

Jenny loves staff nursing. She's worked for a university hospital for twelve years. Recently, the hospital began "educating the staff about patient-focused care and redesign." Jenny likes her job the way it is. She isn't sure she wants to be redesigned.

As Marion stood at the podium, she reflected on the stories she'd heard from these and other fellow alumni as they reconnected with each other at the banquet. As she introduced the speaker, Marion sensed that each of the alumni in the large audience brought unique and personal career questions. She returned to her seat as the speaker began. Marion hoped that her fellow alumni would connect the speaker's remarks with their own personal questions and begin to create the next phases of their career plans. The speaker began to address the audience by referring to the book *Career Planning for Nurses* (Case, 1997).

"'Whether you are responding to changing circumstances and demands or pursuing a dream, you are in charge of your career.' This book contains information about career paths, career choices, and self-assessment. The pieces of information you select and the way in which you combine them will depend on your unique strengths, priorities, and circumstances.

Projections for the year 2005 supply some background for our discussion. In 1994, the United States Bureau of Labor Statistics predicted a need for 765,000 additional RNs to meet the needs of the year 2005. Although the practice of nursing will change as the twenty-first century unfolds, you will continue to find numerous and diverse opportunities to practice nursing."

As you develop your career in nursing or take the skills you developed in nursing to new arenas, many different desires and necessities will pull and push you. Chapter 2 describes some of these influences.

For many years, nurses have functioned competently in the roles and systems designed by their employers. Today's employer no longer provides the security and job definition of the past, however. Particularly for today's professional, career development requires ongoing assessment and redefinition of personal skills, and interests, as well as awareness of the needs of today's health care system. You may choose a change in job or career to satisfy needs and goals unmet in your present situation, to realize a dream or vision, or to adjust to changing circumstances.

Satisfying Needs and Goals

You may experience lessened enthusiasm for your work, lack of challenge or advancement opportunity, or a sense of diminished impact in your work setting. You may find yourself becoming more negative and critical of yourself and coworkers. You may feel exhausted from overinvolvement in your work. You may feel restless, bored, frustrated, or unappreciated. You may dread going to work every day. These feelings signal a possible mismatch between your present situation and your needs and goals (Michalek, 1993).

To respond most constructively to these feelings, clarify your needs and goals. You may be able to make some changes within your current situation that will bring you closer to meeting your needs and goals, thus helping to relieve unpleasant feelings. Even if you decide to leave your current position, the process of clarifying your needs and goals will help you choose a more satisfying future situation.

Most work situations involve some frustrations. According to prominent businessman Malcolm Forbes, "If you have a job without aggravation, you don't have a job" (Sullivan & Gini, 1994, p.25). Clarifying needs and goals and exploring ways to improve the situation without leaving your job can help you determine whether you will tolerate certain dissatisfactions or seek different employment.

Realizing a Dream or Vision

"When you work you fulfil a part of earth's furthest dream, assigned to you when that dream was born" (Gibran, 1923, p. 27). For some, career and life visions emerge with great clarity. For others, such visions take shape gradually through identifying personal and professional passions, preferences, interests, and strengths. Chapter 3 offers some insights into the process of creating a career vision.

Adjusting to Changing Circumstances

Even if you find yourself very satisfied with your current work situation and believe that your current work propels you toward your vision, you need to consider career-development strategies. You may face changing demands as a result of changing personal or family circumstances. Undoubtedly, you will face unprecedented changes in society and health care. As Mary E. Foley, RN, predicted in 1977 when she chaired the American Nurses Association Constituent Assembly, "[the new] reality will assure a new world vision for nurses and a lifetime of career opportunities" (Andreola & Pauly-O'Neill, 1994, p. 4). This new reality has since evolved and, probably in ways not envisioned by Foley in 1977. Nevertheless, inherent in the new reality are opportunities for nurses, including opportunities to shape systems in response to societal needs.

ECONOMIC, SOCIETAL, AND INDUSTRIAL TRENDS

Changes in the economy, in service businesses, and in industry are redefining work in our society. The old rules of work were based on the company being around forever, according to experienced business consultant Gerard Egan (Kleiman, 1994b). A sense of stability, security, and loyalty flourished. Today, however, companies are redefining their missions, services, and products and reorganizing to address those changes. Companies are developing new ways of doing business and are requiring new skills of their workers. Nurses have not always recognized hospitals and organizations that provide health care as businesses and companies. Yet, they indeed are businesses and companies. And they are learning to operate in more businesslike ways. To succeed, companies and their workers must form partnerships to achieve new missions in an efficient and effective manner.

Peters (1994) predicts that the career of tomorrow will consist of a dozen jobs, and that workers will move on and off payrolls of large and small companies in two or three industries. From Peters' point of view, tomorrow's environment redefines stability as continued employability, with flexibility, continued learning, and a reputation for high-quality performance as the required components. Current statistics reveal that a person takes a new job every five years and changes careers three times (Sulski, 1994).

Early in 1994, the United States Bureau of Labor Statistics released projections for the year 2005. The bureau predicted growth in services and decline in manufacturing. Predicted areas of growth include: personal computers, personal services, health care and aging, and secondary education (for both teachers and teacher's aides). One out of three jobs will be in the fields of health, business, and social services. Between the years 1992 and 2005, the department predicts significant growth in the following fields:

- residential care: 150%
- home health aides: 138%
- personal and home care aides: 130%
- computer engineers: 112%
- systems analysts: 110%
- computer/data processing: 96%
- health services: 89%
- child care: 73%
- business services: 71%

Projections include a need for 765,000 more RNs and 594,000 more nurse's aides, orderlies, and attendants.

These projections suggest growing opportunities for nurses in child care and long-term care—opportunities not only in delivering direct care, but also in organizing and managing services and in training and supervising support personnel. These projections also suggest a growing need for managing health care information using computerized systems. Nurses come well equipped with the skills needed in all segments of the high-skill service economy of 2005: curiosity, problem-solving, teamwork, and process skills. Chapter 4 explores application of nursing knowledge and experience in fields outside of the traditional nursing career.

The bureau also projects that the workforce of 2005 will consist of increasing numbers of women, ethnic minorities, and workers between the ages of forty-five and fifty-four. By the year 2000, women will compose 47% of the workforce, and 61% of women will work. Of those entering the workforce between the years 1985 and 2000, 60% will be women. As well as gaining strength in numbers, women are asserting themselves differently in the economy. The number of women entrepreneurs, dubbed the "new American heros" (Silver, 1994), has increased significantly in the past decade. Chapter 13 explores the work of entrepreneurial nurses.

American business has not fully resolved problems such as the "glass ceiling" (limiting promotion of women to high-level positions) and the "mommy track" (limiting advancement opportunities for women who combine careers with childrearing). Yet, such problems present problem-solving opportunities for women in corporate America. As Renee Lerche, a consultant to Ford Motor Company, suggests, "Women need to change themselves to fit the corporation, and then figure out how to change the corporate culture" (Sharpe, 1994). Rosemary Mans, Vice President of Flexibility Programs for Bank of America, proposed her position as a part-time vice president to manage work-family programs. Ms. Mans encourages, "Look for work that needs to be done, shape it and sell it"(Lancaster, 1995).

Women are also gaining a positive concept of themselves in the workplace. According to a 1994 survey, though eight out of ten women worked for financial reasons, seven out of ten reported that they worked to feel good (Associated Press, 1994).

In addition to an increasing number of women and minorities in the workforce, the past decade has seen an increase in the number of African-American women in the workforce and in management positions. In fact, it is projected that African-American women will outnumber African-American men in the workforce in the year 2000 (Johnston & Packer, 1987). In the past decade, African-American women have increased their presence in management positions by 64%, as compared to a 22%-increase for African-American men during the same period (Gaiter, 1994).

Projections for the ways that Americans will work in the future include increases in flexible work schedules, temporary and part-time work, and work at home. In fact, some foresee a dramatic redefinition of the job. In his book *Job Shift*, William Bridges (1994) refers to the traditional job as "a historical artifact created by the Industrial Revolution". This "de-jobbing" trend removes both the boundaries and the securities of the traditional job. Companies expect workers to configure and reconfigure in teams to solve problems with other workers having various skill sets.

Bridges believes that leaders must educate workers regarding these new expectations in order to ensure a productive workforce. In his view, a critical part of this trend is the shift of responsibility to the worker. The job no longer defines the person. Workers must identify and plan to meet their own needs for training, health care, and retirement, because they cannot depend on the company to do so. Workers must prepare to "recycle themselves" in the changing environment by mastering new skills and perspectives.

Many companies are "redeploying" or reassigning workers as new needs and directions evolve. The best candidates for redeployment are those workers who are "de-jobbed," multiskilled individuals who have portable skills. Those who cannot transfer their skills to areas of higher priority and those whose skills are replaced by technology will need retraining. The Department of Labor predicts that three out of four workers employed in the early 1990s will need retraining for employment in the year 2000.

Good candidates for redeployment also know the business of the company from the broadest perspective possible. Executive Andy Grove suggests giving employees a "two hour dump about what's happening to us" every quarter and letting the employees figure out what it means to them in their work (Lancaster, 1994a). The broad perspective assists the redeployed worker to apply skills more quickly in the new situation. Greenberg refers to these individuals as "gold-collar workers" (Kleiman, 1994c). The worker who does not develop additional skills and a flexible approach is likely to be targeted for layoff during reorganization.

As companies redefine their missions and their businesses while focusing on cost savings, some jobs and individuals who hold those jobs become expendable, and layoffs occur. Layoffs became so prevalent in the early 1990s that a number of articles and books were published to assist affected individuals (Harper, 1994; Kirkwood, 1994; Lancaster, 1994b). All such sources of advice urged those who were laid off to take charge of the situation: keep emotions in check while in the work setting, request outplacement and fair compensation; and negotiate the most acceptable circumstances for leaving the company.

The layoff experience is devastating to self-confidence. Grieving and venting in safe surroundings help clear thinking for proactive responses. Planning and maintaining a job-search schedule lend structure to the period of unemployment. Active networking produces potential job opportunities. In fact, 70% of laid-off individuals reportedly find work through contacts (Topolnicki, 1994). Layoff can present an opportunity for reevaluating priorities and exploring new directions. Some new directions and new approaches may emerge by asking former bosses and colleagues for their perceptions regarding why you were selected for layoff.

The job-hunting period may continue longer than you hope. The process of reevaluating priorities and identifying new directions and contacts is time consuming. You can anticipate spending one month job-hunting for every $10,000 of your previous annual salary (Topolnicki, 1994). Although outplacement and job-hunting expenses are not tax deductible for first-time employment or voluntary job change, individuals who have been laid off can deduct these expenses.

Even if you are not laid off, because so many companies are laying off employees, you may find yourself in the position of "layoff survivor," one whose peers or colleagues are laid off. Layoff survivors often experience "survivors' guilt" because the company spared their jobs. Layoff survivors can ensure their continuing value to the company by volunteering for more responsibility and accepting responsibility for streamlining processes and procedures.

As discussed following, economic, societal, and industrial trends offer various career-development opportunities for nurses, both in health care and in the broader marketplace.

Trends in Health Care and Nursing

Echoing the societal trends previously described, nursing leaders urge nurses to consider and reconsider the path of their careers and the nature of their jobs. "The old dependence on routines and stability in the workplace is simply no longer an authentic circumstance. In transformational times such as our current era, people must learn to 'journey' with the understanding that they may never fully arrive. . .. This kind of journeying may mean living more comfortably with adjustment, accommodation, dialogue, negotiation, and compromise" (Porter-O'Grady, 1992, p. xii).

Acute care hospitals have employed the majority of nurses in the past. In the mid-1990s, however, forces are combining to reduce the need for nurses in the acute care setting. These factors include mergers and restructuring of hospitals, shorter lengths of stay, decreased hospital occupancy, increased numbers of nonregistered nurse caregivers, and increased focus on outpatient care. With less need for nurses in the acute care setting, nurses are losing their jobs or finding their jobs redefined. This creates a sobering and shocking phenomenon for nurses who had relied on the stability of careers as hospital staff nurses. As stated by Andreola and Pauly-O'Neill (1994), "Nurses do not lose their jobs. We might resign of our own volition, but *always* of our own volition. Until now. . ."(p. 8).

Nurses need to prepare themselves through continuing education and focused experience for delivering care differently within the hospital, and for delivering care outside of the hospital and in subacute settings. The nurse's caregiver role is changing. Health care policy makers are exploring strategies to reduce cost while increasing access to care and quality of care. Health care organizations are responding proactively by redesigning care delivery. Hospitals are increasingly becoming critical care sites, and subacute care and levels of care previously delivered in general hospital units are instead being provided in the home and in ambulatory care settings.

Hospitals will continue to need critical care nurses. The need for nurses in subacute care, extended care and home health care will also increase. The ever-increasing aging population will necessitate increased geriatric care, extended care, and home health services. Home health and hospice care will serve clients of all ages. Home health care, as described in Chapter 11, will continue to increase in technology and complexity.

The number of advanced practice nurses (clinical nurse specialists, nurse practitioners, nurse midwives, and nurse anesthetists) is increasing. These groups meet the national agenda to provide increased access to care and quality care at reduced costs. Chapters 8 and 9 provide additional information about these roles. Colleges and universities are developing new programs to prepare nurses for these roles. Enrollments in educational programs preparing advanced practice nurses continue to rise.

Within hospitals (Chapter 6), as well as in community-based settings (Chapter 7), the nursing caregiver role is evolving to one of managing care, financial accountability, health care information and systems (Chapter 5), and care delivery using unlicensed assistive personnel (UAP). For nurses, this evolution requires new knowledge and skills related to health care costs, informatics, and delegation. Increased focus on wellness, prevention, out-of-hospital care, and shortened hospital stays highlights the nurse's role in patient education.

Trends in health care delivery also influence the roles of nurses who specialize in education (Chapter 16) and management (Chapter 10). Nurses who educate other nurses, both in academic settings and in health care organizations, face a great challenge in predicting and providing the knowledge, skills, and experiences nurses will need to practice in the future. Enrollment in nursing schools has increased steadily in recent years. In fact, the number of qualified applicants has exceeded the ability of schools to accommodate them, both in terms of faculty numbers and space requirements. In response to the shift toward fewer nursing positions in acute care hospitals, however, admissions to most programs that prepare nurses for entry into practice have levelled off or declined slightly, and admissions to graduate programs have increased (Varro, 1996).

Many hospitals have reduced the RN mix (i. e. ratio of RNs to other bedside caregivers) in staffing. Consequently, experts recommend the closing of significant numbers of nursing schools, as many as 10%-20% (Pew Health Professions Commission, 1995). Some experts predict a return to RN-rich staffing mixes in the future (Curtin, 1995). Regardless of whether the number of RN positions in acute care settings increases, educational institutions will design programs to prepare professional nurses for the future. Schools will prepare nurses for redefined roles, perhaps in numbers lower than earlier predicted.

When a hospital reorganizes delivery of services, the plan often includes reducing the number of management positions. Layoffs have affected more nurses in manager roles than in staff roles. The focus of the manager's role in health care organizations of the future will be the goals of the organization, the needs of those served by the organization, and designing and executing strategies to achieve organizational goals. This differs from the past, when the nursing manager focused on the department or unit and the management of nurses.

SEIZING CAREER OPPORTUNITIES

As a nurse, you can choose among five different strategies for seizing career opportunities:

- Redefine your present job and increase your value to your organization.
- Specialize in a growing specialty or create a specialized practice based on identified needs.
- Prepare yourself for practice as an advanced practice nurse.
- Investigate health care occupations other than nursing.
- Combine nursing with another field such as law, business, or public service.
- Apply your skills in the broader marketplace, outside of nursing and health care.

Redefine Your Present Job and Increase Your Value

Your job will change as your organization redefines its delivery of services. Even if your title remains the same, your role and on-the-job responsibilities and activities will change. You may not be in a position to write yourself a new job description, however, you can develop your knowledge and skills in ways that will increase your value to your organization.

To increase your value to the organization, you need to expand your knowledge of the organization's values. Access as many formal information channels as possible: administrative updates at staff meetings, newsletters, and open-forum meetings. Turn yourself into a sponge for information about your organization and where it is going. Actively pursue information. Interact with employees in other departments. Walk through different areas and departments of the institution by varying your usual routes as you come to and leave from work or as you take your breaks.

Don't hesitate to ask your supervisor for information or clarification. The questions that will give you the most useful information are questions about specific observations, practices, plans, or rumors, rather than big picture questions about the organization's strategic plan. Although you need to know the organization's stated core values, vision, mission, and strategic plan, more specific questions and day-to-day observations of the operations of the hospital will provide you with clues about how to increase your value.

Your information gathering will help you understand where your department or unit fits into the overall scheme and how that might change. The skills that you practice in gathering information (observing and interacting with others outside your immediate work area) are precisely the skills required in the better-integrated, patient-focused health care organizations of the future.

Within your own unit or department, direct your observational skills toward looking for opportunities to improve care and services. Routines and procedures sometimes become so familiar that it is difficult to imagine different approaches. Make an effort to imagine alternate approaches. For example, ask yourself what might make the patient's experience more satisfying or how certain processes could be simplified. You may come up with ideas to make certain hospital systems and practices function more productively and cost effectively. Most health care organizations are searching for ways to reduce costs. To make meaningful suggestions about cost-effectiveness, you need to gain knowledge about the costs associated with various practices.

Whatever path your organization is taking toward the future, your flexibility, ability to take a broad perspective, willingness to work as a team player with others outside of nursing, and willingness to look for and suggest ways to improve care and cost-effectiveness will all be valued.

Specialize

The shift away from inpatient care and the increasing aging population generate the need for more nurses in certain specialties. Health maintenance organizations (HMOs), clinics, extended care facilities, nursing homes, and home health agencies will all need more nurses.

Hospitals will need critical care nurses as the inpatient focus narrows to high-acuity, high-tech care. Subacute care will continue to fill the gap between the hospital and the home. Subacute care serves patients who are basically stable but who require complex technological assistance, such as the ventilator-dependent patient who will be weaned.

Some recommend expanding the nurse's role in performing diagnostic procedures. *The New England Journal of Medicine* reported a study of flexible sigmoidoscopy performed by nurses (Wolfe, 1994). Patients for whom nurses performed the procedure complied with follow-up recommendations more frequently than did patients for whom physicians performed the procedure. The MD author of the article suggests that expanding the nurse's role in the diagnostic process can increase access to care and decrease cost. Not only might nurses specialize in specific diagnostic procedures, but nurses might also develop practices or centers of diagnostic services and contract to provide these services.

Nurses might also expand their roles in patient and family teaching. Increased focus on prevention and shorter hospital stays create increased demand for patient education. President Clinton suggested that standard insurance benefits include health education. Besides emphasizing the patient education aspect of care when caring for patients, nurses can develop systems to address this need. To be effective, systems must go beyond compiling and organizing patient education resources and materials and create processes that ensure that patients and families receive the information they need.

The public will continue to need educational materials and programs focusing on illness, diagnosis, treatment, and prevention. In addition, the public will need education about the health care system and practical matters such as how to choose a health care provider, how to take an active role in one's care, and how relevant to ask questions.

In today's society, people are assuming caregiver roles more frequently. Because of shorter hospital stays, family members often need to provide more care at home than was the case in the past, when patients were more fully recovered upon discharge. In addition, family members are assuming a more active role in the care and supervision of elderly family members, and more fathers are assuming active roles in infant and child care. People need information and skills to function effectively in these caregiver roles.

Nurses are uniquely prepared to develop educational materials and systems to deliver information effectively because nurses have, or can easily obtain, the information. Nurses also have experience in interpreting and communicating information in a manner that facilitates understanding on the part of the patient.

Women's health is a growing field that is full of opportunity for nurses. Developing systems to improve access to antepartal care has significant cost-saving implications. The United States Public Health Service estimates a savings of $21,000 in hospital costs for every infant carried to full term (as compared to those who are delivered prematurely). As one authority said, "The best ICU is the womb" (Millenson, 1993). Infant care also offers specialization opportunities. For example, nurse phototherapists provide care for jaundiced infants in the home environment.

Knowledge about the special health care needs of women during all phases of reproductive life has greatly expanded in recent years. Recognizing these needs and marketing opportunities, many hospitals have developed women's health programs. In addition to physical health needs, nurses can provide services to address the emotional and social needs of women and children who are victims of abuse.

Societal issues, including the AIDS epidemic and the rise of violence, necessitate combinations of physical and psychosocial care, which nurses are well prepared to provide. Investigate the needs of persons with AIDS and their families. Explore the needs of victims of violence and their families. The needs you discover may define some new services.

Industries are recognizing that they can reap savings in insurance and compensation costs by developing and providing preventive and supportive services for their employees. Some industries have developed antepartal care programs and provide the services of lactation consultants. Many industries are expanding their occupational health programs to comply with OSHA regulations, provide workers with a greater sense of safety in the workplace, and reduce costs associated with work-related injuries. Chapter 12 describes the growing field of occupational health nursing.

Alternative medicine, or homeopathic medicine, which includes naturalistic approaches to maintaining health and treating illness, is gaining greater acceptance among those in the health care community, as well as the general public. For example, nurses are practicing therapeutic touch, both as independent therapists and as staff nurses, using the therapy as an adjunct to conventional therapies. While researchers and practitioners debate the merits of therapeutic touch, some nursing schools offer certification programs in this alternative treatment. Nurses need to critically evaluate alternative and adjunct approaches. When convinced that evidence supports the value of selected techniques, nurses might develop speciality practices that offer some of these approaches as alternatives or adjuncts to conventional therapy. Some specialty organizations have emerged to embrace selected approaches, such as the National Association of Nurse Massage Therapists, headquartered in Osprey, Florida.

Nurses' interest in alternative approaches has grown considerably in recent years. The American Holistic Nurses Association in Raleigh, North Carolina, can serve as a resource for exploring this field.

Advanced Practice Nurse Preparation

Advanced practice nurses (Chapters 8 and 9) are delivering services previously provided by physicians. Professional organizations are exploring ways to eliminate legal and insurance reimbursement barriers to expanding the roles of advanced practice nurses.

The Bureau of Labor Statistics predicts that physician employment will grow faster than the average of all occupations through the year 2005. Greatest needs include primary care, pediatrics, internal medicine, geriatrics, and preventive medicine. Geographical areas of greatest need are rural and inner-city communities. Yet, medical schools will fall short of producing the supply of primary care physicians needed during the next decade. Many believe that nurse practitioners can help offset this shortfall, with the added benefits of cost savings, increased access, and improved quality.

State Nurse Practice Acts vary considerably from state to state in defining the scope of practice and privileges of advanced practice nurses. Even within the same state, local and regional demands and the nature of collaborative relationships with physicians vary. Bear this in mind when evaluating opportunities as an advanced practice nurse.

The Gladstone Family Nursing Center, a community-based agency located in an elementary school in Chicago, began with a focus on health promotion and disease prevention (immunizations, hygiene, physical examinations for students, exercise classes, and prenatal care). As it matures, the center plans to expand its programs to address other health needs of the community. Nurse practitioners and a community liaison provide services at the center (Zurlinden, 1993).

Advanced practice nurses also function in acute care settings. For example, Loyola University of Chicago's Advanced Practice Trauma/Critical Care Nursing program prepares nurses to "work with trauma patients from resuscitation through rehabilitation and follow them in the clinic after discharge. Students learn how to manage the critically ill patient, develop physical assessment and advanced technical skills, and develop advanced nursing skills, such as collaboration, research, and legislative/community involvement" (Keough, 1994). In acute care, advanced practice nurses provide some of the care previously provided by physicians and residents. Neonatal nurse practitioners are well established as acute care advanced practice nurses, and growing numbers of advanced practice nurses are developing their roles by linking medical specialties and overseeing the entire patient experience.

Nurse midwives practice both autonomously and as components of physician group practices. The practice of nurse anesthetists is well established in anesthesia departments, and the demand for their services continues to grow. One source (Henneberger, 1994) reports seven job offers per graduate of nurse anesthetist programs.

Investigate Other Health Care Occupations

The Bureau of Labor Statistics projects additional jobs in a number of health care occupations through the year 2000:

- nursing and psychiatric assistants: 616,000
- human service workers: 256,000
- health services managers: 135,000
- medical assistants: 128,000
- psychologists: 69,000
- speech and language professionals: 37,000
- respiratory therapists: 36,000
- occupational therapists: 24,000

The largest increase in jobs is predicted for RNs: 765,000. Growth in health care occupations other than nursing, however, presents opportunities for training such health care workers (e.g., nursing, psychiatric, and medical assistants) and applying nursing expertise to other health care disciplines.

The Adams Jobs Almanac 1994 (Adams, Smith, Brooks, Hale, & Avakian, 1994) projects a much-better-than-average outlook for openings for health service managers. *The Almanac* also forecasts growth in jobs supporting ambulatory surgery, alcohol- and drug-abuse treatment, hospice care, home health care, rehabilitation, and mental health. Extended care is also viewed as a growth field. *The Almanac* suggests that medical group practices and extended care might be good settings in which to begin a career in health services management because competition for these positions in hospitals will be great, and graduate degrees in health care administration may not be an entrance requirement in these settings.

Combine Nursing with Another Field

Nurses who are interested and seek education and training in other fields will find opportunities to blend nursing knowledge, skills, and experience to perform unique roles. Insurance companies rely on the skills of nurses to review claims and supporting documentation. Nurses contribute in a variety of ways to the medical and pharmaceutical products industries. Because of the many legal implications of health care, numerous opportunities present themselves to nurses who combine law and nursing (Chapter 14). The military offers rewarding careers for many nurses, and civilian public service provides opportunities to address and shape health care policy (Chapter 15).

The Broader Marketplace

With enough imagination and motivation, nurses can seize or create an infinite number of opportunities. Chapter 4 examines these possibilities more fully. Nursing education and experience builds expertise in organizational skills, communication, interpersonal skills, critical thinking, problem-solving, and logic. These skills are required for success in many fields. As a nurse, you have a distinct advantage if you seek a job requiring these skills. However, you will need to articulate to any potential employer how you will apply these skills to the job in question.

Carolyn S. Zagury, RN, started the Hence Vista Publishing Company which publishes creative works by RNs. She states, "The nursing process was my solution. It helped me organize my needs and plan an appropriate way to learn the new skills needed for the publishing business" (Zagury, 1994). While Zagury was referring to her learning the publishing business, her statement applies to any new discipline or business that a nurse might pursue. Begin by assessing the expertise you bring to the new situation and the expertise you need to develop. Then, plan to acquire the expertise and implement your plan. Evaluate your newly acquired learning by using the requirements of the new situation as your criteria.

If you choose to pursue a career outside of nursing and health care, your own interests will determine the paths you investigate. Some examples of fields wherein nurses might readily apply their skills include but are not limited to writing and publishing, counseling, and human resources.

Because nursing education and practice require accomplishment in communication, reading, and writing, nurses have some of the skills needed to launch careers in writing and publishing. *The Adams Job Almanac 1994* (Adams et al., 1994) forecasts better-than-average demand for writers and editors and increased demand for technical writers. The field is competitive, and guidance from a mentor experienced in writing and publishing can prove invaluable. In a related vein, nursing and the public can be well served by publicists who call attention to the implications of developments in nursing practice and research. While research and clinical advances reported in the *Journal of the American Medical Association* and the *New England Journal of Medicine* often receive wide media attention, nursing developments are seldom broadly publicized. The public could benefit from new insights into health promotion and maintenance generated by nursing research and practice.

While nurses who specialize in psychiatric nursing may use counseling skills more frequently than do their colleagues practicing in other specialties, most nurses have occasion to assist patients to express and explore feelings. *The Adams Job Almanac 1994* (Adams et al., 1994) predicts better-than-average job outlook in the counseling field, particularly in schools, and specifically, in the areas of substance abuse, crisis prevention and intervention, and sexually transmitted diseases. Some of these counseling roles require further education and certification.

The human resources field offers opportunities for which nurses are uniquely suited. *The Adams Job Almanac 1994* (Adams et al., 1994) projects much-better-than-average availability of jobs in the human resources fields of personnel, training, and labor relations. Citing the complex record-keeping requirements for occupational health, equal employment opportunity, and benefits, *The Almanac* forecasts opportunities in developing and managing human resources systems. *The Almanac* predicts a particularly fertile area of opportunity in human resources consulting firms that develop and administer benefits and compensation for other organizations. Other human resources opportunities relate to the need to develop and implement family-friendly policies and policies and practices to ensure both respect for diversity and equal-promotion opportunity.

A need arising from projections regarding an increasing number of women in the workforce is the development of more and formalized day-care programs, whether independently operated or supported by employers. Nurses, particularly those who specialize in pediatrics, have many of the skills needed to design and operate such programs, although further course work in early-childhood development may be required. A thorough understanding of codes and licensing regulations governing day-care centers is also necessary.

Suzanne Hall-Johnson (1995) suggests that nurses who are interested in creating new opportunities pay close attention to emerging trends and regulations. She urges nurses to think through the opportunities that surround trends. For example, in the shift toward home health care lies opportunity—not only opportunity to practice home health care nursing and manage, own, and operate home health agencies, but also opportunity to develop businesses that support home health care. She suggests that nurses might seize the opportunity to supply medical devices and equipment to the home and provide the necessary education to patients and families.

As an example of opportunity in regulations, Hall-Johnson ingeniously recommends that nurses might counsel persons who are preparing advance directives. Nurses might provide information about various options and assist clients to clarify their own wishes and identify and explore alternatives. She proposes that nurses might perform this service in collaboration with attorneys and that optional services might include videotaping a client expressing personal advance directive choices.

PUBLIC PERCEPTION OF NURSES

In planning to seize and create emerging opportunities, nurses must take account of the public's perception of nursing. In order to enjoy public acceptance of newly developed services, nurses need to educate the public about the unique skills and knowledge that nurses bring to addressing today's societal imperatives.

A national public opinion survey conducted for *RN Magazine* (Begany, 1994) revealed an overall positive perception of nurses along with some misconceptions regarding the knowledge level and diverse specialty practice of nurses. Respondents ranked only physicians and engineers higher in prestige than nurses, advancing nurses two ranks since a 1979 survey. The public highly valued nurses' caring attitude, but only 42% cited clinical knowledge when asked what they thought was best about nurses.

Although 60% of the respondents favored nurses assuming some responsibilities traditionally handled by physicians, most believed that only nurses having advanced training should perform in expanded roles. While 93% recommended giving nurses the responsibility of treating minor illness, significantly fewer recommended allowing nurses to make referrals, perform physicals, and diagnostic screenings, deliver babies, and prescribe drugs. In fact, an overwhelming 80% of respondents opposed allowing nurses to prescribe drugs.

The public showed increasing acceptance of men in nursing, with fewer preferring a female nurse than was revealed in the 1979 survey. Two-thirds found it acceptable for their daughters to become nurses and significantly more men (45%) and women (43%) found it acceptable for their sons to become nurses than was revealed in the previous survey.

Respondents indicated that they formed their opinions of nurses based on first-hand experience rather than on media portrayals. To take advantage of the career possibilities of the future, nurses must communicate with the public as well as with professionals who will purchase the services of nurses.

STRATEGIES THAT WORK BEST

A number of strategies can assist you in developing your career. These strategies include taking charge of your career, being flexible, and seeing the big picture.

Take Charge of Your Career

Taking charge is the first step in developing your career. Until you accept the responsibility for designing your own path, you will probably not find the courage or make the effort to assess yourself and the marketplace. Taking charge does not necessarily mean leaving your present job. You might choose your present job as the best means to actualize your passions, strengths, and preferences. Taking charge means exploring all of your needs and all of the paths that can lead to the satisfaction of those needs.

Be Flexible

Identify the skills, experience, and learning that will prepare you to pursue your chosen career path. You can gain skills and experience through volunteer activities within your organization and in your community. Opportunities may present themselves as new jobs, promotions, or additional duties in your present job. Alfred G. Edwards advises minorities, "Don't turn down a job [or assignment], jump all over it" (Kleiman, 1993). His advice applies to *all* employees. Look for opportunities to develop transferable skills and interpersonal skills. Developing a variety of skills and exposing yourself to a variety of different settings will increase your value in your present job and lead to new career directions.

Don't shy away from the politics of your present situation. Learning and participating in the politics of your organization will give you practice in interpersonal skills and in recognizing the perspectives of others. Workplace politics can work for you. In the past, traditional nursing culture socialized nurses to believe that participating in workplace politics brought the nurse's ethics and integrity into question. By gaining an understanding of the motives of others, however, you can often create and capitalize on win-win situations without violating personal or professional ethics.

With the shift toward seamless organizations and away from rigidly defined departmental boundaries, employees who possess multiple specialty skills, problem-solving skills, and willingness to continually learn increase their value to their organizations.

Increase Your Value

To add value to your organization, imagine different ways to improve processes and practices. How can your customers, including other departments, personnel, and the community, obtain greater satisfaction, quality, and cost-effectiveness from services? Because health care organizations and other businesses in the United States and worldwide are reducing workforces and seeking more efficient processes, you will find a receptive audience for sound suggestions. You improve your situation further by identifying a role for yourself in implementing new or refined processes and practices.

If downsizing in your organization is placing additional responsibilities on you, respond proactively. Propose more efficient procedures to your boss and ask for assistance in setting priorities. When you need to bring a problem to the attention of your boss, offer a possible solution to the problem. As Ireland (1994) humorously recommends in *The Job Survival Guide*, "Don't be the one to say the copier is broken."

Avoid behaviors that your boss may perceive as interfering with accomplishing goals. Hanson (1994b) cites the following behaviors as those that most drive bosses crazy:

- refusing to see the big picture
- showing unwillingness to take on additional responsibility, saying "I've never done that before."
- communicating indirectly
- waffling on decision making

- bogging down the system by consulting everyone rather than gathering only needed information
- covering up mistakes
- failing to ask for help
- repeating confidential information

Use every opportunity to "toot your horn," or let others know of your contributions to the organization. Naturally, you must respect cultural norms for communicating and must communicate professionally and objectively. Keep the focus on how what you have done contributes to the organization, rather than on your individual accomplishments. Use routine reports to highlight your contributions. Quote satisfied customers—not only patients, but also members of other departments, and the community. Don't expect others to know and recognize automatically your valuable work. In the past, the nursing culture encouraged modesty. Today, however, failing to take credit for your contributions can stand in the way of professional growth. For some, in fact, failure to communicate accomplishments and value to those in power has resulted in layoff (Lopez, 1994).

Because today's workplace values teamwork, it is most desirable to frame your accomplishments and value in the context of teamwork. Emphasize your contributions as a team player. Tie your accomplishments directly to organizational goals rather than to victories sustained in competition with fellow workers.

Assess Yourself

Identifying what you enjoy is the single most important aspect of self-assessment for designing a satisfying career path. "If you're doing it for the money, you're in prison waiting for parole" (Lancaster, 1994a). As Clarence Darrow said, "When I was young, I worked on a farm. Then I decided to study law. After that I never worked again" (Sullivan & Gini, 1994). Begin by looking for sources of enjoyment in daily tasks and activities. Or, as a nurse who was interviewed for Chapter 2 says, "Notice what makes you smile and find ways to do more of it" (M. Deck, Personal Communication, February 20, 1995).

Identifying sources of enjoyment begins your assessment process, but there is much more to you than what you enjoy. Maybe other emotions motivate you as well. Anna Quindlen (1994) states that in her career change from syndicated columnist to author of novels, she asked herself, "What really terrifies you that you could do next?"

One of the questions to ask is "What do I want?" As *The Adams Job Almanac 1994* (Adams et al., 1994) points out, you choose not only a career, but also the kind of life you want to lead. Thus, you need also to assess those lifestyle characteristics that you consider desirable and undesirable. Take a full inventory of all aspects of yourself. Write your epitaph. Ask yourself, "For what do I want to be remembered?" According to *The Adams Job Almanac*, "You do what you are" (p. 68).

Another important aspect of self-assessment is identifying the skills, strengths, and knowledge that you have to offer to an employer. Identify the skills you will need in the job or career direction you seek. When you identify discrepancies between your present skills and the skills required, think of as many ways as possible to gain the skills you need. You will usually find some alternate ways to add to your skill set. Exploring alternatives may help you to persevere and not give up prematurely if one option (such as formal education) is not realistic at the moment. Chapter 3 presents some tools for self-assessment.

When you have assessed yourself, prepare to articulate your interests, enthusiasm, skills, and plan to gain additional skills. Employers seek candidates with interests and clear direction. Prior to presenting yourself to a potential employer, however, prepare to network.

Network

Networking can help you discover opportunities for specific positions as well as whole new directions. Furthermore, networking can help you refine your ideas. As a first step, identify people with whom to network. You will increase your chances of networking successfully if you first identify specific individuals with whom to network and then present specific questions to these individuals.

Take a broad view of your present health care organization, college, or university. People who work in departments and jobs within your organization, including fellow students in academic settings, have contacts and marketplace knowledge that may prove valuable to you.

Broaden your search for networking contacts beyond your immediate surroundings. Read newspapers, magazines, and professional literature to identify people and organizations that can help you. Continuing education programs offer many networking opportunities. Study continuing education brochures, even if you cannot attend the offerings. You might identify and contact a speaker who can help you locate further resources.

At public libraries, as well as libraries specializing in health care literature, you can find many networking opportunities to explore. Read journals and literature outside of your usual experience. Look for organizations that might prove helpful.

Volunteer work can also lead to networking opportunities. Fellow volunteers may open a whole new world of opportunities by sharing their experiences, previous backgrounds and contacts. Through interacting with the persons you serve in volunteer service, such as persons with AIDS, you can also identify needs. You might then be able to design services and systems to address those needs.

After identifying persons with whom to network, practice your assertiveness skills. Call someone you've never met and introduce yourself. Present your enthusiasms, strengths, and interests. Identify contacts or information that you have to offer; remember, others will be more willing to help you if you can offer some means of reciprocating. Carry business cards with you even when you don't anticipate networking opportunities. Opportunities often present themselves outside of professional meetings and predictable settings. Be sure to express appreciation for the time and assistance of those with whom you network.

Organize the Search

The job search is an active process and is not simply a matter of reacting to employment advertisements in an effective manner. In fact, employment advertising results in only 8% to 10% of all hiring (Hanson, 1994a).

"The hunt is harder than the job," according to journalist Lynn Snowden (Hanson, 1994c). You may find getting organized for the hunt most difficult of all. Begin with a clear vision of the job (or, at least, of the characteristics of the job) you are seeking. Target your use of resources. Use contacts and friends selectively and purposefully. Narrow down the field of potential employers and contacts. Send résumés selectively and with cover letters customized to the needs of the employer you are addressing.

The more knowledge you gain about the employer and the job, the more likely you are to locate your best fit. Request an informational interview. Begin with an organization that is of less interest to you, so that you can gain some experience and confidence and can revise or create new questions. Do some homework in advance, so that you can ask questions that reflect an understanding of the history and direction of the organization. The human resources department may provide you with some information about the organization. Business publications, newspapers, and business sections of general newspapers contain background information about organizations. As shown in Chapter 3, perusing these publications broadens understanding of opportunities.

Determine the stability of the organization. Have numerous mergers, acquisitions, or executive changes affected the organization? What is the major emphasis of the organization at this time? Has the organization won any awards? Are certain aspects, services, or specialties targeted for expansion or elimination? Are there opportunities for transfer within a corporation or multihospital system? The questions you ask are guided by the features of a job and work environment characteristics that you have identified as being important to you. In formulating your questions, be sure to refer to the list of characteristics you seek in a work situation. Then determine the questions you can ask during an informational interview to obtain this information.

An effective job search requires you to be at your best. Actively searching for a job when you already have a job can deplete your energy. Focusing on your present job allows you to develop and refine your skills as well as learn new directions within your organization. Begin your search only when you are ready, organized, and energized.

Intermediate Steps

Volunteer work affords opportunities to explore new settings, gain experience and become known to a potential employer. However, it is important to limit the time you spend volunteering to allow time for other aspects of your job search—as well as to allow time to earn a living.

Temporary or part-time work offers similar advantages to volunteering and allows you to experience an organization from an employee's point of view. A creative approach might be to propose an internship or residency to an organization such as a home health agency.

If you are interested in developing your career within a particular organization, you might consider starting out in a job requiring fewer qualifications than you currently possess. As workplace expert Carol Kleiman advises, start at the bottom, where the jobs are (1994a).

Maximize Your Résumé

The rule for maximizing your résumé is "less is more." Each word should serve to clarify and highlight those of your accomplishments that are most relevant to the targeted job and organization. If you are sending résumés for differing jobs or to differing organizations, you may need to prepare more than one version of your résumé, customizing each version to emphasize those of your qualifications that are most relevant to the particular job or organization. Make your résumé action-oriented and link your accomplishments in previous jobs to the goals of those employers. For example, you may have participated in planning or opening a new unit, or developing a new service, process, or practice. You may have learned new skills, such as sign language or another spoken language, to better serve patients. Potential employers value not only your skills and experience, but also your willingness to grow in ways that serve the organization. A refined résumé not only increases the chances that an employer will consider you, but may also strengthen your position in setting your starting salary (Melia, 1994). Chapter 3 contains further recommendations for maximizing your résumé.

Interview Preparation

Practice interviewing. Tape record questions and answers, including questions you plan to ask. Role play with another person. If you have any control over the scheduling of multiple interviews, schedule an interview for a position you are less interested in before an interview for a more desired position. Doing so allows you to benefit from the practice and experience of the earlier interview.

Your purpose in an interview is to enhance the positive impression you have created with your résumé and to learn as much about the job and the organization as possible.

To prepare for the interview, keep a file of anecdotes or experiences that demonstrate some of your strengths such as problem-solving, emergency response, or other strengths of practice that you wish to highlight. Review these often as you prepare. Also, review your facts about the organization. You want to appear informed and interested in the organization and, thus, need to formulate some questions about the organization to ask during the interview. Your questions should reflect knowledge and interest in the organization. You should not ask questions that can readily be answered prior to the interview.

To create the best impression, arrive on time. Bring a copy of your résumé. Also bring a sheet of paper or a notebook containing one- or two- word reminders of questions you wish to ask or strengths you wish to describe. Do *not*, however, depend on these notes. Use the same sheet of paper or notebook to make a note or two to document important points and show interest during the interview; but don't write extensively. Preoccupation with taking notes will interfere with communication between you and the interviewer and may make you appear to lack confidence. Show flexibility, but express your own professional goals. Do not make unfavorable comments about previous or present employers. Wait to discuss salary until the employer offers you the job.

Remember that the interview, like all effective communication, is a two-way process. You are assessing whether the potential employer offers a proper fit with your career goals. Plan your questions, and know with whom you will interview. Some questions cannot be answered by a representative of the human resources department, for example, and must instead be addressed to a manager or prospective peer. Remember to design questions to gather information that is important to you in deciding whether a particular job or organization is right for you. With this in mind, some questions you might ask include, "What are the priorities to be accomplished by someone in this job?"; "What is the management style?"; "What are the political and interpersonal relationships like?"; "May I speak with some of the people who would be my peers and colleagues in this position?"; "How do you recognize top performers?"; "Why is this position open?"; and "When will you make the hiring decision?" (Ryan, 1994). Chapter 3 offers additional suggestions regarding the interview process.

Self-Confidence

Self-confidence is key in the job search and the career-development process. Circumstances leading to the job search and the search process itself can diminish self-confidence, however. If you have experienced firing, layoff, demotion, or redeployment, you may feel a lack of self-confidence. Even if you have experienced none of these, you may observe changes in your organization or the health care environment that cause you to question the viability of the future of your job.

Reflect on your past successes. Look for models of self-confidence and emulate them (Rager, 1994). If you experience rejections or a lack of job offers, refine your approach the next time. There is a job or an organization out there that is a better match for you. "Keep reminding yourself that the sooner you go out and get started on your job search and the sooner you get those rejections flowing in, the closer you will be to obtaining the job you want" (Adams, et al., 1994, p. 85).

Get Off to a Good Start

Career development is more than getting a job or envisioning a future course. Succeeding in your new job (and in every job) also develops your career. To get off to a good start, clarify expectations with your manager. Both of you enter the situation with expectations. Be sure you understand your manager's expectations and that your manager knows your goals. Heighten your observational skills to learn the culture you are entering. Look for opportunities to succeed in fulfilling your manager's expectations. First impressions form quickly and are difficult to change. Functioning as a team player is more important in the current environment than ever before. Work hard to establish alliances with coworkers and others in the work setting.

Proactively Address Demotion or Redeployment

Because reorganization is rampant in health care and industry today, you may face demotion or redefinition of your job responsibilities. Should this occur, you must determine whether your newly defined job fits with your needs and career plan. If you decide to explore opportunities outside of the organization, present the demotion or redefinition of your present job in the most favorable light by emphasizing your accomplishments in the new position. If you decide to remain with the organization, address any weaknesses that contributed to your demotion and clarify the organizational direction so that you can most fully contribute to the organization meeting its goals. You may need to develop additional skills. In any case, you must clarify the requirements of the redesigned job and objectively appraise the fit of your skills and interests with these requirements.

Career-Development Resources

Many resources are available to help you develop your career. Self-help resources, career-development centers, and career counselors are examples. This book is a resource. You can find many other helpful books on the shelves of libraries and bookstores. Examples include Carol Kleiman's *The Career*

Coach (1994) and the most recent edition of *The Adams Job Almanac*. These references combine job outlook projections with strategic suggestions for identifying and seizing opportunities that will lead to career satisfaction.

Career-development resources and centers may be offered by the organization for which you work, other health care or academic facilities in the community, or professional organizations. One such center offers a process to identify your opportunities, strengths, career vision, and a plan to accomplish your vision (Argentine, 1994).

If you decide to use the services of a career counselor, be sure you understand the services that the counselor will provide and the counselor's fee structure. Most counselors provide services to assist you in clarifying your vision, your strengths and developmental needs, and strategies for reaching your goals. One estimate indicates that 30 thousand career counselors serve 1 million persons every year. The National Board for Certified Counselors in Greensboro, South Carolina, maintains a registry of board-certified career counselors. You can contact the board at 1-800-398-5389.

Students and New Graduates

"Graduating nurses are still guaranteed a job, but not necessarily at the hospital. We haven't reached a saturation point of our need for nurses. But what they do and how they do it is changing as it should," according to Eli Pick, a subacute care executive (Glanz, 1994). Work experience helps new graduates obtain jobs. Such experience can be gained through volunteer work or work as a nurse assistant, unit secretary, or other position in a hospital, rehabilitation center, community health care center or extended care facility. Junior colleges offer a variety of courses that provide preparation for specialty settings. Seek an initial RN position that provides an internship or a sound orientation program.

A University of Delaware survey found that work experience proved more helpful than grades in securing a job after graduation (Kilborn, 1994). The survey, based on 1993 data, showed that RNs received the highest average starting salary of graduates surveyed ($32,858), displacing engineering graduates, who had received the highest average starting salary according to a previous survey. Findings of the survey also indicated that the percentage of graduates still seeking employment six months after graduation was lowest among nursing graduates (3%).

The National Student Nurses' Association, Inc. (NSNA) offers a variety of programs and services to assist students with career development. The Appendix at the end of this chapter describes NSNA and its programs.

Experienced RNs

When seeking new positions, experienced nurses need to capitalize on how their experience can benefit employers. Experienced nurses command higher salaries than do less experienced nurses. The experienced nurse needs to identify the additional value an employer receives when hiring an experienced nurse as compared to hiring a younger, less experienced nurse for a lower salary. In addition to greater clinical proficiency, the experienced nurse can cite experience in creative problem-solving. The experienced nurse faces the challenge of demonstrating flexibility and assuring prospective employers that curiosity and the ability to imagine new and more effective ways of delivering care have been enhanced rather than squelched by years of experience.

RNs Reentering Practice

In times of nursing shortages, refresher courses abound. Both hospitals and nursing schools developed and offered refresher courses during the 1980s. The nurse who reenters practice today, however, will find few, if any, structured refresher courses to facilitate reentry into practice. Instead, the nurse who seeks to reenter practice today must design and direct a personalized program to refresh and augment nursing skills and knowledge.

To begin the reentry process, find out what you must learn. Many employers have developed lists of specific competencies required for RN positions in their organizations. Compare your skills and knowledge with these competency specifications. Find out whether prospective employers offer orientation, inservice education, and staff development programs and determine the scope of any such offerings.

Although you will probably be unable to find refresher courses, postgraduate and certification courses may be offered. Contact prospective employers, local nursing schools and providers of continuing nursing education to identify such courses.

Volunteer work offers opportunities to reacquaint yourself with the practice setting. While you cannot expect to receive refresher training as a volunteer, you can create opportunities to learn about nursing positions and staff development programs within the organization. You can gain valuable insight by talking with practicing nurses and representatives of human resources, nursing staff development, and staff education departments.

Remember that although you have not been practicing nursing, you have been developing other valuable skills while raising your family, participating in your community, or engaging in other activities. Value your skills and experiences. Clarify and specify the value of your skills and experiences, first for yourself and then for potential employers.

If you have not maintained an active license, contact your state board of nursing or state department of professional regulation to find out how to become licensed to practice.

SUMMARY

Career development in the twenty-first century requires proactive assessment of yourself and the marketplace. "Don't wait for your ship to come in, swim out to meet it" (Sullivan & Gini, 1994). The chapters that follow will assist you to do just that.

REFERENCES

Adams, R. L., Smith, C., Brooks, K., Hale, P., & Avakian, M. (Eds.). (1994). *The Adams Job Almanac 1994.* Holbrook, MA: Bob Adams, Inc.

Andreola, N. M., & Pauly-O'Neill, S. (1994, April 4). Nurse managers: Staying afloat in a sea of change. *The Nursing Spectrum Greater Chicago/NE Illinois & NW Indiana Edition, 7*(7), 4–5.

Argentine, M. (1994, October). *Using conceptual mapping to plan nursing career development.* Poster session presented at the American Nurses Association Council on Professional Development Annual Meeting, Kansas City, MO.

Associated Press. (1994, April 14). Working women feel good about lives, jobs and families, poll finds. *Chicago Tribune.*

Begany, T. (1994). Your image is brighter than ever. *RN, 57*(10), 28–34.

Bridges, W. (1994). *Jobshift: How to prosper in a workplace without jobs.* New York: Addison-Wesley.

Case, B. (1997). *Career Planning for Nurses.* Albany, NY: Delmar Publishers.

Cohen, M. H. (1992). *The power of self-management.* Oak Park, IL: Canoe Press.

Curtin, L. (1995, November). Address to Chicago District of the American Nurses Association, Chicago, IL.

Gaiter, D. (1994, March 8). The gender divide: Black women's gains in corporate America outstrip black men's. *Wall Street Journal.*

Gibran, K. (1923). *The Prophet.* New York: Alfred A. Knopf.

Glanz, S. (1994, December 14). Subacute care is the way of the future. *Chicago Tribune.*

Hall-Johnson, S. (1995). *Decade of the nurse.* Lakewood, CO: Hall-Johnson Communications.

Hanson, C. (1994a, May 15). Working smart. To uncover the hidden job market requires diligent digging. *Chicago Tribune,*

Hanson, C. (1994b, July 24). Working smart. What do bosses loathe most? These 7 employee blunders. *Chicago Tribune.*

Hanson, C. (1994c, August 28). Working smart. Want a new job? How about nine different new jobs? *Chicago Tribune.*

Harper, L. (1994, April 5). Work week. Job-hunt costs. *Wall Street Journal.*

Henneberger, M. (1994, August 21). For nurses, new uncertainties. *New York Times.*

Ireland, K. (1994). *The job survival guide: 365 tips, tricks and techniques to stay employed.* Hawthorne, NJ: Career Press.

Johnston, W. B., & Packer, A. H. (1987) *Workforce 2000: Work and workers for the 21st century.* Indianapolis, IN: The Hudson Institute.

Keough, V. (1994, September 19). Advanced practice nurses in tertiary care. *The Nursing Spectrum Greater Chicago/NE Illinois & NW Indiana Edition, 7*(19).

Kilborn, P. (1994, May 1). College seniors finding more jobs but modest pay. *New York Times*.

Kirkwood, C. (1994). *Your services are no longer required: The complete job-loss recovery book*. New York: Plume.

Kleiman, C. (1993, October 31). Jobs. Tips for minorities. Be part of the system. *Chicago Tribune*.

Kleiman, C. (1994a). *The career coach*. Chicago: Dearborn Financial Publishing, Inc.

Kleiman, C. (1994b, March 13). 'New rules' are key to workplace survival. *Chicago Tribune*.

Kleiman, C. (1994c, December 4). Jobs. Redeployed workers become portable assets. *Chicago Tribune*.

Lancaster, H. (1994a, November 15). Managing your career: You, and only you, must stay in charge of your employability. *Wall Street Journal*.

Lancaster, H. (1994b, December 6). Managing your career: Lessons in surviving layoffs, learned the hard way. *Wall Street Journal*.

Lancaster, H. (1995, January 3). Managing your career: Flexibility can be as good for business as it is for people. *Wall Street Journal*.

Lopez, J. (1994, May 4). Managing your career: Knowing when and how loudly to toot your horn. *Wall Street Journal*.

Melia, M. K. (1994, July 3). Level of skills tied to size of salary. *Chicago Tribune*.

Michalek, M. (1993). Is it time to make a change? *Minority Nurse Professional*.

Millenson, M. (1993, September 19). Prenatal care aimed at healthier babies, bottom line. *Chicago Tribune*.

Peters, T. (1994, August 22). No job description, but great business cards. *Chicago Tribune*.

Pew Health Professions Commission. (1995). *Reforming health care workforce regulation: Policy considerations for the 21st century*. San Francisco: Pew Health Commission.

Porter-O'Grady, T. (1992). Foreword. In C. K. Wilson, *Building new nursing organizations: Visions and realities*. Gaithersburg, MD: Aspen Publications. xi-xiii.

Quindlen, A. (1994, September 26). As quoted in quotables. *Chicago Tribune*.

Rager, P. (1994, October 31). From the desk of, Getting it together. *The Nursing Spectrum Greater Chicago/NE Illinois & NW Indiana Edition*. 7(22).

Ryan, R. (1994). *60 seconds & you're hired*. Manassas, VA: Impact Publications.

Sharpe, R. (1994, March 29). The waiting game: Women make strides, but men stay firmly in top company jobs. *Wall Street Journal*.

Silver, A. D. (1994, May 9). Manager's journal. The new American hero. *Wall Street Journal*.

Sullivan, T., & Gini, A. (1994). *Heigh-ho! heigh-ho!: Quotes about work*. Chicago: ACTA Publications.

Sulski, J. (1994, July 3). Attitude adjustment: Flexibility, openness keys to navigating stormy seas. *Chicago Tribune*.

Terkel, S. (1972). *Working: people talk about what they do all day and how they feel about it*. New York: Ballantine Books.

Topolnicki, D. (1994, March). Down and out? Here's how to go from pink slip to paycheck. *Money Magazine*,

Varro, B. (1996, January 10). BSN enrollment dips as nursing realigns. *Chicago Tribune*.

Wolfe, S. (1994). RN news watch. *RN, 57*(3), 14.

Zagury, C. (1994, June 13). The written word: A powerful tool for change. *The Nursing Spectrum Greater Chicago/NE Illinois & NW Indiana Edition*. 7(12).

Zurlinden, J. (1993, November 29). Grant for school-based nursing center. *The Nursing Spectrum Greater Chicago/NE Illinois & NW Indiana Edition*. 6(23).

APPENDIX 1.1

THE NATIONAL STUDENT NURSES' ASSOCIATION, INC.

Nursing students can get head starts in their nursing careers by participating in the National Students Nurses' Association (NSNA). Nursing students in associate degree, diploma, baccalaureate, generic masters, generic doctoral, or pre-nursing programs can become involved in a national organization and have their voices heard at the school, state, and national levels of the association. Joining NSNA connects nursing students with 40,000 NSNA members, each of whom can take advantage of the many programs and benefits the association has to offer. NSNA's collaborative leadership activities provide: representation in the annual House of Delegates; an opportunity to run for state and national office; a chance to win contests and prizes; and an opportunity to influence the future of the nursing profession. The following is an overview of NSNA's programs and benefits.

IMPRINT

All members receive *Imprint*, NSNA's official magazine published by and for nursing students. Published four times during the academic year, *Imprint* contains articles on current trends and issues in nursing, career development, NSNA meetings and events, membership benefits, association and national news, and job opportunities. *Imprint* is the only publication addressing student perspectives and serving student needs.

CAREER COUNSELING AND JOB SEARCHING

One-on-one career counseling with nurse counselors is available during the Midyear Conference and Annual Convention. The NSNA Career Counseling Center helps students to formulate their career goals and develop personalized plans to achieve those goals.

The *Imprint Career Planning Guide* helps students make important career decisions. The *Guide* contains career opportunity profiles from health care facilities with job openings for graduating seniors. Career-planning articles help students to manage stress, prepare for a first nursing position, pass the NCLEX-RN, explore specialty nursing opportunities, write a résumé, and prepare for job interviews. The *Guide* also contains up-to-date information on nursing organizations.

At NSNA's Midyear Conference, which takes place every November, nationally acclaimed speakers motivate and inspire students to excel in their careers. Programs are offered on taking the NCLEX-RN exam, career and educational advancement, and specialty nursing careers. Also offered is a discussion of new directions in nursing with top nursing leadership.

HELP IN PASSING STATE BOARDS

NSNA members receive up to $25 off the registration fee for the NSNA NCLEX EXCEL!™ courses and a 25% discount for the NSNA *NCLEX-RN Review* book published by Delmar Publishers. The publishers' review book includes an NCLEX practice computer disk.

The NSNA NCLEX EXCEL!™ courses are held at over 200 sites nationwide. Offered through Allegheny University, the NSNA NCLEX EXCEL!™ courses can be conducted at any nursing school. Information is available on request.

To prepare new graduates for the computerized format of the boards, NSNA members receive a discount for the NSNA *NCLEX EXCEL!™ Computerized Q&A*. Discounts are also available for the NSNA *NCLEX-RN Audio Review* on cassettes.

REDUCED RATES ON PRODUCTS AND SERVICES

Being an NSNA member saves students money. Members receive special reduced rates for nursing magazines, computer software, photocopying, and books. Reduced registration rates for the NSNA Convention and the Midyear Conference are available only to NSNA members. Members also receive discounts on NSNA publications.

HEALTH AND ACCIDENT INSURANCE

NSNA members and their eligible dependents can purchase group health and accident insurance provided by the Student Insurance Division of United Insurance Companies. The plan includes a continuation privilege for a period of up to nine months after graduation, if eligible.

PROJECT INTOUCH

Project InTouch, NSNA's "members-reaching-members" contest, gives members a chance to win prizes by recruiting new members. Prizes include NCLEX review books, stethoscopes, subscriptions, textbooks, and reference books.

NSNA PARTNERSHIPS

Through a partnership program, NSNA members can join the American Academy of Ambulatory Care Nursing (AAACN), the Association of Nurses in AIDS Care (ANAC), the Association of Operating Room Nurses (AORN), the Association of Rehabilitation Nurses (ARN), the Emergency Nurses Association (ENA), the National Association of Orthopedic Nurses (NAON), and the Oncology Nursing Society (ONS) for a special rate available only to NSNA members.

Through a joint project with the American Nurses Association (ANA), NSNA members who join the ANA within six months of graduation from a basic nursing program receive a special membership rate and a free set of ANA publications for the nursing professional.

ANNUAL CONVENTION

At the NSNA Annual Convention, which takes place in April, over fifty nationally acclaimed speakers, thirty workshops and major sessions, and a variety of exhibits and social events connect and motivate nursing students, faculty, and leaders.

Hundreds of delegates represent students in schools of nursing throughout the country. The delegates are responsible for the election of national officers and representatives and make collaborative decisions on issues of importance to nursing students. Unify with fellow students by attending NSNA's Annual Convention.

GLOBAL NURSING NETWORK

The NSNA administers the Fuld Fellowship program, sponsored by the Helen Fuld Health Trust, Marine Midland Bank, Trustee. In 1997, Fuld Fellows will attend the International Council of Nurses 21st Quadrennial Congress, June 15 - 20, in Vancouver, British Columbia, Canada. Deans and directors from all schools of nursing are invited to nominate a student for the Fuld Fellowship. One Fellow will be selected from each of the fifty states and the District of Columbia. In addition, nominations will be accepted from Guam, Puerto Rico, and the Virgin Islands.

AWARDS AND RECOGNITION

NSNA members who have contributed to the welfare and advancement of nursing students are recognized annually during the NSNA convention. Members are a part of NSNA's dynamic leadership team through participation in the many programs and competitions sponsored by the NSNA and its contributors.

MALPRACTICE INSURANCE

NSNA members qualify for a low-cost, comprehensive malpractice insurance policy that covers them in school, as hospital volunteers, and as hospital employees.

SCHOLARSHIP PROGRAM

The NSNA Foundation offers scholarships annually to undergraduate nursing students. Members receive points for participating in the NSNA. Scholarship recipients are recognized during the awards ceremony at the NSNA Annual Convention.

AN OPPORTUNITY FOR INVOLVEMENT

NSNA members can get involved in their school chapters and state associations, as well as in the NSNA. Involvement may include community health activities, Breakthrough to Nursing projects, education and practice activities, conventions, educational programs, newsletters, and other self-governance leadership opportunities.

EARN ACADEMIC CREDIT

Through NSNA's Independent Study for Leadership program, NSNA members have access to a model for independent study and to academic credit for participation in NSNA activities. *Independent Study Guidelines* are available.

MORE TO COME

NSNA's membership benefits program is growing. Members are informed of new benefits in the news section of *Imprint* magazine and through special mailings. Members are kept well-informed of the many benefits of belonging to NSNA.

ELIGIBILITY AND COST OF MEMBERSHIP

Nursing or prenursing students preparing for RN licensure in any state-approved program and RNs in programs leading to a baccalaureate in nursing are eligible for membership. Nursing students in generic masters and doctoral programs can also join.

NSNA dues are $30 per year plus state dues. New members each receive a $10 discount for the first year of membership. Students choosing the convenient two-year membership option each receive a $10 discount (total two-year dues are $50 plus two years of state dues).

WHO'S IN CHARGE OF NSNA?

The voting body of NSNA is the House of Delegates, which is composed of nursing students representing NSNA's school and state constituents. The House of Delegates elects the Board of Directors (who are all nursing students) each year to govern the association between conventions. A full-time staff is employed to assist in the implementation of NSNA's programs and projects.

FOR MORE INFORMATION

For more information, write to the National Student Nurses' Association, 555 West 57th Street, Suite 1327, New York, New York 10019. Telephone: 212-581-2211. Fax: 212-581-2368. E-Mail: NSNA.NET@internetmci.com.

Chapter Two

Changing Your Direction

Bette Case and Beth Bongard

INTRODUCTION

For this chapter, a number of nurses who had made changes over the course of their careers were interviewed. The stories told by these nurses as they reflected on their careers, revealed common approaches to career development as well as approaches unique to the circumstances of the individuals. Although these nurses did describe taking advantage of and creating opportunities, for the most part, they developed their careers without using systematic plans. Many commented that "things turned up" or "people asked me to do things."

Although these nurses did not purposefully create all of the opportunities that have shaped their careers, their stories reveal actions that assisted them in seizing opportunities. While these actions do not constitute a planned how-to approach to career change and development, they do suggest strategies that contribute to successful career development. The stories of these nurses also provide some clues for formulating a career plan.

Each individual forms a career plan from the combination of interests, strengths, goals, and skills unique to that person. The experiences of the interviewed nurses provide helpful guides, whether you are developing a career direction or executing a career plan.

 ## Developing a Career and Taking It on the Road

Charlotte earned her diploma from the nursing school of a large Chicago medical center and spent the next thirty years right there! Although she stayed with the same nursing department, the organization changed over those years, and her job responsibilities changed many times. She tells a story of developing her career at that medical center and then taking it on the road.

"I stayed at the medical center for the security and continued promotion opportunities. As a single parent, I needed to grow salary and benefits. All three of my boys have graduated from college. One is an MD.

"I came up through the ranks at the medical center. I worked staff in ortho, med-surg, ambulatory care, and psych. I was among the staff to open the first ICU. I took a head nurse position (as we called them in those days) on a forty-nine-bed med-surg unit. I earned my bachelor's and master's degrees with the help of the tuition-reimbursement program.

"Later, I became a supervisor. Every time another supervisor left, I wound up doing that person's job in addition. Finally, I moved into administration where I was a 'right-hand man' to the vice-president of nursing. I developed the department budget, worked on many special projects, and wrote numerous memos and documents. The VP was a great mentor for me.

"She encouraged me to apply for a VP job at another hospital in the city. I had never interviewed for a job. I couldn't believe it when they called for references the day after my first job interview ever! I took the job and stayed a couple of years. Then the VP of finance took a position at another hospital and asked me to go work there with him. So I did.

"During all those years at the medical center, I always took the attitude that whatever I could learn would be useful sometime, somewhere. I always floated, took on extra duties. I learned many specialties that way, and I also helped a lot of people along the way—everybody from MDs to other nurses to secretaries. When I was getting started in my first VP position, they were all there to help me whenever I asked. I took one of the nurse managers along with me to become my assistant.

"In my second VP position, we opened a skilled care unit, so I got my nursing home administrator's license. A few years later, my father died and I took six months off—my first summer vacation since I was a teenager.

"When I decided to go back to work, I didn't want the top job, mainly because of the stress associated with continuous budget cutting. I saw a blind ad for a nursing home administrator. I applied and got the job. After a couple of years, I wanted to go back to an acute care hospital. I had a condo in Las Vegas and found a chief nurse executive position there.

"I like the challenge of cutting the budget and putting a new plan together. When it's all done, I get bored. It really builds my self-esteem when I come up with an answer that works.

"When I give career advice to nurses, I encourage them to accept that you can't count on job security. Build relationships, don't burn bridges; you never know who can help you in the future. Take advantage of any opportunity. I always gained something, even if I couldn't use it right then. By volunteering to float, I learned more than skills for future reference. I built relationships by solving a staffing problem for the unit staff and nursing administration."

WHAT IS A CAREER?

The term *career* is variously defined in one dictionary as follows: "life work; success in one's chosen profession; a path or course" (Morris, 1980, p.203). The career stories of the nurses interviewed for this chapter chronicle emerging paths defined by choices. These choices that defined their career paths included giving up some dreams, creating others, recognizing strengths and sources of enjoyment, and responding to responsibilities and commitments.

One nurse suggested that a key to her own career satisfaction has been a sense of purpose; "Be able to tell yourself why you're working." The "why" may change with changing stages and commitments in life. At some points, economic necessity and providing for dependents may predominate. At other times, self-actualization needs emerge and drive the career. Often, a blend of concerns and motivators combine to influence career direction. For the individual, periodically addressing the "why" lends a sense of personal control. As career and workplace authority Carol Kleiman notes, "You are the only one in charge of your career and that is both the good and the bad news" (1994). Kleiman recommends spending ten minutes a day over a period of two or more weeks reflecting on career direction and goals.

THE CAREER PATH

Combinations of forces pushing and pulling on the nurses who shared their stories led these nurses to the choices that shaped their paths. Pushes included economic concerns (i.e., salary and benefits) and the need to support a family. The need to reserve time for self and family also drove some choices. Defining personally acceptable parameters for travel (i.e., How often? How far?) determined choices for some. For others, the unpleasant push of losing a job or having one's job eliminated led to considering new directions. Some felt pushed by spouses, family members, and significant others to leave dissatisfying situations or stretch to new opportunities.

The pulling forces of challenge and opportunity moved some to extend themselves to search for the satisfaction of facing challenge and succeeding; to seize the opportunity to develop new skills, contacts, and perspectives: or to reach higher levels of authority, influence, and economic reward. For Charlotte, challenge pulled strongly. She liked the challenge of putting a new plan together, and when it was all done, she got bored. But she also experienced the push of needing to provide progressively higher levels of income and benefits to support and educate her children.

Looking for ways to act on a passionate interest, a personal mission, or sense of conviction drew some into new arenas. One nurse today manages and consults in continuous quality improvement for a quality-consulting firm. She was tapped for a corporate position in quality management in response to her success as a staff development specialist in a hospital owned by the corporation. Her outspokenness regarding her zest for quality led hospital executives to recommend her for a corporate-level position in quality management. While pulled by her conviction, she also identifies concern about the possible elimination of her staff position as a force pushing her toward investigating other possibilities.

A nationally renowned training specialist who began her career as a labor and delivery nurse describes her career path as a constant effort to "notice those parts of my job that make me smile and find ways to do more of those things." Having identified the joy she finds in childbirth education, she pursued a master's degree in adult education and took a position in a nursing staff development department. Later, she became an entrepreneur in the training field (M. Peck, Personal Communication, February 20, 1995).

The love of learning pulled many in new career directions. Because learning itself involves change (i.e., change in your knowledge, values, beliefs or skills), it is not surprising that learning accompanies career growth and change. One nurse attorney who pursued nursing after beginning a career in law states that she "loves going to school and loves to learn." Having blended nursing and law in her career to date, she aspires to become a nurse midwife.

Informal learning opportunities also prove valuable. Charlotte took this approach throughout her climb to her present executive level. Through her willingness to learn, she built clinical expertise ranging from opening the first ICU in a large urban medical center to opening an extended care facility.

Self-assessment and follow-through shaped many of these nurses' careers—not only identifying what "makes them smile," personal passions, and convictions, but also recognizing a knack for certain aspects of the job. Recognizing weaknesses or deficits plays a role as well, but need not automatically close off a pathway. After identifying deficits, you may choose among several alternatives of action, as illustrated by the following comments from nurses.

> "I felt I had to move out of the management/administrative/executive track due to my weak financial skills."

> "I wanted to combine business and nursing. I began to educate myself through reading and talking with people. I saw an ad for a bill auditor with an insurance company, and I took that job while working as a staff nurse on the evening shift."

> "I'm not sure all the skills needed in this job live in one person! I work in partnership with others or select staff to access and make use of those skills I've chosen not to develop myself."

The career path is an individual journey, perhaps without a fixed destination. In fact, career-development authorities encourage a flexible stance guided by goals and self-awareness. A willingness to take risks and learn from mistakes also inspires the journey. As Hugh Prather writes, "My career will form behind me. All I can do is let this day come to me in peace. All I can do is take the step before me now, and not fear repeating an effort or making a new one" (1970).

MYTHS ABOUT NURSING CAREERS

The nurses who told their stories shattered some myths about nursing careers.

Myth 1: You're Either a Nurse or You're Not

Many nurses say, "I always wanted to be a nurse," and many nurses undoubtedly share some common experiences in the educational process as well as the work-place. For each nurse, however, these experiences mesh in a unique way with the nurse's personal and cultural characteristics. And because a nursing career offers so many diverse possibilities, no one nursing identity characterizes the "typical nurse." There are many ways to be a nurse. Many individuals who differ greatly can find success and satisfaction in choosing a nursing career and practicing different aspects of nursing.

Myth 2: You Need Specific Preparation

Although most nursing jobs require some specific education and training, alternatives to traditional preparation may satisfy requirements. One nurse stated that he educated himself in the business aspects he needed to redirect his career toward managed care. The dean of a respected college of nursing selected a nurse who had no previous experience as a faculty member to be his assistant dean. The dean said that her leadership style was more important to him than other traditional qualifications. Courageous nurses who venture into new and unfamiliar career dimensions show the confidence to develop the necessary competence. They approach these stretches with such attitudes as, "How hard can it be?"; "I'll figure it out when I get there"; and "Let's get in there and do this thing."

Formal education does not completely prepare you to function competently on the job. Education prepares you to develop the competencies the job requires.

Myth 3: All Your Degrees Must Be in Nursing

Depending on your goals, you may be better off pursuing advanced-degree work in another field. Any academic degree is a hard-earned credential and a ticket of sorts; before you buy your ticket, know where you're going. Research your options carefully and validate your assumptions about what is available. Colleges and universities are developing new programs every day to address marketplace needs. Academic institutions are offering various blends of business, law, health care, management, and many other disciplines.

Myth 4: There's Something Wrong with Switching Jobs

In today's society, authorities tell us that we can expect the norm to be three changes of profession and six changes of job in a typical working life (Sulski, 1994). In viewing your career as a continually evolving search for self-actualization, you can stay open to new options as they emerge and recognize new personal preferences, interests, and expertise as they develop. The nurses who told their stories described willingness to change as "looking change in the eye," "going against the grain with my eyes shut," "always thinking I'd land on my feet," and "not being afraid to take a risk."

Myth 5: Nursing Offers All the Opportunity You Could Want

Nursing offers numerous opportunities in the many facets of the various specialties and functions that compose nursing practice in the twenty-first century. Nursing can also act as a powerful springboard to launch careers in other fields, however. The nurses who told their stories spoke of their strengths in organizing, communicating, dealing with individuals of diverse backgrounds, and responding to unpredictable situations. Those skills, and others, are highly valued in careers outside of nursing. It is interesting to note that certain career directions within nursing are sometimes viewed as perverse by the nursing mainstream. For example, the nurse who pursued a career in managed care was variously told by respected colleagues and supervisors that he was "a traitor" and was "committing career suicide." Pay attention to what you want. You don't leave nursing; you take it with you.

One nurse, currently assistant provost of an East Coast university, stated that she has occasionally used her nursing skills to respond to urgent requests for assessment in various offices of the university. The services she has provided not only earned respect for her nursing skills, but also helped cement relationships among other departments. She believes that the nursing process and the caring attitude associated with nursing increased her value in her new role at the higher administrative levels of the university.

Myth 6: There's a Career Path

There's your career path, and it's uniquely yours. You choose it, and, in fact, you choose it every day as you recognize your preferences and make the choices that define your career. In years past, there was one career path. It led from bedside nursing to nursing management to nursing administration to the chief nurse executive role, with possible diversions into nursing education. Today, numerous career branches present themselves at all levels. For nurses who choose to practice as staff nurses for their entire careers, there are a host of possibilities for elaborating on the direct care role—not only by cross-training in acute care, but also by venturing into home health, hospice, or ambulatory care. Take charge of your career path; only you can.

KNOWING YOUR WANTS AND NEEDS

The nurses who told their career stories had no real pattern in what they looked for or needed in their work and careers. The good news is that a wide variety of needs were accommodated as these individuals moved through their career paths. These nurses found solutions that fit them, rather than adjusting to rigid patterns of expectations.

As you might expect, several nurses found their former jobs eliminated. Contrary to expectations, however, no two of these nurses responded in the same way or with the same needs. One had two successive administrative positions eliminated and realized she needed independence; she hated being controlled by rules. An affinity for stimulation, variety, and high-pressure situations led her to a career in law.

Another nurse had a strong need for security. She clung to a job in the operating room, although she disliked it. She feared that she could not succeed anywhere else. When administration eliminated her job, however, she found the courage to turn down a management position in another of the hospital's service areas. She made a leap from her hospital job, venturing instead into corporate life. She went to work for a large medical products company, functioning as a sales representative and providing inservice training for the staff of her customer hospitals. She also gained insight into corporate life and corporate career-building. Now awaiting the birth of her first child, she has been working from home on a limited basis. She has not yet decided her next career step. Her need for security still motivates her, but she sees opportunities other than hospital nursing that meet her needs.

Several nurses said nursing offered them the only path they could see that provided financial independence as they sent children to medical school, weathered divorces, or supported families alone. They looked for financial opportunity and stability in their careers.

Several others discussed high-achievement needs—the need to make more and more money as a sign of achievement, to keep moving up and past barriers. One nurse was told he didn't have the right experience to move from his clinical path into utilization and quality management. He had a high need to sidestep barriers and used this as motivation to achieve his goal.

Many of these nurses wanted to care for others. One is devoted to nursing and sees it as a sacred profession. Yet, she had to step outside of nursing to learn techniques to enhance her pain management and "care-for-the-caregiver" practice. Another nurse who originally was motivated by caring for patients now cares for entire systems through organizational development practice. Although she no longer relates to her nursing background, she still sees caring as a continuing need that she addresses through her career.

Others were motivated purely and simply by what they enjoyed. One said, "I paid attention to what made me smile." Another analyzed every job she had for the part she enjoyed most and looked for that aspect in her next role.

Some nurses were motivated by the need to influence on a large scale. One has influence over grants in Washington; another works as an independent consultant in large-scale, core-process reengineering. Other nurses wanted more influence and control over their own lives—the ability to control their hours, have time with their families, or be free of rules.

Some nurses sought variety, continued learning, "something new and different." These nurses turned interests into careers. An interest in "left-brain, right-brain" (i.e., logical, creative) implications in nursing led one nurse to a career as an independent corporate trainer. As a corporate trainer, she provides education, training, and organizational development recommendations to her clients, including a wide variety of businesses and corporations.

Another nurse leveraged her ability to turn learning experiences into interactive games. She now owns her own business, designing learning activities and selling them.

Although no one pattern emerged, all of these nurses actually found what they were looking for. Sometimes, the paths were short; other times, they were long. But each of these nurses found the stimulation, money, prestige, opportunity to influence—whatever it was that each identified as a personal need. Many of them could tell you about jobs they found frustrating or disappointing; yet each of them eventually found satisfaction.

One thing became evident as these nurses talked about what they needed in their careers. Each one had identified what he or she needed and looked for. Not only could they clearly describe it, but they could tell you when they had it at work and when they did not. Furthermore, these nurses were enthusiastic about what they wanted from their careers. And none of them was apologetic. No one felt it disgraceful to mention money, influence, or prestige as a motivator. Thus, while the motivations and needs differed among these nurses, the clarity did not. One thing they definitely had in common was a sense of their own needs. Sometimes this came to them gradually, as with the research director who came to recognize as his career progressed that independence and influence were strong motivators. Others knew all along what they needed, as with the consultant for a big-six accounting firm who discussed her career-long desire for prestige and influence at very high levels. Whether gradually acquired or always present, all of these nurses were at a point where they knew and could clearly articulate what they needed in their careers.

As you work on identifying what you want in your career, take special note of the following messages inherent in these stories:

- Spend time thinking about what you need in your career. The clearer you are, the more likely you are to find it.

- There is room for everyone's career dream. All of these nurses found what they wanted as they pursued their paths.

 ## *Blending Nontraditional Ingredients in Specialty Practice*

Katherine had two brothers who had died—one as a teenager, one as a young adult. She reflects, "Trying to find peace with these deaths influenced my future thinking. I got my master's in psychology and worked in oncology at several Boston hospitals. Then we moved to Los Angeles to meet my husband's career needs.

"I worked at a large teaching medical center as a nurse specialist in a multidisciplinary pain-management service. I assessed patients; contributed to writing pain-management and dying-patient protocols; and worked with dying patients, their families, and the staff who worked with them. I performed as a technical consultant and educator. Gradually, I became more drawn to the nonphysical aspects of pain management.

"When the pain-management service was discontinued, I became a clinical specialist in pain management. At first, I was assigned to oncology and bone marrow transplant units. Later, I became a house-wide consultant. My practice expanded to include running patient and family support groups, facilitating staff support groups, consulting with patients, performing direct pain work, and providing bereavement counseling. Now my practice leans heavily toward care-for-the-caregiver issues.

"I believe nursing is a sacred profession, touching the souls of people in the most personal and meaningful times. This privilege is central to the meaning of being a nurse. My advanced education lies outside of nursing because nursing offered no formal training to best meet patients' pain needs and emotional needs in the dying process.

"I'm constantly called on when traditional medicine has nothing more to offer—even here, in one of the nation's most high-tech environments. I believe patients can be helped right up until the time of death. I've experimented with massage, imaging, variations of pharmacological pain-management interventions, prayer, and anything meaningful from the patient's perspective.

"In my work with staff, I've seen whole staffs depleted from dealing with the trauma of successive deaths. After facilitating ongoing groups for staff, a colleague and I developed a "heal the healer" weekend retreat. In an environment incorporating art, music, movement, and humor, staff members have experienced restored hope and renewed energy.

"I take inspiration from books, historical and philosophical perspectives, and images that stand out in the natural environment. I think about the meaning of my experiences. I allow myself to openly experience new points of view and try new skills in an experiential way. I follow my career as it evolves, rather than preplanning.

"Though I am not a typical specialist, I am squarely in the nursing arena, practicing nursing's mandate of healing. Organized nursing may put up barriers to some forms of nontraditional practice, but these barriers are no different or more severe than the barriers of any administrative system."

MOTIVATORS

When the interviewed nurses talked about their motivations, they identified many and differing personal values. For example, Katherine sought to help others in a nontraditional way, in contrast to another nurse's desire to gain money and prestige. One nurse sought independence from an unhappy marriage, while another nurse continually adjusted her career to fit with family plans. One nurse feared dependence, while another nurse sought steadiness and predictability.

Motivators are specific to the individual and can change over time. No motivator is right or wrong. Motivators are simply needs that compel an individual to act. Energizing factors such as support, encouragement, and specific acts of assistance from others (e.g., mentors, family members, peers, or associates) can also serve as motivators.

You will improve your chances of success if you identify your own personal motivators and brainstorm as many career directions or work experiences as you can think of to satisfy those needs. The personal motivators identified by the interviewed nurses include: wanting to learn, seeking a challenge, relieving restlessness, escaping the boredom of repetition, (whether physical, intellectual, or emotional), hooking someone on an idea, extending sphere of influence, enjoying doing something really well, adding spiritual and psychic skills to nursing, receiving tuition and other benefits for self and family, reducing travel requirements, and the possibility or reality of losing a job.

SOURCES OF HELP

The nurses who told their stories succeeded in making significant career leaps. Only rarely, however, did anyone express complete certainty regarding future paths contemplated or personal ability to succeed. Frequently, in fact, the nurses described feeling apprehensive, doubtful, unconfident, confused, and intimidated. How, then, did these nurses succeed in making such significant changes? As they related their stories, all talked about what helped them get where they wanted to go.

These successful career-changers cited four sources of help: helpful attitudes, helpful skills, help from others, and the help that results from general exploration.

Helpful Attitudes

Certain attitudes assisted these nurses as they made career changes. These attitudes yielded energy and gave perspective to their career-development journeys.

Courage. One nurse said it was his hardest life decision: he took a $6,000 salary cut, left familiar surroundings, and was considered a traitor because he went into utilization review. Another was pursued by her former dean and called a traitor because she sought an MBA. Another nurse who had previously clung to job security chose to leave the security of a hospital position and move into the corporate world. Another left the city where she had lived all her life and where her family lives to relocate 2,000 miles away. Still another chose to commute soon after a new marriage. All described these decisions as requiring great courage. Some made their decisions in the face of vehement counter arguments, the pull of family loyalty, or a leap into the unknown. Yet all the nurses identified these as the best decisions they made in their careers.

Perseverance. Over and over, these nurses advised, "Don't give up." One waited until her son had graduated from medical school and launched his career before relocating. Another was terrified that her position would be eliminated in a corporate takeover; but the terror motivated her to talk to the leadership and convince them that they needed her skills at the corporate level. Another met with frustration after frustration as he tried to move into several different nursing niches, always having to overcome barriers. Many talked of waiting for the right time for their families, persisting through difficult and intimidating educational tracks, and persisting past their own doubts and lack of confidence. Regardless of the challenge and setbacks, however, these nurses never gave up.

Ignore Negative Attitudes. Several of the career-changers ran into hostility and discouragement from peers, bosses, and even family members. Some were asked, "Why would you want to do that?" Others ran into prejudice because they were men. Still others were told that too much math was involved for them to succeed, they did not have the right experience, or any of a number of discouraging remarks. Most of the stories revealed a conscious choice to ignore gratuitously negative attitudes toward their career decisions.

Prepare for Setbacks. Some nurses found it helpful to prepare emotionally for setbacks by telling themselves that "you can't count on anything." They said to have a primary plan and a back-up plan. If you cannot get into your school of choice, have an alternate choice in mind. If you cannot get into critical care in the hospital you choose, seek out a hospital that will let you make that transition. Sometimes, back-up choices open important doors. These nurses' stories depict disappointments and surprises as inevitable events. Expecting surprises helps.

Risk-Taking. "If you don't make a mistake, you're not trying." A number of these interviewed nurses started their own businesses. They put money at risk as well as pride. Calculated risks were inevitable and necessary. The fear or avoidance of risk would have made these career changes impossible.

Many nurses have not developed a tolerance for risk-taking. But without accepting and sometimes even seeking risks, you cannot fully take control and responsibility for your own career. In addition to financial risks, you may risk looking inept, returning to a novice level in a new specialty after achieving expert status in your current role, or actual failure.

Identify your risks. Plan strategies to curtail and manage risks. Obtain help in strategy planning from experienced colleagues, mentors and other support persons.

Love of Learning. Learn all you can about your field: talk to people in the field; read everything you can get your hands on; be insatiably curious. One high-level administrator said she succeeded by learning early in her career that volunteering to float would be helpful to her. She also volunteered for new assignments throughout her career. She learned a great deal, was visible, and was at the right place at the right time. Don't stay within the mantle of nursing; learn from all the disciplines with which you interact. Ask questions. Imagine tasks from other points of view. Show interest and be aware. And the interviewed nurses emphasized, "Read, read, read!"

Increased Awareness. Create opportunities to talk with people outside of nursing. Look for opportunities to meet with other professionals. Business sections and women's sections in local newspapers may list meetings of interest. Use meetings of all sorts—PTA meetings, church groups, committee meetings, and other gatherings—to approach others and learn about their fields.

Enroll in an adult education course. In addition to learning about an area of interest, you may find great resources in fellow classmates.

Learn about trends and be aware of viewpoints other than those of nursing. The interviewed nurses stressed being alert and paying attention to others in the field you plan to pursue.

Self-Directed Preparation for a New Career Direction

Even before entering college, Stephen knew he wanted to get into a medical-related career. "I was working at a hospital when I entered college. The hospital offered tuition payment in exchange for work after graduation." At the time, there was a shortage of nurses. He recalls, "After I graduated from nursing school, I wanted ortho. However, the hospital needed critical care nurses, so I went to critical care. Critical care was exciting, but after a couple of years I felt burned out from the physical and emotional stress.

"I was never sure I wanted a solely clinical role. I was interested in business and wanted to combine clinical nursing and business. At college, we could design our own curriculum. I proposed to substitute business for humanities; my proposal was refused.

"After getting burned out in critical care, I looked for business options. I couldn't get an opportunity at the hospital where I was working. They needed nurses in critical care. Organizations often do not give nurses the opportunity to try something new.

"Quality management or utilization management seemed like logical next steps. There were no chances for me to pursue those roles, however, because there were always so many more-senior personnel who wanted those positions. And I couldn't get a job in those areas on the outside because I had no experience.

"I began to educate myself independently, reading about finance and career movement, talking with people in quality, utilization, and finance. I saw an ad for a bill auditor for an insurance company. I did that job on the side while working 3:00 to 11:00 in critical care. The auditing work provided an entrée for me into business.

"I went into a PSRO (Professional Standards Review Organization) when the opportunity came up. I had to take a $6,000 salary cut. It was so difficult, really hard. But, it was the best thing I ever did. I felt relieved to leave the clinical role. My wife said that I instantly became a different person.

"Some nurses and doctors felt that I was a traitor to practitioners when I went into the financial-management aspect. My boss at the time told me I was committing career suicide. Later, she revised her opinion.

"I got beyond the initial questioning of whether I could do it. My self-esteem grew as I saw that I could.

"For the PSRO, I worked on contracts with several hospitals. One hospital recruited me to code medical records for diagnosis-related grouping (DRGs). I worked there for a year and thought of getting a degree in medical records. The hospital was one of the first to combine utilization management and quality management. They offered me a position managing utilization management. Later, I took over quality and became director of both areas.

"I developed a case management program wherein data was used to analyze practice patterns with the goal of decreasing resource utilization. The hospital was a member hospital of a large, for-profit corporation. I was contacted by the corporate offices to develop case management for the corporation.

"Later, when the corporation reorganized, the quality management department became an independent consulting company. Now, as a consultant with this company, I work with hospitals, accessing their data and comparing it to our database to identify variances and opportunities for improvement.

"A nurse recently told me that she didn't envy me talking with the doctors about case management and changes in practice patterns. But I savor the opportunity. I find the doctors respectful and eager for the information. And I find satisfaction in giving it.

"Through ongoing contact with my mentor, I teach finance and management courses and precept students. I'm looking into external degree programs for a master's degree—an MHA or MBA with a health care focus. I've started master's programs three times, but was unable to finish each time due to family needs and travel requirements of my job.

"My wife also has a career change story. She burned out on staff nursing and wanted more control of her schedule. She started working in telephone triage with an HMO, but missed the patient contact. Now, she works as a surgical nurse clinician/PA (physician's assistant) with a surgeon. She loves her job. When she feels overwhelmed by the stress at times, I remind her that she doesn't have to work to meet our financial needs. She responds that she has to do this work because she loves what she does.

"I strongly encourage nurses to vary from the usual paths—to ask themselves what they've seen others doing that looks interesting. Find out about other roles from those who are working in them. Then you get a more realistic view. I think nurses in general need more knowledge of health care finance and how decisions get made."

Helpful Skills

The interviewed nurses identified certain skills as vital in developing their career paths. Practicing these skills helps further career development.

Interacting Comfortably. The skill of putting others at ease and genuinely enjoying a variety and large number of contacts and gravitating toward such interaction is especially helpful.

Organizing. Career-changers must organize new information and new tasks. You need to set aside old patterns. Decide what is most important now, and plan your time accordingly. Collect information directed toward your priorities. You need to bring order to your new endeavors, whether you are studying, gathering information, organizing a job search, or managing sales contacts. Only you can identify your personal and professional priorities and create the plan to best address them.

Political Sense. Knowing how decisions get made and how to persuade others helps in a major transition.

Communicating Successfully. The nurses interviewed told stories of selling new roles to their bosses and convincing people to take chances on them. They also told of having to adopt quickly and use readily the language of their new fields.

Hard Work. Many of the nurses interviewed said they felt well prepared to develop their careers because they were accustomed to working hard as nurses. These nurses felt that their work habits had served them well.

Business Skills. Several of the interviewed nurses wished in hindsight that they had taken more business-planning courses, and those that had taken such courses were grateful. The skills of analyzing, projecting, budgeting, and using computers were cited several times as being important. The career-changers who had taken business courses or earned MBAs said that the associated skills were vital and that the degrees themselves served to enhance confidence.

Help from Others

While successful career development requires self-knowledge and individuality, healthy interdependence with others, rather than independence and isolation, enhances success.

Mentors. Mentors advised, opened doors, encouraged, and increased the visibility of those interviewed nurses fortunate enough to have them.

"Debtors". Several nurses talked of the help they received from those whom they had helped in the past. Such help came in the form of references, information, networking, and contacts.

Peers. The nurses interviewed told of receiving support from their peers, either in school or on the job. Some developed new peer groups while in school. Others were assisted by peers in their new roles. These nurses received on-the-job coaching and practical help from their new colleagues.

Family. One interviewed nurse spoke of being encouraged, and almost pushed, by her husband to pursue her interests. Other nurses spoke of the emotional support offered by their spouses. Family members also assisted with child care during career transitions.

Unexpected Sources. One interviewed nurse realized that as some people learned that she wanted to move out of nursing, these people no longer viewed her as competing or threatening. Such people became very encouraging, open, and supportive. Another nurse spoke of the "negative example" set by a boss. For this nurse, the negative example served as a constant reinforcement for changing direction—as well as a model for how *not* to perform.

Help from Exploring

All the interviewed career-changers thought exploring was essential to success. They talked about exploring what you like most and understanding your needs and yourself. And they talked about experimenting.

Float to different areas. Volunteer for challenging responsibilities. See what fits and what doesn't. Be open to surprises. Observe what others are doing. Which parts look interesting? When you find a role or work that attracts you, talk with those who do that work to find out what their roles are really like.

Most of the nurses interviewed emphasized that they actually had more choices than they originally thought. They spoke of exploring those choices. Look at trends. Is downsizing an opportunity for consulting, for learning something new, for expanding skills? What legal, financial, and political developments will you be able to leverage for your career? Again and again, these nurses advised to explore trends and roles with everyone you contact.

They also advised to seek out what you need. Look for a mentor. Ask for information. Request new opportunities. Propose a new role. Look for opportunities to gain new skills and exposure. Read a variety of books, journals, magazines, and newspapers. Read about your interests, and find new ones. Keep up with trends, and approach those who are succeeding in your field of interest.

HINDRANCES

Just as these successful career-changers found sources of help in their journeys, they also experienced hindrances. These nurses had to work around or solve problems such as the following:

- Some nurses found that being an RN was a disadvantage in their new careers. "If they find out you're a nurse, they'll walk all over you." A seasoned administrator said that colleagues in the business world told her that she could readily step into an executive position given her skills and experience, but that she would need to emphasize her organizational accomplishments and downplay the titles of her nursing positions.

- Many nurses found limited opportunity in their organizations for RNs to do something new. Nurses found themselves sent where they were needed rather than where they wanted to go.

- Several nurses told stories that reflected a lack of flexibility in academia in general or in specific academic programs. Nurses talked of running into brick walls when trying to either negotiate needed courses into their programs of study or make substitutions.

- Some nurse lacked the financial skills required in their new professions.

- Some nurses lacked the clinical skills needed to make desired changes.

- Many nurses found themselves to be in a "comfort zone," where a sense of security led to inertia. Although they wanted something more satisfying, they were lulled by security.

- Some nurses found that their employers accepted mediocre performance, which, in turn, spawned a general lack of motivation to change systems for the better.

- Some nurses discovered that they had pursued too technical a path in their learning. They needed a much broader education.

- Several nurses felt that their changes were delayed or made difficult because they were unsure of what they wanted. They had a hard time finding mentors because they weren't clear about the areas where they needed guidance and development. Being vague about what they wanted hindered their investigations as they struggled with getting away from what they did not like.

- Many of the career-changers told of a rigidity in nursing. They described the structure as limiting their exploration and their opportunities.

- Some nurses said they were "too busy", or "too panicky" in response to job threats and that this prevented them from envisioning what they wanted.

- Some nurses were held back temporarily by lack of experience in the fields they wanted to pursue; they found it hard to "break in."

- Many career-changers noted that nurses are not encouraged regarding or even informed about nontraditional careers and choices either within or outside of nursing.

- Some career-changers experienced lack of confidence in some of their skills, especially math. Some even spoke of lacking confidence in their overall abilities.

- Some nurses cited jealous or intimidating nursing leaders as impediments. Some career-changers were discouraged subtly for their choices; others were chastised openly.

- Although the interviewed nurses encountered barriers, worries, and even threats to success; each managed to succeed! These career-changers used their contacts, mentors, and other forms of assistance to negate the roadblocks they experienced. When confronted with perceived skill deficits, they found ways to master the skills in question. When they encountered resistance based on lack of experience, they sought out volunteer experience or talked their ways past the barrier. Some had others—such as mentors, network contacts, and people they had helped in the past—talk for them. Some of these nurses used persistence, some sought additional training and education. And sometimes just ignored the problems as they pursued their paths. Each used different strategies, but each succeeded!

WAYS TO SUCCEED

As these nurses discussed overcoming roadblocks and barriers, they collectively revealed a repertoire of useful strategies for success. Each career-changer used a number of strategies to achieve success. Yet, three common recommendations emerged: build your self-confidence, stretch your awareness by exposing yourself to the widest possible array of ideas, and put yourself in the view of those who will make decisions regarding your moving into your desired career.

Build Self-Confidence

These nurses faced new directions with courage and self-confidence. They spoke of "conquering fears" and "looking change in the eye." One nurse attorney who felt "petrified of her first teaching job in a law school" benefited from the support and encouragement of a mentor. Years later when she embarked on a newly defined position at a major medical center, she said, "I don't know what to do when I get there, but that's okay, because I'll figure it out."

Stephen said he "got beyond wondering, can I do it? My self-esteem grew as I saw that I could." Others said, "I never felt at risk. I always felt I'd land on my feet," and "How hard can it be? What's the worst thing that can happen?"

These nurses matured as they succeeded in their careers. Their confidence to develop new competencies grew with their successes. But how did they initially gain that confidence? As often happens when experts talk about their practices, most of these nurses could not exactly describe how they built self-confidence. Take, for instance, the nurse who developed her career as a nationally renowned trainer. She says that she sometimes looks back on paths she has taken and asks herself, "How did I think that was a good idea?" Yet, she also says that if she had it to do over, she would do exactly the same in developing her career.

Psychologists agree that self-confidence builds when individuals receive validation for their feelings, thoughts, and actions. One nurse noted that focusing on what she did very well and doing it repeatedly helped her self-confidence grow. Many noted that their successes fed their confidence. As Charlotte expressed, "Coming up with an answer that worked built my self-esteem." Identifying your strengths, practicing your strongest skills, and seeking feedback and validation from others begins a cycle of ongoing increase in skill and confidence. Several nurses mentioned that they had screened out naysayers and surrounded themselves with supporters.

As you identify your strengths and begin to develop self-confidence, you will also develop confidence in your judgment about your career. When Stephen redirected his career toward managed care, he heard from administrators that he was "a traitor" who was "committing career suicide." Yet he had confidence in his judgment about his own interests and strengths and the growing need for the expertise he was developing. In time, those same administrators changed their thinking about his decision. Another nurse, whose career has included executive positions and high-level consulting, received negative feedback about her decision to pursue a master's degree in business administration rather than in nursing. In reflecting on her career, however, she believes that her MBA has proved crucial in directing her career.

For these nurses, as self-confidence grew, so did the willingness to take risks and the ability to tolerate and learn from mistakes. Our mistakes are our "instructional friends," according to Stephen Brookfield (1994), an authority on critical thinking and adult education. Self-confidence bolsters our ability to view our mistakes as learning opportunities.

The same nurse whom the dean had selected for the assistant dean position despite her lack of traditional qualifications later received an offer to serve as vice president of nursing in a hospital. Although she had not accumulated the conventional qualifications for the position, she felt confident in her successes as assistant dean and asked herself, "Why wouldn't this work in running a hospital?" Not only did she accept the offer, she succeeded brilliantly!

Charlotte built her confidence and her career in the medical center where she received her diploma in nursing. Though she had no experience in job interviewing, she carried her confidence with her to the first job interview of her career—and received the offer of the vice president of nursing. She attributes some of her sense of confidence to a mentor's support, encouragement, and confidence in her ability.

Self-confidence, then, is a key to success. And identifying and capitalizing on your strengths begins an exciting process of building self-confidence.

Become More Aware

These successful career-changers also cited awareness as being integral to their successes. Among the strategies they recommended are the following:

- Pay attention to what you like to read and to what you like to see others doing. Looking for patterns of interest, stimulation, and satisfaction helped these nurses "zero in on" new directions.

- Increase your awareness of the variety of opportunities available. Don't shut yourself off from exposure to other interests. You have nothing to lose by gaining more information and exploring new areas. Open yourself to new experiences.

- Seek out people. Ask them questions about what they do, how they got into it, what barriers they encountered, and how they overcame them. People responded to these nurses, giving them plentiful and helpful information, guidance, and support. Ask!

- Gather as much information as possible about trends and the total picture. What are the opportunities in your area of interest? What is the supply of professionals or practitioners in your field of interest? How will reimbursement legislation affect your new endeavors? What procedures will shift out of hospital settings, thus limiting or creating opportunities for you? What areas of disorganization do you see resulting from major health care changes? How can you leverage trends and the needs they create to your advantage?

- Take off the blinders. If you think a nurse can't do something, rethink it! If one path looks closed, talk to more and more people until you find another path. Don't accept that the way it has always been is the way it will always be.

- Act like the people or the role to which you aspire. Learn the interests and the language of those who are living your dream career. Explore the world from their points of view.

- Pursue study in another field to enhance your nursing expertise. Obtain a broader education than you currently have.

- Expose yourself to what others think of nursing and nursing's viewpoint. You do not have to accept these viewpoints or turn your back on nursing. This information simply gives you options.

- Participate in numerous seminars. Expose yourself to the people in the audience. Open yourself to the differing viewpoints that participants bring to topics. Learn from participants as well as presenters. Use seminars as networking opportunities, not just as occasions for learning specific content.

Gain Recognition

Gaining recognition from those people who can help you meet your career objectives was also key in the experience of these successful career-changers. You can accomplish this in a number of ways, including the following:

- Recognize what you have a knack for and showcase it. Give a class. Mentor someone. Volunteer to write a report or an article. Talk about your interests and talents.

- Ask major players in your field for advice. Call or write to the author of an article you have read or the presenter of a seminar you have attended. Look for connections between your specific area of interest and those of the leaders in the field. Can your work add new dimensions to the field? When you ask thoughtful questions or describe your interests clearly, leaders in the field will usually respond and remember you. Most people *like* to help other people. Your request may flatter authors and speakers. They may respond quickly. Do not be discouraged, however, if your first attempts don't lead to responses. Simply follow up a second time. You may reach your contacts at times more convenient for them to respond.

- Find out who in a seminar audience can influence your career and approach those people. One nurse found the chief operating officer of an organization she wanted to join and laid the groundwork for her career move during a seminar break.

- Stay in contact with classmates and former faculty members as your career progresses. They may have many influential contacts, and, thus, can be a great network!

- Seize opportunities. Expand your role subtly, experimentally. Then build in what you like as a legitimate part of your job. Katherine's story reveals gradual shifts geared toward serving a new market. Gradually, she created an awareness of her presence and skills.

- Leverage projects into career opportunities. One nurse wrote a plan of care adapted to computer use and thus launched her own business and later moved into international consulting.

- Coauthor articles with people in the field you want to enter. This technique led one nurse to a career as a nursing expert in a big-six consulting firm.

Again, each of these nurses interviewed did not use all of these strategies, but each used some of these approaches. And although there was no universal pattern to their needs or their strategies, a common theme emerged from their experiences: persist despite barriers and explore a vision for a new career. Some of the changes they made were gradual and incremental. Some were major leaps. But all of these nurses achieved what they set out to do.

SUMMARY

Many different paths lead to career success for nurses. You will discover the secret to your career success when you create the right mix of education, experience, expertise, interests, passions, and opportunities for yourself.

Two kinds of knowledge will assist you: knowledge of yourself and knowledge of potential opportunities. Getting in touch with your personal strengths, motivators, and passions will help you form a vision of your journey; it may be only your next stop, or it may be an ultimate destination. Ask yourself, "Why am I working? Why do I want to make a change?"

Knowledge of potential opportunities comes from knowledge of the marketplace for the skills and interests you want to pursue. What is happening in health care, industry, and society that creates a need for the services and products you'd love to provide? If you can identify people who are doing the job of your dreams, talk with them to discover what the job is really like and what additional knowledge, skills, and experience will help you get that job. You may discover some new and unanticipated opportunities in the process. When you decide you want to make a change, find a place to go. Shape your goals according to new information you receive about yourself and about opportunities. In the words of one nurse, "Have a goal, but be willing to change it and give up dreams that don't fit."

Drawing on the experiences of nurses who have successfully changed direction over the course of their careers, this chapter described factors that influence career development. The stories of these nurses challenge some myths about nursing as a career. Motivators, sources of help, and hindrances were common variables in the experiences of these nurses. The varied career paths these nurses created, however, demonstrate that there is no one road to career success for a nurse.

REFERENCES

Brookfield, S. (1994, May). Understanding learning organizations. *Creating learning organizations: Moving beyond the competencies.* Seminar sponsored by Marquette University Continuing Nursing Education, Milwaukee, WI.

Kleiman, C. (1994). *The career coach.* Chicago: Dearborn Financial Publishing, Inc.

Morris, W. (Ed.). (1980). *The American heritage dictionary of the English language.* Boston: Houghton-Mifflin Company.

Prather, H. (1970). *Notes to myself.* New York: Bantam Books.

Sulski, J. (1994, July 3). Attitude adjustment: Flexibility, openness keys to navigating stormy seas. *Chicago Tribune.*

Chapter Three

Managing Your Career

Beth Bongard

INTRODUCTION

With each progressing year, fewer and fewer nurses will work in traditional general hospitals. Instead, more nurses will find opportunities with freestanding, nonhospital providers. This trend will continue, keeping pace with changes in health care and society. More nurses will also recognize new opportunities within nursing, expand their job searches beyond nursing, or start independent practices or businesses. To find or create satisfying opportunities in this environment, you must to manage your career.

Your nursing training and background adapts you to the world in a way that you can't fully imagine until you are "standing outside" of nursing. Nurses are wanted for their discipline, knowledge, and ability to handle crisis. Nurses have proven that they can learn difficult and complex concepts, manage intricate and highly intense workloads in a cooperative way, and meet multiple, competing deadlines.

Hospitals may take nurses for granted, but outside employers have a far different attitude. A nurse who worked as a consultant to a prestigious architectural firm says, "The design team insisted on working with a nurse from the very beginning of the project. It was thrilling. I influenced decisions that I couldn't pay a hospital administrator to hear. The architects viewed nurses as the best professionals to articulate the complex interaction of patients' needs, the influence of technology, and the working needs of health care providers. They were convinced that a nurse could help them design a building that's both efficient and livable."

If you're going to get ahead in your career, make plans. This chapter is designed to help you arrive at a plan by looking at yourself as well as at the market. You'll also learn how to best present yourself through your résumé and interview.

ASSESSING THE MARKET

Assess the market through both ends of the telescope. Turned the usual way, the telescope allows you to see small pieces of the horizon and examine them in detail. What changes in technology, health care, and jobs will create immediate opportunities? And how can you profit from them? Looking through the other end of the telescope affords you a broader view of the world. What will be the long-range implications of research, technology, legislation, education, population demographics, and health care reform? And how can you position yourself to profit from them?

For each change, imagine the impact on nurses, doctors, hospitals, patients, vendors, and other potential key players. For example, fiber optics recently changed the treatment provided to hyperbilirubinemic newborns. Many jaundiced babies no longer stay in hospitals and under old-fashioned "bililamps." Rather, they go home wearing vests that deliver light through fiber optic cables. If you had known in advance that this technology would soon be available, you could have benefited in several ways. You could have organized a for-profit unit of the hospital to rent the vests, teach parents how to use the vests, teach parents adjunctive therapy to further clear hyperbilirubinemia, provide for visits to family homes to ensure proper delivery of therapy and monitor the effectiveness of therapy. Or you could have entered into a cooperative agreement with the manufacturer to provide similar services. Or you could have organized your own home health agency to deliver these services. Or you could have worked for the manufacturer to market the vests to pediatricians, home health agencies, and hospitals. Or you could have developed patient teaching materials regarding the vests and sold the materials to pediatricians, home health agencies, and hospitals. Your choice would have been influenced by how you like to work and the risks you are willing to take.

In another example, a nurse developed an independent, part-time practice distributing new AIDS research drugs made available through compassionate-use programs. Because of recent changes made by the federal Food and Drug Administration, promising AIDS drugs are now approved for wider distribution before being fully licensed. But the drugs are shipped directly to the physician rather than to a pharmacy, and the drug manufacturer needs data regarding the patient's condition and laboratory test results. Although the program benefits patients, it requires more time and attention to detail than most of the larger AIDS medical practices can afford. This problem created an opportunity for this nurse, who independently gathers the information, completes the paperwork, and manages the drug distribution. This kind of tiered approval may create additional opportunities to manage other drugs.

LOCATING INFORMATION

Where do you find information about the next merger, demographic trends, research drugs, or the newest technology? Reading is one way to quickly cover a lot of ground. Go to the library and find a newspaper or journal you usually don't read. Make a habit of reading health care management journals, but venture beyond health care literature.

The *Wall Street Journal* has more information about drug approvals, drug companies, hospital mergers, and technology than does any nursing journal or your local newspaper. Many people think the *Journal* is only about numbers and money. It's really about people, however, and its style is very lively and readable. From time to time, also read a large, out-of-town newspaper such as the *New York Times*, the *Los Angeles Times*, the *Chicago Tribune*, or the *Washington Post*. Many times, it's easier to spot a trend in a city where you're less involved in the details. Health care is quickly becoming a national market, and what happens in one city soon affects the rest of the nation. Regularly read the business section of your local newspaper, as well as a local paper devoted to business, such as *Crain's Chicago Business*.

Skim publications in the field you want to enter. Your local reference or serials librarian can assist you in locating pertinent publications. Each profession has its trade journals and association publications. Pay attention to the articles and the advertising. It's an easy way to learn the jargon and identify the issues confronting the profession. Look for themes and trends.

NETWORKING

Network within nursing. Join associations and attend local meetings and annual conventions. Most people get jobs beyond the entry level through their professional contacts and friends. If you work on an association's committee and demonstrate skill and leadership, the other people on the committee learn that you're competent, cooperative, creative, and fun to work with. They will think of you when a position opens that suits your goals.

The best way to network outside of nursing is to be curious. Every new person you meet presents an opportunity to learn. When you meet someone at work or a party who has a career that might interest you, ask questions. People usually love to talk about themselves. Try asking some of these questions:

> "How did you get your position? Where did you go to school?"
>
> "What kinds of experience did you have before obtaining your position?"
>
> "Would people new to the profession enter it the same way that you did?"
>
> "What do you like about you job? What's the most satisfying part?"
>
> "What do you dislike about your job? What's the most frustrating part?"
>
> "How do you spend your days? Do you travel?"
>
> "Where does the position lead?"
>
> "What do you hope to be doing in five years?"
>
> "If you were starting out today, what would you do?"

Although people may hesitate to tell you their salaries, you can usually find out whether commissions or bonuses are involved and to what degree. Instead of playing "twenty questions," show interest and ask open-ended questions. You can probably get answers to important questions without making a person feel quizzed.

You can use the same strategy to talk with your coworkers about the careers of their spouses, brothers, sisters, neighbors, and friends. Phrase your interest in a positive light. You want to avoid giving the message at work that you're unhappy and would do anything to get out. Instead, simply sound interested. You can also tap into your coworker's experiences by asking something such as, "I've always wondered what it's like to work in home health care. Betty, you mentioned you used to do that. Tell me about it." Or you might ask similar questions to learn about the ways your coworkers moonlight.

SELF-ASSESSMENT

Take critical stock of yourself. What are your strengths, weaknesses, preferences, and expectations? You best succeed by either doing what you love or incorporating what you love into what you do. For example, an experienced neonatal intensive care nurse felt drawn to helping mothers who were struggling to continue breast-feeding while their babies were in NICU. Although her colleagues were intrigued by the high-tech challenges of working in NICU, she could see that a baby's health frequently depended on nutrition, and that breast milk made the difference for many babies. Over the course of a year, she investigated the routes to becoming a lactation consultant and carved her niche by helping babies in NICU. She followed her heart, and honored what she did best.

Part of assessment is knowing when it's time to make a change at work. Have you exhibited or experienced any of these warning signs?

- constant complaining that is unrelated to the poor morale of an entire unit
- friends telling you that you've changed
- hating to come to work for more than one week at a time (as opposed to feeling that way on a particular day here or there, which is fairly typical)
- sleeping too much in contrast with your usual pattern
- blaming the system for everything and feeling that you could make a difference
- feeling hopeless, that things will never get better
- feeling bored at work
- wandering mind at work
- feeling drawn to activities outside of your usual job
- feeling like you are being stifled by the way work is structured and that you could do a better job of structuring the work.

Many nurses wait too long before they make changes, endlessly hanging on and hoping that administration will change and that everything will improve. Or they become depressed, assuming that change will never happen. Remember that you are the only one responsible for your career. A hospital is only bricks and mortar. Don't hand over control of your career to someone else.

Make a list of those of your accomplishments that delighted you. When did you feel the most satisfied and invigorated at work? What contributed to that sense of accomplishment? Was it the task, the outcome, or the people you were with?

Methods of Self-Assessment

You might find it helpful to work through the Interest and Skill Assessment exercise in the book *What Color is Your Parachute? A Practical Manual for Job-Hunters and Career Changers* (Bolles, 1988/1995). This exercise helps you pinpoint the things you love and the things at which you are accomplished. After completing this exercise, work through the Interest and Skills Worksheet in Appendix 3.1, Career Mapping Exercise, at the end of this chapter. The Skills Application Form matches skills and interests to career opportunities in nursing. The worksheet walks you through the steps of narrowing your focus and seeking more information. It helps you formulate a plan based on your specific skills and passions.

You can get much more practice in understanding your skills and interests—and how to leverage them in the most advantageous way—by reading other books in the series by John Bolles. I highly recommend the entire series beginning with *What Color is Your Parachute?* and *The Three Boxes of Life and How to Get Out of Them* (1981) and working through to *The New Quick Job-Hunting Map* (1985). An early John Bolles book, *Where Do I Go From Here with My Life?* (Crystal & Bolles, 1974), remains a classic in life and career planning despite the fact that it was written over two decades ago. An actual outline for a college course in life planning, this book is very systematic (as are all of Bolles books) and remains quite useful today.

After you get a fairly clear idea of what you love, and how you have already developed related skills, you might want to consider what style you bring to the work world. Are you thoughtful, and do you work in the world of ideas? Are you extroverted, gregarious, and inquisitive? Do you need definite plans, or do you prefer staying open to possibilities? Do you focus on day-to-day realities, or do you dream about the future and possible ways you could create it? Any of these orientations is a gift that you bring to the world of work to make it a better and more effective place. The best way to approach your gifts is to understand them and not spend time working against them. Don't submerge yourself in a career that demands the opposite of what you have to offer.

An efficient and useful way to learn out about your personal orientation is to take the *Myers-Briggs Type Indicator*®, (Myers & Myers, 1991). This fun and interesting assessment is available at most career-counseling centers and college counseling centers and through many private counseling agencies. It tells you only useful things about yourself and how you work. It does not reveal conflicts, problems, or stresses in your life. Rather, it is a way to understand how to use your strengths and minimize your weaknesses.

After you have explored your skills, interests, and orientation to work and people, spend some time thinking about how you feel about looking for work. Consultants admit that they spend at least 85% of their time marketing their skills and talents to prospective clients. Even when they are working on a particular assignment, consultants are marketing the next phase of work to the same client or networking to gain new clients.

Do you enjoy working alone, or do you thrive on the stimulation of working with others? Nurses who are happy and confident when working alone may want to consider some type of home-based business. Many cottage industries begin—and grow profitable—on the kitchen table. But it may take several years for the business to expand to the point where you hire another person. Home health agencies, publishing businesses, lactation consultant businesses, and other businesses have started this way.

Can you operate on deadlines? Payment for consultations may be contingent on interim or final reports delivered on time. Months of work may be forfeited if anxiety prevents you from meeting a deadline. Do your clients pay on time? Are you dependent upon a weekly or monthly cash flow of a specific amount?

Would you consider moving or long-distance commuting in order to expand your options? The more mobile you are, the more options you have. Nurses who have moved to advance their careers learn that true friends and loved ones are willing to be flexible and creative in order to maintain relationships. Relocating can feel like a great risk. "I have to admit that at first I was afraid to move," says one nurse who chose to relocate "But I kept reminding myself that 'you can always come back; nothing is forever.'"

Before deciding to relocate or commute, assess the financial implications. The more a position pays, the easier it is to relocate or commute. But learn to look at prospective salary in terms of the local cost of living. Pay careful attention to the costs of housing and taxation, and to how the proposed salary compares to other salaries in the locality. Says one nurse who decided against relocating, "I spent the morning interviewing, the afternoon with a real estate agent, and the evening with a friend of mine who's in a similar field. It was a tough decision. After weighing the job responsibilities, the future opportunities for advancement, and the cost of living, I decided that a 40% increase in salary wouldn't put me any further ahead. But until I imagined that I was actually going to live there, I couldn't calculate the cost-of-living equation accurately, even though I had visited there several times on vacation."

Either for financial reasons or because their spouses can't relocate, more and more nurse executives are commuting long distances. They maintain their homes and families in one state while working in another. One nursing director explains, "My husband is very supportive. He knows that when we're together, I'm really there for him, instead of being exhausted after a frustrating day. But I've had to learn to apply much more structure to my life. I work a stretch of twelve-hour days, then fly home for five to seven days. When I'm at work, I'm not interrupted by issues from home. Fortunately, thanks to the time change, it's easy to call him late at night my time. And except for reading on the flight, I definitely *don't* bring work home."

Spend time thinking about how you want to work and what financial support you will need to make your dreams reality. When you learn all of these things about yourself, you will be ready for the practical task of marketing yourself to prospective employers or clients.

PROFITING FROM YOUR RÉSUMÉ

Your résumé or curriculum vitae (CV) alone won't get you a job, but it could lead to an interview and the opportunity to sell yourself in person. First decide whether you need a résumé or CV. Although both formats outline your career and accomplishments, each has its own style.

A résumé is used in the business world as a way to showcase your talents for a specific position. It is intended to summarize your career, and is usually limited to one or two pages. A CV, on the other hand, is more appropriate to the world of academia and is intended to be a detailed record of all your professional activities, including presentations, publications, and history with professional organizations. To illustrate the differences between a résumé and a CV, a résumé might summarize that you "published twenty-five articles in the areas of quality assurance, continuing education, and management," whereas a CV would list a complete citation of each publication. Obviously, CVs can get quite long; but truncating the list is considered professional perjury. If you hope to expand your career in both academia and business, consider maintaining both a résumé and a CV. And regardless of the format you use, make it easy to understand, and keep it in strict chronological order.

In nursing, you want to present yourself in an absolutely pristine fashion. Strive for a résumé or CV look that's classic but highly readable. Look through sample résumés in books. Two brief samples are provided in Appendices 3.2 and 3.3 at the end of this chapter. Choose a style that presents the information in a manner that is easy to understand and that presents you in your best light. While there is no strictly right or wrong way to organize your résumé, do keep these suggestions in mind:

- Use plain white or cream-colored, high-quality paper having no obvious texture or weave, and black ink.

- Choose a common font that has a serif, such as Times Roman. Never use script or clever fonts that look like they might be used on a wedding invitation or menu. Avoid clip art and logos—save the borders, graphics, and creative elements for your nonbusiness stationary.

- Use only copies that have been printed on a laser printer.

- Mail your résumé in a flat, 81/2-by-11 inch envelope. Doing so costs only a few cents more and prevents your résumé from folding up on someone's desk.

- Omit personal information, unless it gives you a special edge or explains something. Note any foreign languages in which you are fluent, but leave out your hobbies. It is not necessary to list your birth date, marital status, and number of children. If you are a naturalized citizen or visiting under a visa, however, include this information.

- Omit your high school education; if you are in or have graduated from nursing school, you must have graduated from high school. Also exclude detailed information about your nursing school courses.

- If you returned to college to take courses that didn't lead to a degree or certificate, describe those courses only if you think they give you an edge. For example, be sure to include computer, writing, or management courses. Continuing education pursued outside of college can be summarized, such as "over fifty contact hours last year in neurological assessment, critical care, and time management."

- If you are looking for your first career position in nursing, by all means include any nonprofessional work experience acquired while completing school. This tells a potential employer that you are serious about work, have a track record, and can manage more than one thing at a time. If you are moving up in your career or changing careers, leave out the details and instead summarize nonprofessional work as follows: "1988 - 1990: Worked a number of positions to support my education. Developed skills in managing deadlines, interacting with the public in high-pressure situations, and eliciting information from reluctant subjects." These skills, by the way, can be obtained in work situations as diverse as paper routes, fast-food sales and telemarketing.

- Include volunteer work or membership on the board of directors of an organization if this information gives you an edge, and especially if related to the field in which you hope to direct your career.

- Explain obvious absences from the workforce, such as military service or volunteer work in the Peace Corps. Absences that are family-related (e.g., raising children or attending to family obligations) should be saved for the interview.

- If you are switching from another career into nursing and want to use your business experience to obtain a unique nursing position, be sure to briefly explain the duties and responsibilities of your previous positions, because these may be unfamiliar to nurses. For example, "1988 - 1990: District Manager, Acme U.S.A., Limited, Chicago's leading manufacturer of VCR remote controls. Supervised a ten-person sales force that exceeded sales goals each year by 35%. Received District Manager of the Year Award in 1989."

- Some recruiters recommend using a functional (i.e., categories such as management, teaching, or research) rather than strictly chronological format. If you choose to do so, however, be careful not to confuse the reader or raise the reader's suspicion. The reader might suspect that you are attempting to conceal periods of unemployment by organizing your résumé in categories and not chronologically. Also, be sure to include a brief list of your jobs.

- For each position you've held, include at least one accomplishment: for example, a suggestion you made that improved the unit. Demonstrate that you were faced with a dilemma and helped solve it. For example,

"1988 - 1991: Staff Nurse on adult medical-surgical unit, General Hospital, U.S.A. Served on the patient education committee and developed patient teaching guidelines for diabetes mellitus, hypertension, and lowering dietary cholesterol. Advanced through the clinical ladder program to the top of the ladder." Or "1990 - 1993: Charge Nurse on oncology unit, St. General Hospital, U.S.A. Career Highlights: (1) contributed to hospital policy concerning safe handling and disposal of chemotherapeutic drugs, (2) established guidelines to assess and manage pain in post-operative mastectomy patients, and (3) completed annual performance evaluations for staff nurses on the evening shift."

- If you are a student looking for your first job, highlight a project you completed in school that would differentiate you from your peers, such as, "Developed series of learning experiences for preschool children on handwashing, germ theory of disease, and basic nutrition. One hundred twenty children completed the series."

- Check, recheck, and check again for spelling, grammatical, and punctuation errors.

- Ask someone outside of nursing to read your résumé. What does it say about you? How might it compare to résumés of other people in the field where you hope to direct your career?

- Keep your résumé or CV current.

One last note regarding résumés: a cover letter should always accompany a résumé. The cover letter notes the position for which you are applying and serves as a forum for conveying your enthusiasm and drawing attention to a few highlights about yourself.

A cover letter should be one page in length, refer to the position you are seeking, explain how you found out about the position (such as through a newspaper advertisement, at a professional meeting, or through a mutual colleague), and *briefly* highlight a pertinent skill or interest. For instance, perhaps you have worked on an article in the field or successfully completed a related project. Make brief mention of such facts. Finally, establish a time frame for contacting the recipient of your résumé to follow up. And then do it; Follow up with a call to track the progress of your application.

Following are some further tips regarding cover letters:

- Use the same quality of paper and type design as used for your résumé.

- Ensure pristine grammar and typing.

- Use the best standards for a business letter.

- Use the full name and title of the person whom you wish to receive your résumé. Never send your résumé to a department or a general address.

- Never use a boilerplate cover letter. Always compose a new letter specific to each application or contact.
- Personalize the letter and say something specific about the position you are seeking and the organization with which you are interested in working.
- Follow up in the time frame you specify.

You will find a sample cover letter for an advanced position in Appendix 3.4 at the end of this chapter. Books of sample cover letters can also be found in any library. Make sure you use such resources only to get an idea of how you can personalize your cover letters, however. Make your cover letters reflect your enthusiasm by composing each one specially for each position you wish to explore.

INTERVIEWING

Your networking and your résumé have landed you an interview. How do you showcase your strengths, make a professional impression, and learn whether the prospective position suits you (i.e., your skills and your career goals)? During an interview, you have a unique opportunity to both sell yourself and to assess the prospective position firsthand. Keep in mind that few people are offered jobs during first interviews, but many candidates blunder their ways to guarantees of never being called back.

Interestingly, most staff nurses with experience solely in nursing have never had more than perfunctory interviews. Because of the nursing shortage, hospitals and home health agencies have traditionally hired almost anyone who fills out an application and looks qualified. This severely underserved market has been characterized by minimal background checking and higher-than-average risk-taking. Frequently, any interview amounted to little more than a tour of the unit and a general description of the expected duties. With fewer nursing positions to fill, the process has become more rigorous.

Also in business or in highly sought-after positions outside the mainstream of hospital staff nursing, competition can be fierce. Employers can easily afford to be choosy, preferring to leave a key position vacant rather than hastily hire a person whose personality and qualifications don't match the job requirements.

If presenting yourself in an interview is a new skill, read through both the basic and advanced sections following. If you already have interviewing experience, and are primarily looking to hone your interviewing skills, however, skip to the advanced section.

Basic Interviewing

- Arrive five minutes early, never late. Be aware that arriving too early can put off prospective employers by making them feel rushed. If you happen to arrive more than five minutes early, walk around the block, have a cup of coffee, or relax in the lobby.

- Pay attention to your attire. Never wear a white uniform or scrubs. As a rule, you should dress in a similar manner to the person who is conducting the interview. It's better to err on the side of being simply or classically dressed. Don't let your appearance distract the interviewer. Remember, you're not making a fashion or a political statement.

- A woman should wear a clean, well-fitting, conservative skirt, blouse, and jacket or conservative, tailored dress. The skirt should be long enough so that you don't have to worry about how you sit. Keep jewelry to a minimum, use make-up moderately, style hair conservatively, and wear hosiery and low-heeled, conservative shoes appropriate to your attire. Carry either a small handbag or a briefcase.

- A man should wear a white shirt, a tie, and a dark nonpatterned jacket. As a rule, do not wear earrings, chains, or bracelets. Be freshly shaven and neatly groomed. While a manicure may be suspect, clean nails are a requirement.

- Wear something that makes you feel confident and assured. If you need to buy a new suit just for interviews, it's a worthwhile investment.

- Both men and women should avoid wearing fragrances. Many people are allergic to or offended by a quantity of perfume that a regular wearer hardly notices. People who are accustomed to wearing fragrances often forget that previous applications can still permeate clothing.

- Don't smoke before or during the interview. Health professionals are judged more harshly regarding their bad habits than are others.

- Excitement and high energy are contagious. Don't try to hide your enthusiasm.

- Anxiety and nervous agitation are also contagious. If you are nervous, your interviewer will be nervous about you. If you're afraid of the unknown or of being judged, find out more information about the interviewing organization prior to the interview. Also, practice. If you become nervous, concentrate on slowing your breathing. Briefly pause before you answer the next question, and think soothing thoughts, such as, "This isn't my first interview; I can do it. These people have talked to thousands of people; I'm not the worst one."

- If you are applying for a nursing position, bring your nursing license and pertinent certificates with you.

- Prepare your own set of questions, and order them by priority. The interviewer will conduct the interview to gather information about you, and may leave little time for your questions.

- Practice responses to questions that you hope you'll never be asked. One way to do this is to write the answers to such questions and then critique your answers several days later. *Never* say anything bad about a former employer, no matter what the circumstances were. And never discuss "personality conflicts." You'll be labeled as a crank or a malcontent.

- Describe the reasons for leaving positions in specific yet positive terms. "I was in that field of nursing for five years, and I could see that I needed fresh challenges. While I was there, I learned a lot about delivering care to patients. Now, I want to plan and manage care." Or if you're forced to explain a sudden departure, you might explain, "The hospital was reorganized, and I felt that the new director was leading my unit to accomplish goals that I didn't entirely share." Unless you were fired, you rarely are forced to acknowledge exactly why you left a bad situation.

- Never lie.

- Don't withhold information about being in an impaired professional program (a substance abuse treatment program). An interviewer should not ask for this information, however, and you needn't volunteer it. A counselor within the impaired professional program can explore this issue with you and help coach your answers.

- Don't expect to talk about salary, working conditions, or hours during a first interview. In any event, wait for the interviewer to raise these issues.

- Follow up with a brief thank-you letter that mentions one aspect of the interview or the position that excited or interested you, and that serves to highlight one of your strengths.

Advanced Interviewing

- Be certain to answer the question. In no more than three sentences, enlarge on the question by providing useful information about yourself, for example, "Yes, I've worked in teams. At first it was difficult because we lacked a sense of direction. But by the end of the year, we had accomplished our goal of a reducing turnaround time for medication ordering by three hours."

- Bring evidence of your accomplishments, such as copies of professional publications you've authored, an extra copy of your résumé, letters of recommendation, and organizational charts showing your previous positions. Use a briefcase rather than a knapsack, to carry these things.

- Some people are concerned about appearing boastful. However, using emotional language to describe your accomplishments is desirable. For example, saying, "I was very pleased to be part of the planning team for remodeling the OR, and I'm sure I can use those skills in other situations as well" is perfectly acceptable. Boastfulness is more often conveyed by the tone of your voice rather than by what you say. Avoid sounding arrogant, dismissive, or judgmental regarding your former coworkers. Don't try to make yourself appear more important by demeaning others.

- Find opportunities to describe how you worked with others and to compliment the accomplishments of others. For example, you could say, "One of the staff nurses suggested that we change the way we manage turning schedules for immobile patients. I helped her organize a small working group to make recommendations. It was a pleasure to watch her grow through that experience. They came up with an excellent plan that we soon implemented."

- If this is a new clinical area for you or you've been away from clinical nursing for a while, be honest, and admit your unfamiliarity with new technology, medications, or diagnostic routines. At the same time, stress that you have extensive experience in solving problems, managing in a crisis, and knowing how to assess and meet your leaning needs.

- Describe your day-to-day work experiences in terms of your underlying abilities, such as organizing, managing multiple deadlines, and competing demands for time and resources, or reducing costs without sacrificing service or quality. Be prepared to cite at least one specific example to illustrate each ability.

- For each position you've held, be prepared to describe the outcomes you accomplished in a quantifiable way.

- Be prepared to describe how you have been able to respond to changes originating both within the organization and outside the organization (e.g., those that are market or regulatory related). Flexibility and ability to manage change are highly desired skills.

- If you're trying to switch professions, find out as much as you can about people already in the profession you want to pursue. Go to conferences they attend. Ask them what to expect both in the profession and in a job interview. Ask them how to best prepare for an interview; what the hardest part of the interview will be; what interviewers are looking for; and what will be most attractive and least attractive about your being a nurse, from the interviewer's perspective.

- Know the key jargon used by and key issues of concern to insiders.

- Come prepared with a set of questions such as, "What do you see as the challenges of this job for a nurse?"; "What accomplishments do you expect within the first year of performance?"; "Where do you see this position a year from now?"; "Where do you see this position ultimately going?"; "What are the interfaces within the company?"; "Who depends on this position?"; and "On whom does this position depend for success?" Ask questions that are astute yet not threatening. You want to demonstrate that you are tracking and thinking about what is being said in the interview.

- Conclude by asking something along the lines of "What's the next step?"; "Do you have a sense of your time frame for filling this position?"; or "Do we need to schedule another interview?"

You can gain experience by practicing with a friend, colleague, instructor, or prospective employer. Through practice, you'll gain poise and confidence, and you'll learn to "think on your feet." A friend can also give you feedback regarding your body language and the way you come across to others. Be careful about practicing with prospective employers, however. You don't want to gain a reputation as the person who is always looking for a job but who never qualifies.

If you decide after the interview that the position is a poor match for your skills and interests, formally withdraw from consideration. If you have developed a relationship with the interviewer or seemed close to being offered the job, telephone to withdraw, and follow up with a letter. Otherwise, write a letter to withdraw. Think of the letter as a variation on a thank-you letter. Highlight at least one of your skills and at least one thing that appealed to you about the position while at the same time being honest—in a general way—about why the job would be a poor match. Even a withdrawal letter can help you network for future positions.

Accept only these jobs that you intend to take. Some nurses accept jobs and then fail to show up for orientation. Not only is this extremely unprofessional, but it virtually guarantees that you won't be taken seriously in the future.

FINDING GREATER SATISFACTION IN YOUR CURRENT POSITION

Although you may be looking for a new position, it is possible to increase your satisfaction with the job you currently hold. There may be many reasons why you must stay in your present position for a while, even though you have made the decision to move on in your career. For example, results of your assessment may indicate that the market isn't ready for your skills or that it will take time to develop the skills necessary to take full advantage of the market. How do you still work toward your dream and find satisfaction in your current position?

When you are dissatisfied at work, it is helpful for you to find ways to feel like you matter, can make a difference, have influence, or are gathering necessary skills and information for your eventual career or life change. You can accomplish any or all of these things in your current job, in volunteer assignments outside your paying position, or in your personal life away from work.

At work, participating on hospital committees may increase your satisfaction, as well as expand your opportunities. Committee work allows you to evaluate problems and, more importantly, to help determine policies addressing those problems. It also moves you closer to the sources of power. Instead of being the person always affected by decisions, you can be in the position of contributing to the decision-making. You also can make contacts, learn about roles other than the one you hold, and gain access to other opportunities. Many nurses on products committees, for example, have developed relationships with vendors, leading to careers in sales, product evaluation, and marketing.

Other in-hospital strategies include cross-training to broaden your skills, contributing to policies you consider important, volunteering to educate colleagues about subjects in which you excel, and offering to interface in staff development. All of these activities increase your exposure, make you feel valued, and help people see you in a new light.

If the thought of extending yourself further at work is too unpleasant, you can always find opportunities to make a difference in your community. Volunteer to sit on local boards, (such as the library board), municipal committees, local American Heart Association committees, the PTA, or other organizational committees of interest to you. Do anything that exposes you to skills and people you find fascinating. You will find the access easy and rewards great. It won't be long before you experience a marked increase in self-esteem, as well as in skills. Not only will you be making changes, but you'll also be gaining an understanding of how many systems work. Furthermore, you will be meeting people who may very well be able to help you in your eventual transition. But most importantly, you will be offsetting the frustrations you experience at work, thus decreasing their importance in your life.

Your personal life also offers many opportunities for increasing your feelings of satisfaction.

- Take a community-college course for fun and enjoyment: maybe painting, maybe computers, maybe exercise. Learning something new is engrossing, and it enhances your opinion of yourself.

- Take stock of yourself. Are there areas on which you'd like to work? Perhaps improved nutrition and an *achievable* physical activity plan could help relieve some stress.

- Learn to meditate.

- Get in touch with the spiritual, philosophical, or otherwise "deeper" side of yourself.

- Renew relationships with the most meaningful and supportive people in your life.

- Limit involvement with people who deplete your energy and discourage you.

- If you are harried and frenzied, simplify your life. Eliminate the clutter, and focus on basics.

- If you are isolated and lonely, reach out to people and groups. Build bridges to relationships that will provide meaning and sustenance.

Spending time focusing on yourself and enhancing your strengths puts work-related frustrations in a different perspective. You feel less powerless in general, a benefit that carries over to work. As you feel more enhanced and less depleted personally, you will eventually begin to see avenues for movement and change.

AN ONGOING PLAN FOR SELF-MANAGEMENT

To initiate an ongoing plan for self-management, write down your goals, and tell them to a friend or loved one. Doing so makes your goals real on an elementary level. Acknowledge that you have a dream and that it may be unique. Seek support from people who validate your dream. Avoid people who refuse to accept that you can attain success.

Start with your ultimate goal and work backwards to recognize the stepping stones that will get you there. This helps you welcome change and recognize opportunities as they occur. The clearer and more vivid your goals, the easier it is to recognize opportunities to move you closer to attaining them.

Divide large goals into tasks that can be accomplished in short periods of time. For example, if one of your goals is gaining new skills by going to school, you must evaluate programs, decide on a school, take Graduate Record Examinations (GREs), register, and arrange a work schedule that allows both going to and paying for school. Each of these tasks can be easily accomplished if managed separately. Develop a time line, so you can see how each task contributes to your goal.

Maintain as much flexibility as possible. Broaden your skills, your awareness of opportunities, and your support network.

Daydreaming can be one way to promote success. But not all daydreams are helpful. Imagining that no action is necessary because you will be rescued by some form of white knight will prevent you from taking the responsibility of managing your own career. Likewise, although daydreams of escaping to an idyllic paradise may help reduce your stress level, such daydreams won't move you closer to achieving your goals. Instead, daydream about your career goals—about what it will feel like, look like, and sound like to be in your ideal position. Don't be afraid to dream the big dream. Picture yourself successful, and you will recognize the opportunities that will help get you there.

Don't share your plans with everybody. Select your confidants carefully. A close friend can give you courage to follow your dreams, even when success appears remote. But many coworkers will feel abandoned or degraded by your plans to leave. They may give up on you long before you're ready to leave. At some point, they may no longer offer the help and support you need. And managers expect your mind and commitment to be on the work at hand, not on preparing for your next career.

On the other hand, developing a partnership with someone to help you manage your change can be transforming and motivating. If you are able to find such a relationship, stick with it.

Some people recommend approaching your career search as if it were a job. Spend a part of every single day working on it. Many colleges, communities, and agencies have support groups for job-seekers. Members encourage each other to keep motivated, share strategies and leads, and celebrate successes. Find such groups in your area, and access them.

Finally, keep in mind that your successes thus far give you unbelievable advantages. You chose nursing, got through the rigors of licensure, entered into practice, and navigated the turbulent health care market. Bravo! You have already succeeded, and other employers are eagerly awaiting the strengths, discipline, intelligence, and complex management skills you have developed as a nurse. What you have gained from your nursing experience is eagerly sought after. You just have to package it and take the first step!

SUMMARY

Managing your career requires both knowledge and skill. You must know about the marketplace, yourself (your strengths, passions, and skills) and appropriate job-hunting techniques. When you have the needed knowledge, you must then focus on the needed skills—the skills of interviewing, packaging your unique blend of talents and experience, and making the correct contacts in the most effective way.

Armed with the best information, well-managed contacts, and well-honed job-hunting skills, you can take your career places you never imagined!

REFERENCES

Bolles, J. (1981). *The three boxes of life and how to get out of them*. Berkeley, CA: Ten Speed Press.

Bolles, J. (1985). *The new quick job-hunting map*. Berkeley, CA: Ten Speed Press.

Bolles, J. (1988/1995). *What color is your parachute? A practical manual for job-hunters and career changers*. Berkeley, CA: Ten Speed Press.

Crystal, J. C., & Bolles, R. N. (1974). *Where do I go from here with my life?* Berkeley, CA: Ten Speed Press.

Myers, P. B., & Myers, K. D. (1991). *The Myers-Briggs type indicator®*. Palo Alto, CA: Consulting Psychologists Press, Inc.

APPENDIX 3.1
Career Mapping Exercise
Skills Application Form

Skill Clusters	Career Opportunities within Nursing
Machine and Manual Skills	Dialysis, ICU, central supply, technical training, equipment demonstration, product representation for technical products
Detail and Follow-through Skills	Cost analysis, research, financial administration, staffing projection, general management, policy coordination, regulatory compliance (JCAHO, Public Health, etc.) overseeing OR scheduling, staff dispatching/coordination
Numerical/Financial/Accounting/Money Management Skills	Consulting to administration, budget forecasting, budget analysis, financial administration, supplies and equipment analysis, OR equipment management
Influence and Persuasion Skills	Recruitment, internal organizational development consulting, contract negotiating, policy making, training, legislative work with nursing organizations, grantsmanship, funding/development management or consulting
Performing Skills	Training, program development (films, A-V production), advocacy
Leadership Skills	All forms of management, self-employment, rural practice, regional or national leadership in nursing organizations
Development, Planning, Supervising, Management Skills	First-line and middle management, teaching, consulting, group work, staffing coordination, supplemental agency management, committee leadership, project leadership
Reading, Writing, Communication Skills	Creating journals or newsletters, publishing articles, policy and procedure work, fund-raising (development work), public relations, private consulting for scientific or trade publications, grantsmanship
Instruction, Guidance, Educational Skills	University education, staff education, preceptorship, learning resources and packages development, educational consulting
Service, Helping, Human Relations Skills	Counseling/advising, direct patient care at all levels, psychiatric nursing, supervising/mentorship, organizational ombudsman, independent therapy, management (if in possession of the related technical skills)
Institutional and Innovational Skills	Inventing, program development, program consultation, Chief Executive Officer, sales (if persuasive), for-profit-agency work marketing people, skills, or products
Artistic Skills	Art or music therapy, self-employment creating packages for educational use, directing activities in various settings, consulting to theatre, TV, or film producers
Observational and Learning Skills	Work in high-pressure areas like ER and ICU, counselor training, political action work, graduate school faculty, research (both basic and applied), recruitment, placement agency work
Research, Analysis, Systematizing Skills	Nursing research, systems development, work-process redesign, consulting, negotiating, academic work, grantsmanship, quality management, analyst in consulting firm, computer analysis, project management

INTEREST AND SKILLS WORKSHEET

   I. My skills clusters seem to be in the areas of:

      1.

      2.

      3.

      4.

      5.

  II. Based on this, I have a tentative career interest in:

      1.

      2.

 III. I need more information about these opportunities and can seek it by (for example: library searches, calling people who hold those jobs, calling schools and asking their placement counselors, etc.):

 IV. I need to work to acquire the following skills in order to advance toward my career interest:

      1.

      2.

      3.

  V. Ways by which I might be able to achieve the skills I have identified in the previous step (for example; school, in-service classes, a mentor, internship, etc.):

      1.

      2.

      3.

APPENDIX 3.2
Sample Basic Résumé

FULL NAME, RN
1234 Pleasant Street
Anywhere, Illinois 60000
Telephone: (123) 456-7890

OBJECTIVE: Position as an RN in an acute care setting

LICENSE NUMBER: State of Illinois #_____

**PROFESSIONAL
EXPERIENCE:**

1992 – present   **St. General Hospital and Medical Center**
                      Chicago, Illinois

                      Position: RN, medical oncology unit
                      Provide direct care as a team member on a 36-bed unit. Work
                      in cooperation with nonlicensed team members. Manage nurs-
                      ing outcomes using assistive personnel. Obtained BCLS
                      instructor certification through CHA. Organized BCLS
                      recertifications on unit and shift. Obtained certification as a
                      bone marrow transplant nurse through in-house program.
                      Helped develop policies related to transplant care. Developed
                      a standard care plan for the care of patients with nonHodgkins
                      lymphoma. Received three letters of commendation for patient
                      care delivery.

1987 - 1992   **City Teaching Medical Center**
                      Any City, Illinois

                      Position: RN, general medical unit
                      Provided direct patient care on a 25-bed medical unit. Gained
                      experience caring for pulmonary, cardiology, and geriatric
                      patients. Participated in mock arrest drills. Helped develop
                      unit procedures for shift rotation. Participated in an average of
                      12 hours of continuing education contact hours per year.

EDUCATION: **Local University, This City, Illinois**
                      Completed 24 credit hours of course work in BSN prerequi-
                      sites, focus on physiology and psychology.

                      City Community College
                      Associate of Arts Degree (Nursing), 1987
                      Class representative to faculty council

**RELATED
EXPERIENCES:**   Organized BCLS training for local PTA group
                      Lectured twenty-five preschool students on keeping healthy,
                      repeated program four times

AFFILIATIONS: Member, ANA
                      Member, Oncology Nursing Society

REFERENCES: Available upon request

APPENDIX 3.3
Sample Résumé for
Advanced Skills

FULL NAME, RN
1234 Pleasant Street
Anywhere, USA 60000
Telephone: (123) 555-7890

OBJECTIVE:

Financial and administrative systems executive position in a large, complex medical center or health system, supporting department of nursing, or a combined patient-care services function

LICENSE NUMBER:

State of Illinois # _____

PROFESSIONAL EXPERIENCE:

1993 - present

Administrative Services Director, Department of Nursing
Medium City Medical Center
Omaha, NE

Initiated position responsible for budget analysis, computerization of the department, and supply management. By developing new control systems, was able to reduce supply expenditures by 18% in first year. Manage pharmacy committee, improving pharmaceutical charges by 21% through automated delivery systems. Manage project teams for patient-records automation and nursing MIS. Projects are on target and on budget.

1989 - 1993

Nurse Manager, 42-Bed Oncology Unit
Medium City Medical Center
Omaha, NE

Managed busy unit through a transition to patient-focused care. Developed computerized expense-tracking system that provided information daily rather than biweekly. Increased accuracy of reports, resulting in tighter financial controls while maintaining levels of care. Chaired nurse manager group. Served as a member of organization-wide systems reengineering committee.

1985 - 1989

Staff Nurse, then Assistant Manager, 25-Bed Medical Unit
St. Small Hospital
Randolph, IA

As a new grad, learned to manage patient care in cardiology, pulmonary, and geriatrics. Precepted new employees, developed learning modules for orientation, and represented unit on the policy committee. Promoted to assistant manager in 1987, managing scheduling, first-line discipline and day-to-day budget compliance.

EDUCATION:

MBA, State University, NE 1993
Accounting specialization, with focus on financial operations.
Internship in finance department of Acme Pharmaceutical, a national pharmaceutical supply corporation.

EDUCATION **(continued)**	BSN, Midwest University, IA, 1985 Besides core course work in nursing, pursued computer classes and business systems classes. Senior project focused on using computers for staff self-scheduling.
RELATED **ACTIVITIES:**	Keynote speaker, 1994 Business Managers in Nursing Networking Group Annual Conference Internship Development Committee, Business School, State University, NE
REFERENCES:	Available upon request

APPENDIX 3.4
Sample Cover Letter

Ann Jones
1234 Pleasant Street
Anywhere, USA 60000
April 24, This Year

Ms. J.W. Winston
Best Careers, Inc.
2000 Lofty Lane
Big City, New York 60000

Dear Ms. Winston:

I am following up on our conversation last week at the Annual Meeting of the Executives in Medical Enterprises in Denver. We discussed the Vice President for Operations Support position at Western States Medical Center, for which you are recruiting. I am still very interested in that opportunity, and, as you suggested, I am submitting my résumé for the position.

My solid background in patient care and, especially, my positions managing patient-care units have given me a strong understanding of the systems needs at the bedside. At the same time, my restructuring and systems backgrounds have given me access to the tools needed to manage patient-care environments in a tremendously competitive business climate.

My progressive background renders me well-suited for the position you describe: developing a new division that supports management at all levels in the organization by providing the systems, information, and technology needed by Western States Medical Center to maintain its leadership position.

As we discussed at the meeting, I bring the ability to innovate (such as providing cost-effective support to nurse managers by designing business-school internships in the department of nursing), as well as to see old problems in a new light (as evidenced by my reengineering background).

The position seems exciting, and I look forward to talking with you more about it in the first week of May.

Yours truly,

Ann Jones, RN, MBA

Chapter Four

Creating Your Own Job: Using Nonlinear Strategies to Reach Your Career Goals

Beth Bongard

INTRODUCTION

Finding the right career for you involves more than following the rules you learned in nursing school. One of the most valuable strategies you can use involves "thinking out of the box"—or looking at the same old thing in a brand new way. This is called *nonlinear thinking*. It is the cornerstone of creativity, and everybody does it once in awhile.

This chapter provides examples of nonlinear thinking and outlines some nonlinear job-search strategies. It is meant to help you assess your own level of nonlinear thinking as it applies to your career. A number of exercises designed to stretch your nonlinear thinking "muscles" are also provided.

A Fable about Friends

Annmarie had just returned from the fifteen-year reunion of her nursing class. She had not kept up with the careers of her fellow graduates since moving to another state right after her graduation . What she learned surprised her.

Of course, many nurses were doing just what Annmarie had expected. As reflected in nursing demographics all across the nation, many of Annmarie's classmates were either working part-time or staying home with their families after having worked for several years in in-patient nursing. Some were working as staff nurses in the same hospitals with which they had affiliated right out of nursing school. Others had become nurse managers, clinical specialists, or educators. And many were staff nurses who had moved from one clinical area to another, thus increasing their skills and experience. Also as Annmarie had expected, a number were in school, completing degrees or pursuing graduate work. Some had even given up nursing completely; but far fewer than she had expected.

Also as was happening all over the country, Annmarie found that many of her classmates had taken on intriguing, unconventional, and even surprising roles.

Cathy, for instance, had started a one-nurse business offering home assessments and narrowly defined diabetes-oriented interventions. She was performing these services in a very large, assisted-living system for a group of physicians whom she had carefully selected. Her classmates were most surprised because for many years, Cathy had worked at far-below-market salaries in doctors' offices. In her new venture, not only had Cathy tripled her income, but she had gained something she had always sought most: control over her worklife.

Pam, although she worked in home health, had a fascinating part-time activity lobbying and raising money for international health causes. Annmarie learned that, after spending five years in Thailand working with Cambodian refugees, Pam had negotiated with the Thai military, the United Nations officials who handled refugee affairs, and the Cambodian leaders of the camps. Her skills gave her the confidence to lobby government officials all the way to the U.S. Congress.

In contrast, Pat was working for a national consulting company, managing health care compensation clients. She was now a group head, specializing in merging health care organizations. Incidentally, she was making $170,000 annually, plus bonuses.

Jim was doing graphic design for technical publications. Rita was working as a lawyer specializing in insurance fraud. Jenny, while working primarily as a clinical specialist in a teaching hospital, had provided consultant services to three Hollywood studios over the past ten years. She has proved quite valuable in ensuring that movies and TV series reflect actual hospital practice. Brendan was working as the chief official in his state's family mediation service. And Lynn was running for mayor of her middle-sized city; having already served as alderwoman, she was favored to win the mayorship.

As Annmarie listened to the stories of her colleagues, something became clearly apparent. Although most of their unconventional positions were outside of nursing, all of her classmates believed their backgrounds in nursing were instrumental in their career successes. Specifically, these holders of unconventional careers believed that nursing had provided them with access they might otherwise not have had, and that nursing had developed in them the discipline needed to follow through on their career plans.

Annmarie was amazed. All of these nurses had started out in traditional, hospital-based nursing positions. How did they make the moves leading to lobbying, fundraising, independent business, or Hollywood consulting? Where did her colleagues get the ideas that led them to consider politics, law, and design?

LINEAR CAREER PATHS

Although the story about Annmarie is a fable, the stories about her nursing colleagues are real. The names are different, as are several small details; but the stories are true. In this vignette, Annmarie was unprepared for the unconventional careers of her friends because she, like most every nursing student and career nurse, had been thoroughly exposed to *linear* career advancement. Linear careers progress just as the name suggests: in a predictable line. Annmarie, as most of us, had been socialized to look at careers in a linear way.

Linear nursing careers unfold in the following ways. A nursing management career starts with a staff nurse position; moves through a charge nurse, assistant manager, nurse manager (supervisor, if that position exists), and division director (such as head of critical care nursing); and culminates with vice president of either nursing or patient-care services. An academic nursing career progresses along a well-defined tenure track, from assistant professor to associate professor to full professor. The rules for teaching and publishing are stringent but well known, and progress occurs in orderly steps if your work is favorably judged. A nonmanagement nursing career might begin with a staff nurse position, move through a unit preceptor to a clinician, and, finally, culminate with clinical nurse specialist, depending on the hospital's complexity.

Linear career advancement sometimes requires further education (for example, a Master of Science in Nursing is usually required to become a clinical nurse specialist). Generally speaking, however, such education is usually in a nursing discipline or one of several narrowly defined and related fields, such as education or management.

In each of the linear nursing career paths then, the steps follow in order; one step leads to another. These career paths are common paths, steeped in tradition. Most nurses have seen their peers progress through the steps and most nurses know the "rules".

NONLINEAR CAREER PATHS

The career paths encountered by Annmarie at her reunion are called *nonlinear* career paths. Nonlinear career paths are highly unpredictable and draw on all aspects of a person's life and experiences rather than solely on job-related experiences. For example, a nurse who is an avid rock climber in her personal life might, over time, incorporate this personal interest into her professional life. By becoming a search and rescue professional, for instance, she could meld her nursing knowledge and experience with her passion for adventure activities.

A somewhat more mainstream example might be the nurse in neonatal ICU who realizes that mothers want to breast-feed their infants but are very intimidated. This nurse learns as much as possible about breast-feeding to help these mothers. As she becomes increasingly successful and satisfied in this work, this nurse becomes a sought-after resource by the mothers. Her fellow nurses, however, see this enhancement and application of her"soft" skills as rendering her less and less able in the high-tech business of neonatal care. Eventually the nurse's alienation from her coworkers leads her to pursue a career as a lactation consultant specializing in complex feeding problems. A true story, this nurse was motivated first by concern, then by interest, then by the pain of alienation, and, finally, by the success itself. She is now a lactation specialist working in a group practice that serves a multistate region.

Nonlinear careers allow nurses to create their futures by "patching" together their interests, their experiences outside of work, and their nursing skills. The drawback is that there are no maps as there are in linear careers. On the plus side, however, the paths can be so surprising that even those doing the hiring are caught off guard. The nurse-on-the-move can use this to great advantage. Thus, what nonlinear career-seekers lose in the comfort of predictable steps and rules, they gain in the advantage of surprise.

Nonlinear career-seekers use persuasion, networking, creativity, and seizing the moment to a greater degree than they have been taught in the traditional nursing environment. The unusual nature of the positions these career-seekers design catches employers off guard, often intriguing them. This gives the nonlinear career-seeker openings to experiment and demonstrate, openings that the linear career-seeker rarely gets. In this way, the balance of power is shifted slightly away from the hirer and slightly more toward the job-seeker than is typically the case in an interview scenario. And anything that shifts the traditional balance of power is an advantage to the job-seeker.

Why a Shift Toward Nonlinear?

Had the fable about Annmarie continued, she would have heard dramatic stories from her classmates regarding rapid and repeated shifts in their work environments. Such stories, however, are not fables; they are the reality of health care in this decade.

Although the majority of nurses still work in in-patient settings, these nurses are witnessing rapid changes, including empty beds, consolidated units, and restructured care. In short, the shift is toward the need for fewer hospital positions in nursing. Many nurses are having to move to new units because their current units are experiencing surpluses of RNs, and, thus, no longer need them. These nurses are not necessarily seeking new experiences. Other nurses are being laid off as their positions are eliminated, and other nurses are even seeing their hospitals closed.

Nurses are witnessing an upsurge in geriatric patients—and fewer allowed hospital days to treat their problems. Over the past decade, nurses have seen patients sent home with IVs, on ventilators, and with numerous chronic care considerations. Nurses everywhere realize that there are plenty of health care needs, but that these needs are increasingly being handled outside of hospitals. This results in far fewer traditional, in-patient staff positions.

Managerial nursing in hospitals, a traditional career path that was both visible and available in past decades, has also been affected by these rapid changes. Most nurses have witnessed the elimination of supervisor positions—and, thus, of a traditional promotional opportunity—over past years. Fewer units and fewer hospitals mean fewer managers needed. Mergers mean consolidation of entire hierarchies.

Although many nurses are aware of the squeeze on traditional positions, many of these same nurses remain unaware of the opportunities outside of traditional, hospital-based care that have replaced the disappearing positions in hospitals.

The nonlinear job-seeker does not approach the job market by looking for a specific job, such as manager, dialysis clinician, or staff development instructor. Rather, these job-seekers look for ways to profit from their passionate interests (e.g., breast-feeding), to leverage highly individual talents (e.g., rock climbing), and to tailor positions to meet their interests and needs. They see things differently.

By seeing things differently, they are better able to see opportunities where others see dead ends. For example, a merger is always a potentially frightening experience in losing that with which you have become familiar and comfortable—be it leadership, the expectations placed on you, or even your patient population. Nonlinear thinkers, on the other hand, see a merger as an expansion of their hospital—as a chance to move around in a bigger pond.

Are Nonlinear People Born or Bred?

As you observe colleagues who push past the traditional, you may wonder whether they were born looking at things differently, or whether they learned this skill. The answer is; a little of both.

Some people are creative by nature; they look at a brick but see a sculpture. Others are traditional; they look at a brick but see a building element. Yet others fall somewhere in the middle. They have learned that bricks make buildings, but, out of necessity have used bricks to make bookshelves; then they wonder how else they can use bricks.

Most people probably fall in the last group; they start in one place and move in steps and small leaps to another place. Nonlinear thinkers, on the other hand, move not incrementally but in large leaps. And this way of thinking can be learned by most people.

You might think of linear thinking as a continuum running from the staid to the impulsive. There are those who hold on for dear life no matter what; they do not even realize that the ship is sinking (or the unit closing, or the hospital is being acquired, etc.). Then there are those who jump ship without a plan or reason—because they are bored, frustrated, angry, etc. Most productive, however, are those who suspect a trend, understand and accept their interests and strengths, have passion for something, and, through planning, put it all together in personal and unique ways.

For example, one psychiatric nurse found herself in a hospital where the major admitting physician left. The service was in chaos. For the first time, she hated work. Her solution was to combine her passion for music with her background in psychiatric nursing to become a music therapist. Holding on to her psychiatric nursing job through school, she eventually was in a position to control her career in a way that made her happy and buffered her from the problems inherent on the patient-care unit.

Listening to her story, her career move may seem an obvious evolution. But to her, it was a major leap. Nothing in her nursing background had prepared her to figure out how to incorporate music into her livelihood. She figured it out in a burst of insight; but first, she had to trust that music could be pivotal in her future.

YOUR CURRENT PLACE ON THE LINEAR-NONLINEAR CONTINUUM

In order to move toward a more nonlinear way of thinking, it is helpful to assess where you currently fall on the linear-nonlinear continuum. Are you most comfortable staying put for long stretches, moving only when you must?

Or do you often leave your friends and colleagues wondering how you arrive at and implement such great new ideas?

Following is a set of questions to help you explore your place on the linear-nonlinear thinking continuum. These questions relate to scenarios rather common in nursing today. Following each scenario are four potential courses of action. For each scenario, circle the course of action that most closely reflects your gut response. Do not try to figure out the *best* approach—just circle the response that seems most like what you would do.

1. You are just finishing nursing school and have not received a job offer despite a three-month search. You thought getting a job in pediatrics in your university hospital would be a breeze because you have good grades and great clinical references. You now know what reengineering, mergers, and managed care have done to the availability of positions in your area. It's grim; none of the recruiters are at all encouraging. Your fellow students all seem to be experiencing the same problems. What do you do next?

   A. You exhibit an impressive amount of energy, perseverance, and strategy. Calling every hospital within fifty miles, you ask about any available openings, emphasizing your flexibility and availability. After you're done, you start over to see whether anything has changed and to remind your contacts that you are still interested.

   B. You realize the job market is too tight, and, so, go back to school, believing more education (i.e., a master's degree in pediatric nursing) is the best way to get a leg up on the competition. Although you aren't crazy about school, it seems the right thing to do. Maybe in two years the market will be more receptive to you. You are willing to go through the hoops.

   C. You notice that the nursing journals are full of ads for camp nurses. You loved camp as a kid, and worked at one during the summers during high school. Now, you look for camps for kids with renal problems, especially large camps. You know you would be working with experienced colleagues if the camp is large enough for several nurses. Although the pay would be low, the job would give you pediatrics experience, as well as the chance to network with renal professionals, an advantage when you go back to your job search after the summer ends.

   D. You acknowledge that you *hate* looking for a job in this environment; it's completely depressing. While in school, you were sure there would be a job waiting for you upon graduation. Although nursing is OK, you really loved your English classes. You decide that your nursing education can never hurt you, but that you'd actually like to pursue a career teaching; you love it, you're good at it, and it will only take six months to get your teaching credentials.

2. You have been a dialysis nurse for eleven years, and in that time, you have become an expert practitioner. Unfortunately, there has been tremendous turmoil in your unit during your tenure. Recently, your unit was "bought" by a national system of dialysis care units. What do you do?

   A. You stay put. You've seen a lot and survived. You do not know what else you would do. While this change is unsettling, you remind yourself that you are good at your job, and you resolve to ride out the latest changes. You are sure that things will eventually be on an even keel.

   B. You stay put and pull together information on all the classes you've given, projects you've handled, and situations you've successfully managed. The manager resigned during the turmoil, and you plan to apply for the job. You've carefully lined up your credentials, and the manager position is the next step in your career.

   C. You stay put. You haven't been this excited in a long time. You have a wealth of teaching experience, both at work and as a part-time health instructor in adult education classes. This chain is known for its education program, and you have great references. You see this as an opportunity to move around in a very large system, without losing the security of a home base. You plan to start talking to the educator in the sister unit across town by the end of the week.

   D. You stay put just until you get the job in graphic design that you've been pursuing. Nursing is OK, but this turmoil has soured you. You've illustrated children's books for years, and now you have an opportunity to design textbooks. You have great contacts, and it looks promising. Finally, this split in your activities would be over, and you would be able to concentrate full-time on design. It would be a pay cut, but you need to break into the business.

3. You have been a critical care nurse for seven years. Your children are all in school, and you have finally finished your degree. You like critical care, and you certainly have seen a lot. But, amazingly, your favorite experience was participating in the legal issues workshop last year. You played the role of plaintiff, which really made you look differently at your work. Now that the demands on your time are easing, what do you do?

   A. You decide to take it easy, really grateful for everything you've learned, especially in that legal issues workshop. You feel you'll be a better nurse because of it. Although you can perform the care in your sleep, there is no other unit that interests you.

   B. You decide to look into management. A nurse manager is the next obvious career step, and you feel that with your education and expertise, you are ready to progress. You examine the job postings and start getting ready for the application process. Although you can't get that legal workshop off your mind—it was so interesting—you can't figure out what to do with it. So you continue to ready yourself to apply for management. It seems the practical thing to do.

C. You recognize your excitement regarding the legal issues workshop. Knowing you now have time and energy for school but not knowing where to begin, you start talking to lawyers you meet through your activities in your village. You also read about nurses in law and ask questions whenever the opportunity arises. Finally, you commit to law school.

D. You decide against doing the same thing, even for one more day. You liked being a nurse but are now ready for a change. You loved the stimulation of the legal workshop; it really got you thinking. You plan to quit your job and start writing legal thrillers. You're confident that your college writing course along with the writing seminars you pursued on your own time will be real plusses here!

4. You are a staff development coordinator. You have your BSN and are half way to completing your master's. Your hospital has just merged with the local university hospital. As the least senior member of your department, you know your job will be eliminated when the departments from the two hospitals merge. What do you do?

A. You investigate other options at the hospital. You like staff development, but you get along well in other areas of the hospital. You have significant hospital-wide seniority and wide-ranging experience. You see yourself as adaptable. You make an appointment with human resources and see what positions they offer you. You find the situation stressful but figure you can make the best of it.

B. You investigate your seniority status and are relieved to find out that you rank fairly high. Your hospital's policy states that you can bump into your previous position. You decide to go back to being an assistant manager in geriatrics, a position that is currently vacant. From there, you plan to complete your master's—but in the management sequence. You plan to keep accruing seniority and apply for the next manager's position to open. You suppose these positions to be less vulnerable to layoff.

C. You really hate to see your job end! You were good at it and brought all your experience to bear on it. Toys and games have been a fascination and hobby of yours for years; you've even developed numerous simulations at work as an outgrowth of this interest. Your interest in games led you to pursue educational technology, where you've earned a reputation as a gaming whiz. Although the departmental consolidation is a setback, you have many contacts and quite a reputation. You plan to take an evening clinic position, complete your master's degree, and take steps to start your own company developing and marketing medical simulations.

D. You are fed up. You've been thinking about branching off into sales for years. Your family has a distribution business and you cut your teeth on sales. In fact, you miss the adrenalin rush that accompanies competition! You still have numerous contacts in sales, as well as experience in the plastics field. You plan to let your contacts know you are available and to get back into the business environment. Although you like hospitals, you are tired of the turmoil. You want a job where your performance is all that counts!

The preceding was by no means a "test" to reveal anything hidden in your thinking. The answers you selected, however, can prove useful in exploring your typical responses to career dilemmas. With that in mind—and, again, this is not a test—do the following patterns accurately reflect your current career-management style?

If you answered two, three, or four A's, you may have a tendency to stay put and let fate or circumstances outside yourself have a strong influence on your career. You approach your job looking for continuity and how to fit in at work. Your strength is your belief in your resilience. You do not manage your career as such, but manage events on day-to-day basis, aiming for maintenance as a goal.

If you answered two, three, or four B's, you may readily see the need for change in your career, but you are likely to look to traditional models to prepare you for your next step. You may be most comfortable with a traditional education and career path. If you have strong interests outside of nursing, you probably do not seek to integrate them into your job. One potential drawback associated with this approach to career management is that you may have to wait longer for traditional opportunities to present themselves than have others in the past. Among the advantages are that the career paths are generally already mapped out, and there are plenty of resources to guide you through the steps—from teachers to books and journals to mentors.

If you answered two, three, or four C's, you have passions and interests that motivate you. You see opportunities to combine these interests with your current nursing background. You understand how nursing is a great building block and source of leverage, and you use this background to give voice to your interests. You are likely comfortable letting all of your life experiences and interests guide you to the goal best suited to you.

If you answered two, three, or four D's, you have strong interests and are passionate about things outside of work—perhaps so much so that you don't see the relevance of your nursing background to achieving your goals. This may lead you to totally leap into exciting endeavors—or to overlook the wealth of experience and skill brought by your nursing background. You are likely to be comfortable with strongly unconventional directions and paths but may be unable to see ways to use your current skills as leverage or a bridge to those paths.

Moving on the Continuum

Wherever you currently fall on the linear-nonlinear thinking continuum, it is possible to change. A completely or mostly linear-oriented career-seeker can become more of a divergent thinker. Likewise, a radically divergent (i.e., nonlinear) type can find ways to use a current skill set to leverage a passionate interest into a career—in other words, to become a little more linear-oriented for a while.

If you chose mostly *A*s in the preceding thinking "assessment", you probably do not incorporate any nonlinear thinking processes into your career planning, perhaps because career changes do not tend to be your choice. If you find yourself in the position of needing to make a choice, being armed with some nonlinear-thinking skills may prove very helpful, however. You may find that exposing yourself to some of the vast array of careers available to nurses is a great first step. Even hearing the stories in this chapter may help to jog your creative side. Learning to understand how your hobbies, interests, and outside strengths can set you apart in the job market could give you an advantage over others, if you ever need it.

If you selected mostly *B*s, you are fairly well acquainted with traditional career mobility. Becoming aware of your strengths and using nonlinear thinking could give you an advantage in selling yourself in a crowded field of candidates.

If you selected mostly *C*s you are likely comfortable using nonlinear thinking strategies in your career planning. You are able to balance moving out past the obvious and retaining the advantages of your current nursing experience. Reviewing the strategies that follow may help to reinforce your confidence as you move forward in your career.

If you selected mostly *D*s, not only are you comfortable with nonlinear thinking strategies, but you may verge on being radical. Although this can be a strength, you should be aware of this potential tendency and exercise it deliberately. You might benefit from exploring the role that your hard-won nursing skills could play in advancing you toward your career goals. These skills are already yours; you may as well use them, if they can be helpful. You may have difficulty seeing their relevance, however. A little practice in recognizing and using the skills and experience you have gained from your nursing background might be helpful to you, even should you choose to move out of nursing.

BEFORE PRACTICING NONLINEAR THINKING

Before you start practicing techniques for nonlinear thinking, it helps to focus on *why* you are doing this. The following items constitute *prework* designed to bring your current career, your strengths, and your support network into sharp focus.

Understand How You Feel about Work

Take some quiet time to think about your feelings regarding work *now*. Do you look forward to going to work every day? Why or why not? Are you more or less happy at work than your coworkers seem to be? Do you spend a lot of time complaining? Are you still enthusiastic about patient care? Do you drag at work, or are you energetic? Can you think of what you get from your job, other than money? If the answers are not positive, how long have you been feeling this way? When did it start? Can you identify a cause and fix it?

This process may take a little time. If you feel great about work, isolate and focus on the reasons why. If you do not feel so positive, try to understand what you need more of—or, perhaps, less of—at work. What could you contribute that you have not. What opportunities don't you get?

Write down your answers. Put them away and look at them in two weeks. Ask yourself the same questions and see whether your answers vary.

Take Inventory of Your Work Skills and Experience

If you don't have a resume, create one (see Chapter 3). If you have one, review and update it. Collect all of your awards, evaluations, and thank-you letters. Review them to refresh your memory about your strengths. List your committees, projects, contributions, and ideas that have made a difference at work. Go through the process outlined in the latest edition of *What Color is Your Parachute.* (Bolles, 1995).

Take Stock of Your Interests and Hobbies

Think about the last few years. What did you do for fun? What skills does it take to do those things? What church- or civic-related activities did you love? What have you learned from them? Of which projects in your life are you proudest? What would you like to spend more of your time doing? What makes you happiest when you are outside of work? What activity has been closest to a lifelong interest for you? What do people ask you to do with great frequency, (such as advise them and about what, play music at events, sing, demonstrate craft skills, write for community publications, etc.)? Do you like to do those things? What skills are involved?

List all of your answers to the preceding questions. Review your answers. Circle any answers that you have an especially strong feeling about, whether they be interests or skills. Are there any patterns? What picture about you emerges?

Identify Your Support Network

Think about your bosses, coworkers, friends, and neighbors. Bring to mind the groups to which you belong, perhaps classmates, club officers, church officials, civic-group leaders. Of these people, who do you know admires you? Write down why they do. Who has thanked you recently? Why? Call to mind the favors you have done for them. Whom have you helped, gone out of your way to support? List these people, and the reasons they value you. Review the list in a week to see whether more people belong on it. If so, add them to the list.

Look Further into Your Past

Think about school and the things you did as a child. At what were you great? Of what were you proudest? What did friends and teachers admire about you? What do you wish you had kept doing—in sports, academics, clubs, or other areas? Do any of these things fit in as a pattern with previous lists? Is there anything that stands out as very different? Why is it still not part of your life? Would it make you happy if you could build it back in?

Review Your Lists

Look over all of your lists. Highlight anything to which you have a strong positive emotional reaction. Write down why it is so wonderful. Go over the list again. Are there any patterns to what makes you feel good—strengths, skills, supportive people, passionate interests, major successes?

Collect Examples of Jobs Held by Current or Former Nurses

In newspapers, novels, communication with colleagues, notes from your alumni association, radio or TV programming, trade publications—anywhere you can think of—make note of references to jobs held by current or former nurses. Write these down or cut them out, and put them in a file. Ask your friends or coworkers about the most unusual jobs that they know of nurses holding. Try to learn about professional activities performed by RNs, not necessarily for pay. Do any serve as unpaid lobbyists, civic leaders, writers, advisors to significant groups or people, members of speakers' bureaus (and on what topics)? Ask your friends, coworkers, and former teachers. Attend your reunions and research the career trajectories and volunteer activities of fellow alumni.

After one month, review all your findings in one sitting. Refer to a newspaper after reviewing your findings. List as many additional related careers as you can find. Next, make a list of things that you find notable because they are *not* listed.

Review your new list, as well as your original findings. Highlight all those career activities that sound interesting or arouse your curiosity.

TECHNIQUES FOR PRACTICING NONLINEAR THINKING

Nonlinear thinking is the backbone of creativity. It is a process of taking leaps, using your imagination, and suspending judgment. Nonlinear or creative thinking *can* be learned. And the more you practice it, the more you can draw on it to help you in your career.

Most of you have already been exposed to exercises in brainstorming, a process that encompasses nonlinear strategies. Nearly everyone is familiar with the exercise that asks you to think of as many uses as possible for a brick or a coat hanger in a five-minute time frame. At first, the ideas tend to be linked: hang clothes, hang scarves, hang belts, drip dry clothes. Then, they diverge slightly: prop open doors, open locked car doors, beat rugs. Next, the ideas tend to get "stranger": twist into a sculpture, make a frame for a kite, use as a tool for painting abstract art. Finally, the ideas depart from reality, as people struggle to make a huge list. At this stage, however, everyone is amazed to discover that some of the most "unreal" ideas are among the most novel ideas. It never fails! Therefore, this is a good place to begin practicing nonlinear thinking.

■ *EXERCISE 4.1: What Can You Do with a...?*

Look around the room and list the first five objects you see, each on a different page. On one of the pages, list as many things as possible that can be done with that object. Time yourself for five minutes. Work very quickly. Don't worry about usefulness, practicality, or anything else. You are the only one who will see this list, so the wilder the ideas the better! Be crazy, ridiculous, break the rules!

Next, count the items on the list and write the total in big numbers at the top of the page. Then, highlight at least five items that did not stem directly from the items preceding. Finally, note any feelings you had while doing this exercise: foolishness, joy, boredom, frustration, challenge, etc. Put this page in a folder. On each of the next four days, repeat the process with one of the remaining pages. On each day, challenge yourself to come up with more entries than on the previous day's page. At the end of the week, look at your lists. Did the feelings evolve? Did the lists get longer?

■ *EXERCISE 4.2: List That Career!*

Review your lists made for the "Before Practicing Nonlinear Thinking" section (beginning on page 98). List two of your hobbies or interests, two of your skills, and two of your high school activities, each on a different page. On the first day, take one of the hobby/interest pages and list as many jobs or careers as you can think of that will allow you to use that hobby or interest. The careers do not need to be related to nursing in any way. Work as fast as you can for fifteen minutes. Quantity is your goal. When you are done, count your entries and write the total at the top of the page.

On day two, repeat the process with the other hobby/interest page. This time, your goal is to exceed the previous day's total. Proceed through your lists until all six are completed.

After you have completed the lists, count all of the career options, eliminating duplications. Put the grand total on the first page. Review your work. Did it seem to get easier? Was it stressful? Was it fun? Did you allow yourself to be ridiculous? Did you think of things to add to your lists throughout the day? Did you experience the creative process as continuing in fits and starts throughout the day and night? Did you allow yourself to continue to imagine even though you were not actively doing the exercise? If so, congratulations! The process of imagination seems to come naturally to you.

■ *EXERCISE 4.3: What's Your Angle?*

From the list of nursing careers that you amassed in the month-long activity described on page 99, select the three most appealing occupations you found to be held by nurses. Put the title of each of the selected occupations on a separate page. Adapted from *A Kick in the Seat of The Pants*, (von Oech, 1986).

On the first page, work through the following activities:

1. Write down how this occupation is like planting a garden.

2. Write down three ways you can make fun of (parody) this occupation.

3. Write down at least two jobs that are opposite of this occupation.

4. Write down at least two ways to combine or somehow connect this occupation with a nursing background.

5. Write down two famous people who would be well suited to this occupation. Complete these activities for each of the occupations you chose, but do so on a different day for each. When you have finished, review what you wrote. You have just completed an exercise in viewing a subject from different angles.

■ *EXERCISE 4.4: Putting It Together*

This exercise is closely related to your career. Take as much time as you need; do not try to complete the exercise in one sitting. Review the lists of favorite activities, skills, and supportive people that you made for the exercises beginning on page 98. List your two most favorite activities, your three best skills, and two supportive people. Then complete the following tasks:

1. List three occupations that incorporate both of your favorite activities and your three best skills.

2. List five of your nursing skills that will support each occupation. (This will result in three separate lists, one for each occupation.)

3. Pretend you are each of your two supporters. From each of their points of view, write a brief letter of recommendation stating why they believe you to be an excellent candidate for each of the three jobs.

KEEPING THE CREATIVE JUICES FLOWING

Although the preceding exercises were closely related to nursing careers and interests, you do not think about your career every waking moment. However, you do experience countless opportunities to be playful, creative, and nonlinear. As you wait in line at the grocery store, for instance, imagine the opposite of every item that the person in front of you is buying: peas are corn, hamburgers are buns, mustard is ketchup, onions are candy—the more ridiculous, the better. Or as you wait for a bus, think of flowers that would make a *terrible* combination for a garden. Or sometime when you are put on hold, imagine the consequences of rain falling up. Or on a rainy afternoon, sit with a young child and invent a silly card game. The more often you look at things a little "off center", the easier it will be to see the ordinary parts of your work life in a new way. It takes practice, so make it a habit.

Following are some additional ways to facilitate nonlinear thinking:

- Seek out creativity courses. Check your community college, adult learning programs such as the Learning Tree, park district programs, or flyers that come from nursing organizations. Suggest that your staff development department sponsor a creativity workshop. Sign up for more than one such course, then practice what you learn on your friends.

- Talk to everyone you can about their careers. Get as many ideas as possible, write them down, and throw them in a box. Periodically take out the box and review the contents. As you look at each idea, ask yourself which of your treasured skills or interests would make that a better job and why. Repeat this process many times over; it will keep you mindful of the contributions you can make.

- Buy creativity workbooks such as *A Kick in the Seat of the Pants*, (von Oech, 1986) or *A Whack on the Side of the Head* (von Oech, 1983). Work through the exercises. They're lots of fun, and they really work.

- Spend time every week imagining yourself using your favorite skills. What are you doing? Who is there? How did you get there? Be as elaborate as possible in your thoughts.

- Familiarize yourself with your library's career section. Browse through books on career development, and read articles on inspirational career switches.

- Most importantly, keep doing the things that you love to do outside of work. As you do these things, remind yourself of why you love them. Make a commitment to work them into your career.

SOME FINAL WORDS

It is widely known that the Chinese symbol for *threat* is the same as the one for *opportunity*. Health care and the world of work will continue to change, sometimes at a frightening pace. As a nurse, however, you are pivotally positioned to launch yourself in many interesting and lucrative directions as you ride the waves of change. In addition to your nursing skills and experience, your way of looking at the world will help determine what opportunities are available to you. As you enhance your ability to think in a nonlinear fashion, you will be better able to see how your personal attributes link with your nursing attributes; you will see opportunities sooner and seize them more readily. You will be better prepared to make yourself happy throughout your worklife, and you will be able to turn threats to your advantage.

SUMMARY

You can learn to look at what you do, what you want, and what you know in new ways. The more perspectives from which you are able to view your career and your options, the more your choices. Nursing does not always teach the skill of nonlinear thinking, yet this skill is critical to establishing your best advantage in the marketplace.

Nonlinear thinking can be learned. It is fun, and it will help you expand your career horizons. But, as is true of all skills, nonlinear (or creative) thinking takes practice. Working through the exercises in this chapter offers you a good beginning on the road to broader career choices. Good luck!

REFERENCES

Bolles, R. N. (1995). *What color is your parachute? A practical manual for job-hunters and career changers.* Berkeley, CA: Ten Speed Press.

von Oech, R. A. (1983). *A whack on the side of the head: How to unlock your mind for innovation.* New York: Warner Books.

von Oech, R. A. (1986). *A kick in the seat of the pants: Using your explorer, artist, warrior and judge to be more creative.* New York: Harper Row.

systems in health care are becoming increasingly complex, as movement toward the computerized patient record continues. Although standardization of both health care information systems and communication between systems is still under development, some levels of standardization do exist, such as Health Level Seven (HL-7). HL-7 is a standard designed to allow applications to communicate between each other to share data; thus, the laboratory system can communicate with the accounting system to bill for tests and with the pharmacy system to notify the pharmacist of significant laboratory tests such as toxic antibiotic levels. In addition, this standard is designed to allow an information system at one agency to communicate with an information system at another agency, so that a patient record can follow the individual from one health care system to another.

A universal health record is far from a reality, and many problems can be anticipated before such a record is implemented. However, this potential change is a major issue in health-related informatics. Development of such a system has the potential to dramatically change health care delivery. If and when universal health care records become available, the role of informatics specialists will expand. Major issues include what the record will include, how the record will be developed technically, and how privacy will be maintained (considering confidentiality and security). Current work on developing standards and guidelines for the electronic universal health care record is underway and being led by the Computerized Patient Record Institute (CPRI), an interdisciplinary group comprising health care professionals (from medicine, nursing, pharmacy, and other disciplines), vendors, and other interested parties.

Changes in access to information also are occurring exponentially. Computerized references, available both locally in health care settings and through the Internet and World Wide Web, demand new skills in information retrieval and provide new challenges in authenticating information and maintaining data security for the health care agency. When a health care agency is connected to the outside, not only can staff retrieve information from the outside, but internal information may be vulnerable to tampering. This raises numerous ethical and legal questions, many of which yet remain unresolved as agencies strive to balance needed information access and service to their customers (including physicians' offices and patients' homes) with maintaining data security and integrity. Technical developments in information availability and retrieval can be expected to continue.

Practicing nurses interact regularly with computers. Many nurses routinely document and plan care using the computer. Some nurses are currently using point-of-care systems to update and document plans of care at the bedside. Computers are also integral parts of many types of patient care equipment and monitoring systems.

Changing Printed Information to Improve Care Delivery

In one agency, unit census material from the information system was made available in printed form for nurses to use in taking report on groups of patients. The initial form of this printed material was insufficient, however. Not only was the format crowded, leaving little space for notes, but information such as diagnosis, intern, code status, diet, and NPO status—all of which were kept in the information system for all patients as part of normal business—was absent. This information was subsequently added to the "nursing report sheets", making them much more usable by nurses on a daily basis. In addition, the white space was increased to allow for notes, and separate sheets, with names and room numbers, were made available for technicians to use in taking and recording vital signs.

This change made use of information already available in the system to save time in reporting; nurses no longer have to write this information. And seeking these changes did not require specific programming skills. Instead, the nurses communicated their information needs to others who could make the necessary system changes. Receiving the information was a nurse informatician who knew the system, could validate the need for change with other nurses, and could then communicate the needed changes to the programmers. Two nurses, then, were instrumental in this information system change: one whose primary responsibility was to patient care, and one whose primary responsibility was to the information systems department. The result was an improvement in the delivery of care; nurses are now aware of code status, interns to call in emergencies (and the interns' beeper numbers), and other information. The nurses assigned to patients now have a clear picture of the computerized information and can easily validate the accuracy of this information.

Opportunities to Impact Information Systems

As illustrated in the preceding example, nurses need to be vigilant in looking for opportunities to impact information systems. As systems are introduced into agencies, the nurse needs to question the effect of that system on nursing. Too often, for example, nurses are not included in consideration of the pharmacy system, into which they will need to enter orders, or the laboratory system, from which they will need to retrieve information. Although nurses may not have primary impact on system selection, they may impact modifications to the predesigned system so that it facilitates rather than complicates patient care from the nurse's perspective.

The nurse representing the informatics department of an agency has the responsibility of communicating with nurses in all areas and at all levels to learn the specific information needs of each area and level. This nurse both educates users and communicates users' needs to programmers. Nurses involved in systems development need a clear understanding of the system design process and of needs assessment. In addition, these nurses must be keenly aware of management concerns regarding resource use, financial responsibility, and the enterprise (systemwide) goals of the institution. The informatics nurse is not focused on a specific unit or patient population; rather, this nurse represents the total institution and balances the information needs and resources of one area with those of other areas. These nurses must take a global view of the information system and other resources and use that information in communicating both to nurses and to programmers or systems analysts.

Preparation and Characteristics

Practicing nurses who function as informatics communicators must be aware of the information systems changes occurring around them and to consider the implications of these changes to their practice. These nurses must identify possibilities and be open to alternate approaches to providing care. A willingness to learn and change are, thus, important characteristics for the nurse communicator. Special preparation may involve exposure to new developments in the world of computers. These nurses must seek out such learning opportunities.

The informatics-based nurse becomes aware of current systems and future plans by virtue of his or her position in the informatics department. This nurse may have advanced preparation in information systems design, systems analysis, and needs assessment. This nurse also must be able to recognize opportunities for change and be open to new possibilities. In addition, this nurse must be knowledgeable regarding business plans and organizational issues. Ideally, information systems personnel are involved in the strategic planning of the organization and, thus, are cognizant of and can contribute to both long-term and short-term goals. Communication skills are vital. The informatics nurse communicator must listen carefully to nurses in the clinical areas so as to identify the information system needs in these areas. This nurse must then incorporate these needs into the information plan for the agency and develop teaching plans to educate users on new information systems developments.

The Future

Future possibilities in computer-assisted nursing practice are limited only by the imagination. For example, handheld computer technology has expanded and improved dramatically (Mossberg, 1996), as evidenced by a 1996 conference cosponsored by the American Nurses Association (ANA) and called "The Forum for Handheld Computing in Health Care". This three-day conference focused solely on mobile data management at the point-of-care/point-of-contact.

The role of nurse as communicator will be key in maximizing computer applications. Nursing expertise and insight will refine these systems, resulting in management of information in the most effective manner. Nurses' input will also guide development of systems and hardware that are "nurse friendly" and that complement quality care. Nurses in the communicator role have the opportunity to shape an important dimension of future nursing practice.

NURSE AS PROGRAMMER

Nursing informatics specialists who are programmers develop specific programs for use in patient care, administration of patient care, or education. These nurses use programming languages to modify or develop programs that fulfill these needs. These informatics nurses combine their knowledge of nursing and of specific programming languages to develop programs that can be used by other health care providers. Examples of programs developed by nurse programmers include computer-assisted-instruction materials, programs to format papers according to American Psychological Association (APA) style, scheduling programs, decision making programs, and other computer-based programs.

Health care management relies on computer-based programs to manage information and project into the future. Computer-based programs serve as valuable tools for clinical databases, financial accounting and planning, and quality improvement. Nurses who develop programs must have a clear understanding of either specific programming languages or specific applications, such as expert systems packages, authoring packages, database programs, and other software. These nurses also must have a clear understanding of the nursing component, whether involving education, pediatric nursing, administration, or finance.

Today, nurses may pursue careers in programming after completing specialized education and training. As a related career option, nurses may create and design computer-assisted software. Current computer programs use the graphical user interface, pull-down menus, and readily available help programs to assist the user. As computers became faster with more available memory, programs became more sophisticated and made more help available to the user. The changes seen in word processing packages alone illustrate this dramatic change. Most adults are familiar with the standardized interfaces seen in either the Apple or Microsoft Windows environment. After a user becomes familiar with one program, basic applications in another program can be learned fairly readily. Similar changes have occurred in more complex computer programs, facilitating the development of database applications, decision support tools, and other computer-based applications. Therefore, nurses interested in informatics—even if they wish to develop programs—no longer must be able to use binary language, which reduces everything to either 0 or 1. Advanced application language provides an interface between the user and the machine.

How the Role Has Changed

Pioneers in nursing informatics had strong skills in either programming or computer-based applications. As computer technology advanced, however, so too did the applications available to the potential author to develop computer-based programming. And as programming became more sophisticated, so too did the tools authors could use to develop applications. Specific syntax became less important as the process of writing code was automated through the use of high-level languages. In the past, nurses who used databases needed to know specific command languages such as prolog and structured query language (SQL). Today, however, programs guide the user in defining fields, field type, length, and other characteristics. Users can select from a group of commonly used commands and implement them without using specific words in a given order and with exact punctuation. As computer programs and applications became more user friendly, the applications available to the nonexpert computer user grew.

 Programming Progress in Word Processing Packages

Early word processors required the user to push the *control* key, the "*k*" key and, the "*r*" key to insert a file. Users then had to type in the name of the file exactly as saved on the disk. To implement specific text enhancements, such as bold-facing, underlining, and italicizing, the user was required to insert specific codes both before and following the text to be enhanced. Users either memorized such commands, developed cheat sheets listing the commands, or consulted the manual each time a command was necessary. Today, however, the user moves the mouse to and, clicks on *Insert*, selects *File*, and selects from a list of available files to insert into the current document. Specific text enhancements appear as choices on the screen, and the user can see which words are enhanced (and how). Users can easily go from using Word Perfect for Windows to using Word for Windows to using other Windows-based applications designed for composing simple documents.

Preparation and Characteristics

The nurse interested in programming must have expertise in nursing and skill in using a programming language or a specific application. Programming requires orderly, methodical thinking and problem-solving skills. The author of a program must ensure that the program works reliably and as planned, and that any problems are resolved. Solving programming problems requires orderly examination and modification of the program to locate and fix the problem. The nurse programmer should have the credentials necessary to convince potential customers that a given program's outcomes are reliable and valid. Depending on the content area of the program, this may mean credentials in administration, clinical practice, or education. Potential nurse customers are more likely to scrutinize credentials in the content arena than in the programming field. Customers who are primarily information systems professionals, however, will require credentials and demonstrated competence in the programming field.

The Future

Future changes in computer programs will likely make use of research in human-computer interaction, with the goal of designing user-computer interfaces that enhance productivity, are easy to learn, and are easy to use once learned. Learnability and usability are major areas of information systems research. Movement will continue away from a text-based interface, which presents the user with a blank screen on which he or she writes specific, and syntactically exact commands, and toward a graphical interface. The movement to make technical specificity somewhat transparent to the user will continue. When this is accomplished, the user will see the interface and the result, rather than the specific command sequence used to achieve the result. In the future, nurses who wish to develop programs may be able to do so with less technical knowledge. Conversely, because programs are becoming ever larger and the graphical interface ever more complex, the nurse who wishes to program "from scratch" will have a much more difficult challenge.

THE NURSE AS VENDOR REPRESENTATIVE

The nurse who works as a vendor representative frequently travels and assists specific agencies in selecting information systems products, modifying those products to meet agency needs, and developing implementation plans to introduce the systems into the agency. This nurse also assists in staff development and in troubleshooting during the implementation process.

Besides working with agencies that purchase from the vendor, this nurse represents the vendor at demonstrations, in competitions with other vendors, and at trade and professional meetings. This nurse, therefore, needs to be well aware of the strengths and weaknesses of the product, how the product compares with other available products, what the agencies are seeking in an information system, and how to overcome any weaknesses in the system. As the representative of the vendor, the nurse also needs to provide the vendor with feedback regarding those things that an agency is seeking in an information system, any modifications that are desired, and ideas for product improvement. This nurse, then, serves not only as a salesperson, but also as a problem-solver who helps the agency identify how and why a particular system will meet its information needs. The latter role is crucial because agency personnel may not have a clear understanding of the benefits and possibilities associated with a given information system.

How the Role Has Changed

As information systems have become increasingly complex and sophisticated, so too have agency demands and expectations. To do their jobs well, nurses who represent vendors must keep current on all systems, both those they represent and those of the competition. Users are becoming more sophisticated and expect more from vendors. As systems become more expensive, demands on the seller expand. Just as home consumers have become more demanding with regard to home information systems, so too have professional consumers. Vendors' representatives must therefore commit themselves to customer service.

One Nurse's Vendor Rep Experience

When her hospital introduced the new computer-based patient-care system, LaToya represented medical-surgical nursing on the planning committee. She had enjoyed playing with computers since high school and, so, seized the opportunity to tailor this system to the nurses' needs.

During her service on the committee, she met Sheila, the vendor's representative. She and Sheila worked together to collect and organize information about nursing care delivery and requirements related to the information system. Sheila was impressed with LaToya's enthusiasm and encouraged her to look into a job with the vendor.

LaToya was ready for a change and followed up on Sheila's suggestion. After training with the vendor, she began a series of relationships with hospitals that were introducing the vendor's system. Two years later, she was working at a hospital that was a member of a large hospital corporation. LaToya's expertise and respect for the hospital staff's concerns attracted the attention of nursing administration.

Based on the recommendation of nursing administration, the corporation offered LaToya a position on the corporate information systems staff. LaToya accepted the position and subsequently became active in the Midwest Alliance for Nursing Informatics. Through this organization, she learned of an opportunity with a consulting firm composed of a group of nurses who consult with hospitals to help their clients analyze computer-systems needs. After three years with the corporation, LaToya is now considering taking another step in her nursing informatics career.

Preparation and Characteristics

As previously stated, vendor representatives must be knowledgeable about *all* information systems, including those of the competition. Sales skills are also important as are the ability to determine exactly what consumers want and need in a system and the ability to design and modify a system to meet those needs. Current needs must be addressed and future needs must be anticipated. Other necessary skills include being able to interact well with others and, especially, with strangers and new acquaintances. Knowledge of the various needs of health care agencies as well as of the specific aspects of the vendor's product is essential. The vendor representative also works with agency personnel in designing an implementation process to ease transition into the new system. This requires skill in educating new users to use the system optimally. Thus, the vendor representative is a combination of salesperson, change agent, and educator.

The Future

As health care information systems expand, so too will the demand on the vendor representative to be knowledgeable about a variety of information needs. Furthermore, increasing amounts of information will be needed in order to implement information systems. As financial resources shrink, purchasers of information systems will require evidence of positive cost-benefit ratios. The vendor representative will also need to be able to communicate the positive results of installing a system.

Vendors will be able to offer the nurse a variety of positions including salesperson, trainer, developer, consultant, demonstrator, and programmer.

OTHER OPPORTUNITIES IN INFORMATICS

Informatics opportunities are not limited to the major roles of communicator, programmer, and vendor representative. Hospitals, professional schools, freestanding consulting groups, and hardware and software manufacturers all offer opportunities in nursing informatics. Hospitals and other health care organizations have needs for data managers, system administrators, analysts, clinical consultants, and information system managers. Professional schools may have positions in computer learning labs or may offer opportunities to consult with faculty who are developing computer-assisted learning materials. Freestanding consulting groups offer full ranges of services to clients who are in various phases of implementing computer-based systems. Consulting groups may specialize in systems for particular applications such as administration, clinical, quality management, or finance. Manufacturers may have a broad spectrum of positions available, from marketing and sales to authenticating online reference data to developing computer-assisted learning materials. Investigate such opportunities by contacting health care organizations, schools, hardware and software manufacturers, and professional organizations. Explore online resources and nursing journals for additional opportunities.

Preparation and Characteristics

Nursing skills transfer well into a career in informatics. Informatics requires skill in data gathering, planning, organizing, delegating, and evaluating outcomes. Interpersonal skills are also important, because informatics requires interacting with system users to identify and respond to their needs. Finally, nurses know the roles of the multiple departments and disciplines within the health care agency, and they know how these variables work together. This knowledge is valuable in anticipating and understanding the needs of system users.

EDUCATIONAL PREPARATION

Nurses wishing to prepare for practice in informatics can obtain education in many ways. Some roles lend themselves to self-education, such as clinical nurses who identify implementation possibilities on their nursing units. Nurses who have extensive experience with a vendor's product may be good candidates to represent that vendor, if the nurse also has skills in sales, selection of new systems, or implementation of new systems. Further academic preparation can be pursued at the baccalaureate, master or doctoral level. Nursing programs are expanding the informatics content in their basic curricula. Graduate-level study focusing on informatics is available in both nursing and nonnursing programs. Certification as an informatics nurse by the American Nurses Credentialing Center (ANCC) requires course work in nursing informatics or experience and continuing education in the field. Certification examination topics include the following:

- system analysis and design
- system installation and support
- system testing and evaluation

- human factors
- computer technology
- information/database management
- professional practice/trends and issues
- theories

Specific guidelines can be obtained by telephoning ANCC at 1-800-284-CERT.

Information about accredited graduate programs is available from the National League for Nursing and from several programs with tracks in informatics nursing. Nonnursing course work is available either through business programs, programs in information systems, or other programs. Course work in computer science is geared more toward the technical aspects of systems rather than the interaction with the user.

Printed materials, conferences, and the Internet are other potential sources of information about nursing informatics. One overview of informatics is contained in *Introduction to Nursing Informatics* (Hannah, Ball, & Edward, 1994). Other information sources include the American Medical Informatics Association annual meeting and conference and the Healthcare Information Management Systems Society meetings. These are large meetings that incorporate research results, practical guidance (e.g., "what worked for my agency"), and numerous vendor demonstrations.

NURSING ON THE INTERNET

On the Internet, the discussion groups Nrsing-L and Nursenet provide opportunities to discuss issues related both to informatics (Nrsing-L) and general nursing. The World Wide Web (WWW), contains many "pages" (sites of information on the Internet) related to health care. You can find informatics-related pages by searching on "nursing informatics" as key words. Some such pages are linked (connected) to other sites of interest. Each site has a specific address and can be located using that address.

This author established a WWW home page in January of 1995 and has been updating it regularly since. The biggest challenge is updating the page to reflect the most current information. The URL (uniform resource locator, or Internet address) is http://www.nursing.ab.umd.edu.

A WWW search as of September, 1995, revealed 975 documents with the word "nursing" (Goodwin, 1995). Goodwin notes that she personally knew of additional home pages that had not yet been included at the time of her search. The Internet is a rich resource for networking with colleagues, investigating career opportunities and asking specific questions of other professionals to learn from their experience. Professional organizations and schools display information about their programs, services, and ongoing projects on the Internet. And nursing schools sometimes list faculty members and their interests. You can discover a wealth of useful information by employing search engines such as Webcrawler to search on key words.

RESOURCES FOR FURTHER INFORMATION

American Medical Informatics Association Nursing Informatics Working Group (Newsletter available online at abbott@gl.umbc.edu)

American Nurses Association
Council for Nursing Services and Informatics
600 Maryland Avenue SW
Washington, DC 20024-2571
Telephone: 202-651-7000

Midwest Alliance for Nursing Informatics
P.O. Box 9313
Downers Grove, IL 60515
Telephone: 708-923-4535

SUMMARY

Nursing informatics is an ever-changing field; the informatics nurse thus must grow in terms of knowledge and skill as the field changes. In this way, nursing informatics certainly offers a challenge. As the demand for health care information and for health care information systems expands, so too does nursing informatics as a field. Preparation can involve both formal, academic study and practical experience. Informatics can be combined with other nursing areas. For example, the nurse who is primarily interested in a specific clinical specialty can incorporate informatics in that practice as well as represent that specialty to the information systems department. Conversely, a nurse can focus on the informatics component and use nursing skills to communicate with nurses and other health care providers regarding information systems needs. As with any expanding field, the pioneers are defining the practice!

REFERENCES

American Nurses Credentialing Center. (1996). *Informatics nurse certification catalog.* Washington, DC: ANCC.

Ball, M. J., Hannah, K. J., Newbold, S. K., & Douglas, J. K. (1995). *Nursing informatics: Where caring and technology meet (2nd ed.).* New York: Springer-Verlag.

Goodwin, L. W. (1995). Nursing and the World Wide Web. *Nursing Informatics,* 6 (2).

Hannah, K. J., Ball, M. J., & Edwards, M. J. A. (1994). *Introduction to nursing informatics.* New York: Springer-Verlag.

Mossberg, W. S. (1996, March 28). Personal technology. *Wall Street Journal.*

Chapter Six

The RN in Redesigned Organizations

Bonnie Wilson and Rose Pfefferbaum

INTRODUCTION

As a profession, nursing has traditionally responded to changing health care needs and the environment in which health care is provided, continually adapting to and guiding system changes to help ensure delivery of patient care. It should come as no surprise, then, that nursing is taking a lead in the redesign of health care organizations.

In most redesigned health care organizations, economic forces have driven the redesign effort. Redesign efforts intend to make the most efficient and effective use of resources. RNs are a costly resource. Redesign efforts focus on creating a role for the RN that fully uses the RN's unique expertise while minimizing use of RN power for duties that lesser-prepared caregivers can perform. Redesign efforts also focus on more direct and decentralized delivery of services to patients. Delivering services more directly creates the potential for increased quality and satisfaction for patients as well as caregivers. Although financial factors have driven most reorganization efforts, redesign efforts in some organizations have emerged from quality-improvement initiatives.

To understand changes in the role of the nurse, it is important to understand basic changes in the health care delivery system. Within redesigned hospitals, nurses typically work as members of cross-trained, multidisciplinary teams that serve a specific number of patients. The RN manages care for assigned patients by providing only selected aspects of care directly and delegating other aspects to cross-trained caregivers. The skill sets of cross-trained caregivers include basic nursing care and certain other competencies that, in the past, have characterized particular departments including respiratory, physical and occupational therapy, phlebotomy, and EKG. Care is taken to the patient whenever feasible, rather than taking the patient to the various departments to receive care. Hospitalized patients are sicker than ever before, and the environment is more cost conscious.

Nurses are increasingly employed in home- and community-based settings, which are equally cost conscious. Case management by a nurse (or, sometimes, by a social worker, in community-based care) is increasingly common in any setting, as is increased reliance on alternate, sometimes multiple, sources of care. In hospitals as well as in home health and community-based settings, redesign has focused attention on client outcomes.

While redesign changes are not made easily and there is still confusion and serious disagreement about direction as well as substance, the RN is nonetheless central to any redesign effort in health care.

IMPLICATIONS OF REDESIGN FOR THE RN

Nursing is, and must continue to be, concerned with those factors that have given rise to redesign. These factors include cost containment; access to and quality of care; rapid changes in technology; informatics; emphasis on holistic care, wellness, and prevention; case management; and the aging of the population. These factors have created a health care environment characterized by decreased lengths of stay; decreased number of hospital admissions, visits, and procedures; decreased need for nurses in acute care settings; increased reliance on home- and community-based care; interdisciplinary teams, and nonnurse caregivers; increased severity of illness at virtually every level of care; and a focus on patient outcomes.

If nursing is to help shape health care of the future, nurses must continue to rethink their role and position themselves to make optimal use of the strengths of the profession. Nursing practice will continue to involve critical thinking, therapeutic communication, and technical skills, but with new emphasis and within new contexts.

Critical thinking encompasses collecting, processing, and interpreting information. The nurse must be able to identify and access information;

store, sort, and select it; and, finally, retrieve and analyze it. This process is increasingly complicated by an ever-increasing amount of information (only some of which is relevant), technological change, greater patient acuity, cost and quality of care, and ethical considerations. In redesigned organizations, certain aspects of critical thinking are especially important: rapidly assessing and adapting to new situations, thinking in a flexible manner, and accommo-dating change.

Therapeutic communication, involving the use of verbal and nonverbal messages to convey thoughts and ideas, is typically goal directed. In working with clients in redesigned, patient-focused health care settings, it is important for the nurse to know the patient's goals and to help shape those goals so that they are consistent with reasonable expectations based on data. Chronic con-ditions, for example, typically require the focus to be more on maintenance of functional level and healthy adaptation rather than on cure. The nurse may need to help patients who have grown to expect cures to understand that care, rather than cure, is the more appropriate expectation under certain cir-cumstances.

The technical skills required for clinical practice are growing increasingly complex and are interwoven with assessment and evaluation. While some basic tasks can be safely delegated to assistive personnel as part of a multidis-ciplinary team approach to patient care delivery in redesigned organizations, it is important to remember that increased reliance on high technology and pharmacology make the health care setting more sophisticated, more power-ful, and, therefore, potentially more dangerous than in the past. Competent RN practice in redesigned organizations, then, requires nurses not only to perform technical skills, but also to delegate tasks safely and to assess the competence of assistive personnel.

While nursing practice will continue to require critical thinking, therapeu-tic communication, and technical skill, the role of the nurse is evolving along with the health care environment. Changes in the role of the nurse arise as a result of the focus on patients; an emphasis on outcomes; the need for better collaboration among service providers; the use of cross-trained, multidiscipli-nary teams; greater reliance on unlicensed, assistive personnel; and attention to the bottom line. To some extent, these changes are as much a matter of degree as substance. To a large extent, they have resulted in increased respon-sibility and increased accountability for the nurse.

Patient-Focused Care

Redesigned organizations typically characterize themselves as providing patient-focused care. For the hospital, this has come to mean decentralizing services, with cross-trained teams providing care at the patient's bedside whenever feasible. In describing her hospital's redesign efforts, one nurse executive succinctly characterized the meaning of patient-focused care:

"There are no demeaning tasks when it comes to taking care of patients. A prime principle in patient-focused care is to never pass over something you can do yourself" (Brider, 1992, p. 28). For the RN, this does not mean doing all the tasks for every patient, but, rather, ensuring that all needs are met. On the patient-focused care team, all members are responsible for responding to the needs that come to their attention. That may mean locating the proper person to take action. Assistive personnel need to know who to call on for the many different needs, requests, and problems that patients and their families communicate to them. Assistive personnel also need to know exactly which tasks they can perform and under what circumstances. To work most efficiently and effectively, RNs must delegate duties to assistive personnel and, thus, free themselves for assessing needs, planning, and managing care.

Though "there is no acceptable professional standard for the safe or optimal amount of time nurses should spend on direct patient care" (Hendrickson, Doddato, & Kovner, 1990, p. 32), a number of studies suggest that hospital redesign can result in increased time spent by the nurse on direct patient care. This may be accomplished through greater use of assistive personnel and support staff, cross-training, teamwork, decentralization, and greater reliance on computers (Brider, 1992; Hendrickson, et al., 1990).

For the health care system in general, patient-focused care generally leads to community-centered care—that is, to providing quality care in the least-restrictive yet medically safe environment. While the downsizing of hospitals has occurred in direct response to reimbursement issues, the increased supply and utilization of home- and community-based services is in large part the result of a preference for deinstitutionalization of care. For nurses, this means a greater number of employment opportunities in a greater variety of settings, as well as opportunities to perform in a greater variety of capacities including entrepreneurial endeavors, case management, program development, health promotion, and education.

Regardless of the setting in which care is provided, patient-focused care emphasizes the patient and the patient's goals to a greater extent than has historically been true. It is typically the nurse who helps the patient understand health needs by providing, interpreting, and clarifying pertinent information. It is the nurse who helps the patient formulate meaningful goals and strategies for accomplishing those goals. The nurse is increasingly able and obligated to help the patient formulate goals and strategies that are appropriate for that patient.

The nurse's role as teacher and advocate is of particular importance to quality care in redesigned organizations. Shorter hospital stays mean that patients must function independently and at higher levels of acuity, find caregivers in the home or community, or be placed in nursing institutions or residential care settings. The nurse must prepare the client for these possibilities by teaching the necessary procedures and skills and by serving as advocate for the client in accessing appropriate services. Under such circumstances, the nurse is likely to be working with families, friends, and other professionals, as well as with the client.

Focus on Outcomes

Health care in general has become increasingly focused on outcomes. This is true with respect to regulation, oversight, and reimbursement, as well as with respect to the delivery of care itself. By choice or by necessity, redesigned organizations operating in redesigned communities of care also now focus on outcomes.

The nurse, too, must focus on outcomes. This may be a challenge for the traditional nurse whose training and practice have emphasized the nursing process. Nurses in redesigned organizations have to look at desired outcomes and manage backwards, identifying interventions to secure those outcomes. This does not mean the nurse should disregard the nursing process. It does, however, require a change in emphasis. It is not an issue of outcomes instead of process, but of using outcomes to determine process.

The focus on outcomes requires the nurse to identify and address multiple goals and outcomes. Nurses in redesigned organizations are expected to consider the patient first, but to consider also the payer, the organization, the delivery system, and the community. The nurse must help the patient identify appropriate goals and may help articulate and interpret goals for the payer, the organization, and the community. The nurse should know the vision, mission, and goals of the organization, which typically reflect its culture. Because the nurse works closely with a variety of stakeholders, the nurse may be able to bring consensus among stakeholders who have divergent goals. In this respect, great importance attaches to the role of the nurse as communicator, interpreter, educator, advocate, and, even, negotiator.

Recognizing the multiple stakeholders (including patient, payer, organization, delivery system, and community) with various and sometimes contradictory concerns, and the change in focus from process to outcomes may permit the nurse to see new approaches in managing and delivering care. At times, these approaches may challenge existing practice. Even so, nurses are in a pivotal position and will increasingly be expected to exercise creativity in case management, particularly when such creativity leads to favorable outcomes for the organization as well as the patient.

An outcomes orientation is facilitated by the development of data-based expectations, standards of practice, and informatics. Nurses in redesigned organizations must be able to access, analyze, and use information with relative ease. The focus on outcomes heightens the nurse's role in terms of critical thinking and creativity.

Health-related outcomes, particularly for the patient, are often difficult to measure. Indeed, the traditional focus on structure and process in the evaluation of health services owes as much to the difficulty in measuring outcomes as to any inherent advantage to structure and process variables themselves. Structure and process measures, however, are likely to translate fairly easily into organizational goals. The successful nurse will recognize the importance of such goals and help move the organization toward achieving them.

Collaboration, Teamwork, and Multiskilling

Patient-focused care and the emphasis on outcomes frequently result in decentralization within hospitals and an increasingly complex, but more substantive, continuum of care within communities. The intent of such redesign is to facilitate the delivery of care from the patient's standpoint. Barriers to care are lessened by bringing care to the patient's bedside in hospitals and by making care available in clinics and homes for clients who reside in the community.

The result of these changes is a need for better collaboration within and across institutional boundaries and greater use of cross-trained, multidisciplinary teams in the delivery of care. The nurse in such settings frequently assumes the role of case manager, overseeing the delivery of care to the client. This clearly requires a thorough knowledge of and the ability to access resources—whether within a hospital or the community—and a proficiency in working with multiple specialties, service providers, and third-party payers. It requires an appreciation of, if not agreement with, the patient's goals. It also requires that the nurse become the patient's advocate, even to the extent that the nurse may need to negotiate on the patient's behalf.

Patient-focused organizations frequently rely on interdisciplinary teams, with members cross-trained to perform multiple tasks. The multidisciplinary approach potentially brings greater expertise to the patient care setting and, when combined with cross-training, helps to reduce departmental and administrative barriers. The nurse must be able to work with multiple disciplines in settings characterized by flatter organizational charts, serve as a role model for other caregivers, and coordinate and oversee the delivery of care.

Cross-training permits a more timely and efficient response to immediate patient needs—a natural concern for redesigned, patient-focused organizations. According to one nurse, cross-training and multiskilling are "ways of sharing skills to the patient's advantage" (Brider, 1992, p. 32). Cross-training also should enable nurses to spend more time on activities for which they are uniquely qualified—that is, to spend more time being nurses. Ideally, the use of interdisciplinary, cross-trained teams frees the nurse for case management, permitting the nurse to focus greater attention on assessment, teaching, and advocacy.

The team approach to care and the cross-training of staff typically rely on as well as permit greater use of unlicensed, assistive personnel. Though still controversial, the increased use of unlicensed caregivers appears to be here to stay in hospitals and in home- and community-based health care organizations. The nurse is an essential component of the multiskilling process, in terms of facilitating its acceptance, training the staff, and overseeing the delivery of care.

To be successful over the long term, multiskilling requires involvement of and consensus among affected professions and regulatory boards (American Health Care Consultants, 1993). The nurse is certainly a key player in recognizing the need and potential for, as well as the major implications of, multiskilling. The nurse in redesigned organizations must identify and work with the major stakeholders, helping to resolve disputes in what is often a heated decision making process.

Multiskilling requires training that is consistent with the level of responsibilities to be assumed and dependent on the specific roles the trainee will play (Weinstein & Sobota, 1989). Nurses will be involved in identifying training needs and designing training materials. Some nurses will be directly involved in the training itself. At the very least, nurses in redesigned organizations will be involved in ongoing assessment and evaluation of the performance of the caregiving team. This is essential for the delivery of high-quality care.

Multiskilling focuses on assistive personnel performing certain tasks other than professional decision making. Professional decision making remains in the domain of the nurse. For RNs, in redesigned organizations that employ unlicensed, assistive personnel as part of multiskilled care teams, skills in critical thinking, problem-solving, team building, delegation, and supervision assume greater importance.

Cost-Consciousness

Never before have nurses been so required to operate within fiscal constraints and to focus on cost containment. The trade-offs are particularly difficult. Nurses perform a delicate balancing act with regard to care quality, organizational integrity, and the bottom line. Establishing an acceptable balance among these variables is complicated by the interrelationships among the variables themselves and by the preponderance of ethical dilemmas associated with modern health care.

Nurses must be knowledgeable about health care costs, reimbursement criteria, and alternate resources and sources of care. This knowledge and the critical thinking skills associated with decision making under increasingly severe constraints are central to case management in redesigned health care settings. Case management today focuses on "making established services more economically efficient within critically monitored populations" (Giuliano & Poirer, 1991, p. 52). The nurse case manager is responsible for "assuring effective use of available resources, maintaining established standards of care, and meeting outcomes within appropriate" time frames (p. 53). Increasingly, the nurse case manager must assist clients in identifying informal sources of care (that is, services for which there is no charge) that may be available within the client's personal social support system. This is particularly important with respect to institutional discharge planning and home- and community-based care settings.

One of the most attractive features of using cross-trained personnel is the potential cost effectiveness. Cross-training increases an organization's human capital without increasing the size of its workforce. It also creates "a workforce which can be more flexibly deployed to meet unpredicted surges in demand." Cross-training personnel may be less expensive than hiring additional staff during times of high demand. This is particularly true to the extent that cross-trained personnel are already oriented to the work setting, are part of the organization's culture, and are knowledgeable about organizational policies and procedures (Lyons, 1992). Nurses in redesigned organizations must be open to the use of cross-trained personnel, whether cross-training is a requirement for the nursing staff itself or whether it is applied to assistive personnel.

Optimal resource utilization involves considering the variety of available human and nonhuman resources, their alternate uses, and the potential for resource substitution. Attention must be given to both time management and waste management. At some point, even the most routine tasks and processes must be evaluated with respect to budgetary implications. Continually confronted with a tension between cost and desired outcomes, nurses in redesigned organizations must learn to deal appropriately with that tension, incorporating cost concerns into decision making.

CHARACTERISTICS AND SKILLS NEEDED IN REDESIGNED ORGANIZATIONS

In any setting, nursing relies on critical thinking, therapeutic communication, and technical skill. In any setting, the nursing process—consisting of client assessment, diagnosis, intervention, and evaluation—is valid. Redesign, thus, has changed the emphasis more than the substance of what the professional nurse does. In doing so, however, it has expanded and complicated the nurse's role.

The use of cross-trained, assistive personnel permits nurses in redesigned organizations to spend less time on routine tasks, clerical activities, and housekeeping chores and more time on case management, problem-solving, and client teaching. There are requirements, however, for successful adjustment to the restructured role. The nurse must be skilled in team building. The nurse must also recognize the potential and the limitations of individual team members and empower each accordingly. The nurse must diligently and continually assess the competency of unlicensed staff, respond to the training needs of the caregiving team, and delegate and supervise adeptly.

Responsibility and accountability are often greater for nurses working in redesigned organizations. Not only must the care needs of patients be met, but these needs must be met under increasingly severe budget constraints.

Cost considerations now attend virtually every decision regarding care. The nurse must be an expert when it comes to health care costs and reimbursement criteria. In the redesigned organization, the nurse manages resources as well as cases.

Although patient acuity is typically greater in redesigned as opposed to traditional organizations, patients also tend to be discharged sooner from these settings. In any given case, the nurse may be involved prior to the patient's admission and after discharge, requiring the nurse to be knowledgeable about the variety of resources that compose the continuum of care. The nurse also must prepare patients to assume greater responsibility for themselves.

Today's health care environment is fraught with legal and ethical problems associated with providing health care to an aging population in an environment characterized by complex technological advances. These problems are exacerbated by increased patient acuity, cost-conscious decision making, and reliance on unlicensed caregivers. Nurses in redesigned organizations must be attentive to the legal and ethical implications of their decisions and actions. They also must be committed to professional nursing standards and be determined advocates of high-quality care.

The nurse must be flexible and able to adapt to an ever-changing environment. Effective accommodation to change requires comfort with technology and informatics, sensitivity to context, and an innovative approach. The nurse who practices effectively in redesigned roles will help redefine the role of the nurse over time.

In short, redesign requires a nurse skilled in delegation, supervision, and team building. Communication and teaching skills are essential, as is proficiency in working with multiple specialties, service providers, and third-party payers. Critical thinking alone is not enough; the nurse also must become a creative problem-solver able to access and analyze information with ease. Driven by the bottom line, restructured organizations place greater emphasis than ever on patient outcomes and consumer satisfaction. At best, such organizations establish a delicate balance between quality of care and fiscal restraint. When they are unable to do so, not only are safety and professional standards threatened, but the nurse may be ethically defenseless and legally vulnerable.

Redesigning Viewpoints toward Work

Two nurses, newly employed at a redesigned hospital, were overheard discussing their jobs one day at lunch. They spoke in the hushed tones of professionals, but if you listened very carefully, you could hear their great frustration and pining for the "good old days", when they felt secure in their roles. The sense of security attached to the good old days was probably due as much to the fact that the nurses understood the expectations associated with their positions and had learned to meet those expectations. They hoped that the same would soon be true of their new positions.

Hilda acknowledged that when she took her new job, shortly after moving from a traditional hospital in the Midwest, the personnel director had told her that she would be working as part of a team. It would be different, she was told, from the team nursing with which she was familiar.

Pat seemed surprised that they were still practicing team nursing anywhere: "Gee, I thought this state was behind the times! I haven't practiced team nursing in years. We did primary nursing at the hospital I came from across town."

Pat went on to describe primary nursing to Hilda. "You know, each nurse has full responsibility for a certain number of patients. You do it all! Now that makes sense—at least you have some control over what's happening to your patients," Pat enthused. "Not like now, with all these unlicensed people running around, supposedly helping you," she lamented.

Pat continued to whine about the increased patient load. She repeatedly expressed distaste for the use of multiskilled, cross-trained, unlicensed personnel. "It's impossible to know what they're doing to your patients. Cross-trained? I don't think so. They call these folks multiskilled, and they use that as an excuse to increase my patient load! Don't they know that it only makes my work harder?"

Pat was becoming more and more upset thinking about the changes inherent in the new position, obviously yearning for the time when nurses worked basically alone and could "take pride" in the care they gave. "I sure long for the days when my patients knew I was their nurse. You could really bond with your patients then. They were mine and I was theirs. Now, many of my patients don't even know I'm the nurse. They think all these unlicensed people are nurses, too!"

"Yeah," said Hilda, "and what's this stuff about outcomes? I spent years learning the nursing process. Now they want me to forget all about it and worry about outcomes!"

"To be honest," interjected Pat, "I don't think they want us to forget the nursing process. They just want us to focus on the outcomes and go from there—manage backwards, as someone said."

But Hilda wasn't ready to concede. Much of the problem, as she saw it, was that "you can't manage backwards as easily as they think. And what does it mean, anyway, to manage backwards?"

Apparently growing tired of the grousing and nearing the end of the lunch break, Pat redirected the conversation toward some of the advantages to "this new way of doing things". "At least people at the hospital seem more concerned about the patients. And I love it that they have decentralized the place. We used to have to go through all kinds of hoops to get help from other departments."

"You've got that right," affirmed Hilda. Showing obvious appreciation for bedside care, she went on to admit that "it's a lot easier to have services brought to the patient than to take the patient to the services."

But Hilda couldn't let it end on a positive note. As she and Pat were heading for the elevator, Hilda was heard to utter: "If only they didn't make you watch every penny. Sometimes I feel more like an accountant or a banker than a nurse!"

THE RESTRUCTURING CONTROVERSY

As illustrated by Pat and Hilda's story, hospitals are in various stages of development in terms of the RN's role. To a large extent, primary nursing replaced team nursing in the 1970s and 1980s. Primary nursing typically entails greater accountability and continuity of care, but is a luxury when there is a significant shortage of RNs (as is often true in rural areas, for example). In some localities, therefore, hospitals still practice team nursing.

The current redesign movement has met with considerable resistance in some areas; in others, it seems to be taking hold with relative ease. Redesign, in some form, will eventually be required of virtually all health care organizations because the conditions that fostered the redesign movement—such as rising costs and an aging population—are fairly widespread and are expected to persist.

Much of the controversy regarding redesigned roles centers on concerns about quality, safety, and professional nursing. Though opponents of redesign may deny it, some of the dialogue about professionalism is really about maintaining nursing's domain. Nonetheless, the arguments raised by dissidents cannot be dismissed as merely turf protection in disguise. The concerns are legitimate and deserve careful attention. Redesign done poorly can have major negative consequences.

Nurses need to be alert to the manner whereby their organizations approach redesign. Approaches that enhance quality, safety, and the professional RN role involve RNs in the preplanning and planning of new caregiver roles and care-delivery systems. Effective systems are supported by intensive initial training and ongoing change management—not only for assistive personnel, but for all team members.

At its best, redesign permits nurses to be nurses. It can result in increased time for direct patient care, more effective and efficient responses to patients' needs, and improved case management, assessment, and client teaching. Accrual of these benefits, however, typically requires increased use of assistive personnel, support staff, and computers; multiskilling; teamwork; and decentralizing of traditional departmental functions. It requires nurses skilled in delegating, supervising, and team building—nurses who appropriately empower team members.

Redesigned organizations rely heavily on the RN's expertise in critical thinking, problem-solving, and professional decision making. Perhaps ironically, however, restructuring generally entails a reduction in nursing staff. Because they favor the employment of more nursing assistants and other ancillary personnel as substitutes for nurses, reconfigured staffing patterns pose a threat to safety and quality.

Nurses in restructured organizations are expected to find an appropriate balance between safety, quality, and professional standards on the one hand and increased patient acuity, greater reliance on unlicensed support personnel, and cost containment on the other. Nurses who oppose redesign are not convinced that such a balance exists, and they are unsure whether the implied trade-offs are acceptable. Concerns about restructuring's threat to safety and quality, in fact, have led the American Nurses Association to undertake efforts to increase awareness among the public, as well as among nurses, regarding the implications of cost containment and reductions in nurse staffing (Marulto, 1995).

Many nurses and nursing organizations have joined the American Nurses Association in questioning the redesign movement. Change as profound as that which accompanies redesign is difficult. It challenges vested interests and creates insecurity and chaos. But unless it can be clearly demonstrated that safety is significantly compromised, redesign will be the norm for the future. Indeed, redesign may become a continual process—one of the few constants in an ever-changing environment.

RESOURCES FOR FURTHER INFORMATION

For current information about redesign and the nurse's role, contact the American Nurses Association and its state affiliates. The official publication of the American Nurses Association, *The American Nurse*, comprises articles addressing various issues of interest to nursing.

The National League for Nursing is vigilant in its examination and promotion of nursing. It is a major force in defining roles and ensuring the preparation of qualified professionals. State constituent leagues operate with varying degrees of sophistication, often focusing on state and regional interests.

The State Board of Nursing in each state is an essential resource for every nurse. At the very least, nurses should contact their boards anytime questions arise relating to scope of practice, delegation, and educational requirements. The board for any given state should also be able to provide information on legal responsibilities associated with nursing practice. There also is a National Council of State Boards of Nursing, which can provide summary information about nursing in all states.

It is important that nurses, especially those working in redesigned settings, comply with minimum standards of practice as set forth by appropriate professional organizations (such as the American Organization of Nurse Executives) and accrediting bodies (such as the Joint Commission on Accreditation of Healthcare Organizations). It is only by virtue of the members upholding the standards of a profession that any profession exists.

Restructuring is fairly new, and jobs in restructured organizations are, thus, often poorly defined. Titles may not convey uniform understanding of roles or the requisite education and training needed to perform them successfully. Written job descriptions that clearly describe the roles and responsibilities of RNs and other members of the caregiving team are, therefore, particularly important. Insist that the employer provide them. They can be surprisingly useful when questions arise or doubts occur; and they may provide legal protection.

SUMMARY

Professional nursing routinely changes along with changes in the environments in which nursing is practiced. Small, incremental changes often occur virtually unnoticed. Not so, however, with the changes arising as a result of redesign. Changes associated with redesign appear monumental, and so, too, do the associated changes in the role of the nurse. For better or worse, these changes involve a focus on patient outcomes; case management via multidisciplinary teams; cross-training; greater reliance on unlicensed, assistive personnel; increased collaboration within and across institutional boundaries; and cost-conscious decision making.

In a health care environment that is increasingly market driven, nurses must be resource managers as well as case managers. They must be innovative in terms of resource utilization. They may need to consider new, revenue-generating strategies and investigate new models of practice. It is no longer sufficient for nurses to deliver quality care. They must deliver quality care in an environment that is significantly constrained by economic, legal, and ethical realities.

At this juncture in time, nurses are the most respected members of the health care workforce. Nurses are the caregivers. They are the teachers, the ones who will answer even the dumbest of questions, the ones patients trust and naturally turn to for help. In order to maintain that esteemed position, nurses may have to relinquish some control. Paradoxically, it may be only through relinquishing control that nurses are able to maintain their status and stature.

Nurses are arguably better equipped than any other member of the health care team to successfully meet the greatest challenge of health care delivery in the coming years: ensuring optimal patient outcomes while containing costs.

REFERENCES

American Health Care Consultants. (1993). Cross-train cautiously to assure legal, regulatory problems do not derail PFC plans. *Patient-Focused Care, 1*(1), 1–7.

Brider, P. (1992, September). The move to patient-focused care. *American Journal of Nursing,* 26–33.

Giuliano K. K., & Poirier, C. E. (1991). Nursing case management: Critical pathways to desirable outcomes. *Nursing Management, 22*(3), 52–55.

Hendrickson, G., Doddato, T. M., & Kovner, C. T. (1990). How do nurses use their time? *Journal of Nursing Administration, 20*(3), 31–37.

Lyons, R. F. (1992). Cross-training: A richer staff for leaner budgets. *Nursing Management, 23*(1), 43–44.

Marulto, G. (1995, June). Letter to Marjorie Beyers, Executive Director of the American Organization of Nurse Executives in *The American Nurse, 27.*

Weinstein, S. M., & Sobota, E. R. (1989). *Restructuring the work load: Methods and models to address the nursing shortage.* Chicago: American Hospital Association.

Chapter Seven

Nurse Case Management

Joan Stempel, Jean Doerge, Karen Van Wie,
Vicky Mahn, and Judith Combs

INTRODUCTION

Managed care is greatly impacting delivery of health care services. The concepts of managed care and case management are growing in significance for all practicing nurses. This chapter describes the part played by managed care in creating case management roles for nurses and the roles that nurses employed as nurse case managers are performing in today's health care arena. Also, individuals currently working as nurse case managers describe the unique aspects of their work with targeted populations.

MANAGED CARE

In recent years, the number of nurses calling themselves "case managers" has rapidly increased. These nurses perform a wide variety of functions, from authorizing services to providing hands-on care. To understand the reasons for the sudden emergence of nurse case management as a field, it is essential to understand managed care and its impact on the health care system.

The health care industry is facing a new set of challenges in the decade ahead. These challenges include: (1) finding ways to provide quality care at reduced costs, (2) designing systems to meet the needs of high-risk populations such as premature neonates or chronically ill elders, and (3) shifting the setting for providing medical services from the acute care hospital to community settings whenever possible.

The idea of cost containment is not a new one to the health care system. In the 1980s, the Health Care Finance Administration (HCFA), that department of the federal government responsible for administering Medicare, began to limit reimbursement amounts going to hospitals for services provided to Medicare recipients. Under this payment system, the amount of money hospitals receive is predetermined according to diagnostic related grouping (DRG). With some exceptions, the reimbursement received by a hospital for the care provided to a patient with a myocardial infarct, for example, is the same amount whether that patient's hospital stay is five days or ten days. Under this system, hospitals often are forced to absorb the cost of prolonged stays and, thus, must assume more financial risk.

The DRG system reflects the basic premise of managed care insurers: costs can be controlled by putting a ceiling, or cap, on reimbursement for services. Managed care attempts to control how much a patient costs the system, (Cipe, 1995). As hospitals and medical providers experience shrinking reimbursement for their services, managed care systems have emerged as a means of controlling costs.

A managed care system is a system of health care services. The focus of such a system is to reduce and/or control costs by controlling the utilization of services and providing services in a cost-effective way (Cipe, 1995). These systems provide mechanisms that attempt to match medical and nursing services to client need in a cost-effective manner. Cost and quality outcomes of care are then evaluated as monitors of managed care performance.

Managed care systems may be payers and providers of care, as is often the case with health maintenance organizations (HMOs), or may link hospital and physician providers under a business structure called a physician hospital organization (PHO). In a managed care system, the payer shares financial risk with the hospital provider. PHOs or HMOs also may share risk with the hospital. Sometimes, all three structures together share this risk, as systems become integrated into care-delivery networks encompassing payer, provider and professional services.

Ideally, managed care provides clients easy access to care at the lowest possible cost while still providing quality. In order to achieve these aims, many managed care firms are developing continuums of care. Many care modalities traditionally provided in the acute care setting—such as IV therapy, rehabilitation, and total parental nutrition—are now being provided in less costly settings such as skilled nursing facilities or patients' homes.

THE OPPORTUNITIES FOR NURSES

Across the country, nurses are assuming the role of nurse case managers, managing the risk represented by groups such as high-risk perinatal patients, costly open-heart-surgery patients, or chronically ill elders, all of whom have the potential to consume large amounts of health care resources and dollars. At this time, a substantial portion of the country has not experienced significant managed care penetration; however, if projections are correct, up to 55% of Americans will be enrolled in managed care programs by the year 2000 (Cipe, 1995). With such rapid expansion of managed care, nurses who are willing to assume a high level of accountability and implement cost-reduction strategies can position themselves to create new roles as nurse case managers (Michaels, 1992).

THE PROCESS

The most familiar application of case management in today's managed care environment is the utilization review/gatekeeper model. But the scope of nurse case management is much broader than one of gatekeeping. In addition to being employed by insurers in a utilization management/discharge planning role, nurse case managers may work as clinical experts in the hospital setting, coordinating programs relating to specific client populations. They also may function independently in the community setting. If you are considering employment as a nurse case manager, it is important to first understand the general process of case management, and then learn how this process is uniquely applied in different settings.

Managed care provides a system, or a structural umbrella, for addressing cost, quality, and utilization issues. Case management is the actual *process* of coordinating care and services (Cohen & Cuesta, 1993). In all settings, case management shares common elements based in the *nursing process* of assessment, planning, coordination, implementation, and evaluation of nursing care. Functioning autonomously, assuming responsibility for the coordination of care, and being accountable for integrating costs and outcomes of care are features of the nurse case management process in all settings (Cohen & Cuesta, 1993).

NURSE CASE MANAGEMENT MODELS

Models of case management come not only from nursing theory, but also from public health nursing, social work, rehabilitation, and behavioral health. From these varied disciplines, differing models of case management have

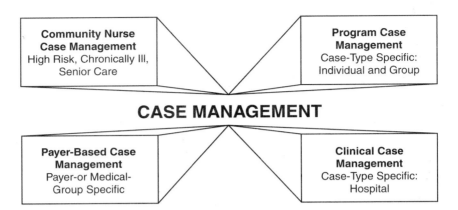

Figure 7-1

developed. Each model primarily reflects the setting where the case manage-ment services are provided and the type of services delivered. Figure 7-1 illus-trates these four types of case management as they relate to nursing: clinical case management, payer-based case management, program case management, and community case management.

Following are descriptions of these case management models along with case studies designed to illustrate the unique applications of each model. It is important to realize that these models are continually evolving and changing and that in practice, different models of case management may overlap.

Clinical Model

In the acute care setting, several models of case management have evolved. In the staff nurse model as manifested in the New England Medical Center model, the primary care nurse coordinates a client's care through an episode of illness within the acute care setting. This model has successfully demon-strated shorter lengths of stay and improved clinical outcomes for certain case types such as pediatrics (Zander, 1991).

In contrast to the staff nurse model, clinical case management is a profes-sional nursing role in which a clinical nurse specialist is assigned to a popula-tion of high-risk patients to optimize clinical and cost outcomes (Mahn, 1993). These outcomes are achieved by partnering with patients and families and facilitating interdisciplinary process improvements along the continuum of care (Mahn, 1994). The role is self-guided and self-directed. In addition to demonstrated clinical expertise, this role requires critical thinking, analytical skills, and a knowledge of continuous quality improvement methods.

The Carondelet St. Joseph's Hospital's Clinical Case Management program incorporates a type of role developing across the country for advanced prac-tice nurses. Vicky Mahn, a master's-prepared nurse whose area of clinical expertise is the cardiovascular population, was chosen to further define a

"Within-the-Walls" case management model for Carondelet. The program endeavored to make a cost and quality impact on high-risk groups who receive care in the inpatient setting. The Vice President for Patient Care required that quantifiable cost/quality outcomes be demonstrated in the first year in order for the program to continue.

After reviewing the literature as well as established models of clinical case management, the target population was determined. This population met the criteria of high-cost, medically complex, and frequently admitted conditions that demand heavy use of resources. In addition, the need for improved teamwork and coordination of care required interdisciplinary collaboration and facilitation. Information from the financial department was analyzed to identify both high-cost client groups and baseline cost measurements in order to determine the impact of the case management role. Patients undergoing DRG 107, elective coronary artery bypass grafting, were selected as the initial target population for the pilot program.

The nurse case manager established outcome measures of the program, including clinical indicators such as adverse medical outcomes, blood utilization, and unplanned readmissions. Cost indicators included length of stay, number of critical care days, and lab, respiratory care, and pharmacy costs. Finally, customer satisfaction was measured for patients, staff, and cardio thoracic surgeons. Data was collected from the hospital quality information system, the cost account system, chart audits, and interviews with patients, staff, and physicians.

The clinical nurse case manager analyzed the process of care delivery for coronary artery bypass graft patients, from preadmission to postdischarge. She identified problems and opportunities for improvement prior to implementation of the project, which involved actually going through the entire process of care with several coronary bypass patients and observing redundancies in systems and practices that were wasteful or unnecessary.

Areas for intervention by the clinical nurse case manager were planned. According to the plan, this nurse would develop comprehensive physical, psychological, and social assessments, as well as conduct focus interviews with cardiothoracic surgeons. The goal was to improve communication and coordination of care preoperatively and postdischarge by developing a health management plan for patient and family education and by smoothing the process of transition into community care. Additional interventions included follow-up phone calls and home visits for high-risk clients who were not authorized to receive home health services.

After the six-month pilot, the project was evaluated in a comprehensive manner, and the findings were presented to the administration and physicians. The result was a program that permanently changed the way care is delivered to coronary artery bypass patients at Carondelet St. Joseph's Hospital. And, interestingly, cost savings were substantially greater than the first-year start-up costs for the clinical case management position (Mahn, 1993).

Special Features. The Carondelet example illustrates the different facets of the clinical nurse case manager role. The clinical case manager is accountable to the hospital to reduce the financial risk of identified target populations by applying advanced practice nursing knowledge and expertise. Advanced practice skills, education, and experience with patients in an area of specialty are important, but equally essential is an understanding of the research principles used to assess, plan, implement, and evaluate program intervention. In addition, organizational expertise is needed in order to successfully obtain data from multiple sources, facilitate implementation of changes in the process of care, and communicate program results.

A nurse filling the clinical case management role must be creative, flexible, and credible as a clinical expert. A master's degree often is required for success in this role. One trend emerging across the country is for clinical nurse specialists to assume clinical case management of high-risk groups in hospital settings.

 ## *One Clinical Case Manager*

Mr. Bowen was scheduled to have a coronary artery bypass graft procedure. His surgeon's office manager notified the clinical case manager, advising her of the scheduled date of surgery and of Mr. Bowen's birth date, insurance carrier, and phone number. The clinical case manager then phoned Mr. Bowen to schedule a preadmission visit. She explained to Mr. Bowen that the purpose of the visit was to prepare him and his family for the open heart surgery, review his medication regimen, complete any necessary lab or diagnostic studies, perform a physical exam, and complete the consent forms for the upcoming surgery.

Two days prior to the scheduled admission, the clinical case manager met with Mr. Bowen in the preadmission office. Prior to this meeting, she had reviewed his medical records to familiarize herself with Mr. Bowen's past medical history and the findings from his cardiac catheterization. She interviewed Mr. Bowen regarding his past medical history, medication regimen, and history of activity tolerance. During this part of the interview, Mr. Bowen divulged that he had a severed phrenic nerve, which prevented him from taking deep breaths. This information was not previously disclosed, either in the medical history or during the physical.

The clinical nurse case manager performed baseline incentive spirometry volume assessment and noted that Mr. Bowen's maximum inspiratory volume was insufficient for his height and weight. She recorded this information on the open heart preop assessment worksheet and faxed the worksheet to the surgeon and the intensive care staff to alert them to potential alterations in postoperative pulmonary function. Following standard preoperative protocols, the clinical case manager ordered a type-and-crossmatch and a urinalysis. Because the findings for the remaining preop lab tests were all within normal range when measured as part of the lab work for Mr. Bowen's cardiac catheterization the week before, she did not order these tests to be duplicated.

During the preadmission visit, Mr. Bowen expressed concerns regarding who would take care of his invalid wife while he was in the hospital. Without twenty-four-hour care for his wife, Mr. Bowen was unwilling to undergo the bypass procedure. The clinical case manager first reviewed options of family support, and then notified Social Services of Mrs. Bowen's needs. She collaborated with the patient and Social Services to arrange for home assistance to provide forty hours of inhome care for Mr. Bowen's wife. Mr. Bowen's daughters agreed to stay with their mother during the evening and night hours.

The clinical case manager then followed Mr. Bowen throughout his hospital stay, making daily rounds in the intensive care unit and, later, in the step-down telemetry unit. During his third postop day, Mr. Bowen's temperature rose to 100.8° F., and he started complaining of severe pain in his left chest wall. He also informed the staff RN that the oral analgesia was not providing sufficient pain relief. The clinical nurse case manager and the staff RN assessed Mr. Bowen's status and determined that his inspiratory volume was only one-half his baseline volume. Although the morning x-ray report had not yet been interpreted, the cardiopulmonary assessment revealed that Mr. Bowen's respiratory excursion on inspiration was markedly limited on his left side.

The clinical case manager and staff RN together reinstituted intermittent positive pressure breathing (IPPB) treatments with normal saline for Mr. Bowen, according to the standing protocol. The nurses implemented a plan to medicate Mr. Bowen with a stronger dose of analgesia thirty minutes prior to ambulation. They decided to increase his ambulation frequency to five times daily, but to decrease the durations. They entered a brief note as part of the multidisciplinary progress notes for the surgeon's review. The chest x-ray later confirmed substantial atelectasis in the left lower lung.

Mr. Bowen was discharged on Sunday morning following a six-day stay. Mr. Bowen's insurance provider did not authorize home health care because he had not met the criteria for skilled nursing intervention. Because Mr. Bowen was anxious to return home to his wife, he was dressed and packed before the staff RN had the opportunity to complete a thorough physical assessment.

On Monday, the clinical case manager called Mr. Bowen to inquire about his home recuperation status. Mr. Bowen reported that he was constipated and that he had lost his instructions for a low-fat cardiac diet. He also reported that he had "two threads with metal tips" sticking out of his chest wall, and he asked when these would be removed. The clinical case manager scheduled a home visit to Mr. Bowen's for later that day.

Upon arrival, she verified that Mr. Bowen had been inadvertently discharged with his pacemaker wires and chest tube sutures still in place. In addition, Mr. Bowen's blood pressure was 160/90 after five minutes of ambulation. She also noted that his ankles were slightly swollen.

She next reviewed Mr. Bowen's medication and noted that he had not resumed taking the diuretic he had been taking to control his blood pressure for the past four years. From Mr. Bowen's home, the clinical case manager notified the surgeon of her findings. On the surgeon's orders, the clinical case manager removed the wires and sutures without incident. She told Mr. Bowen to resume his diuretic as directed and to self-administer an oral laxative to relieve his constipation. Finally, she again instructed him about his cardiac diet. Together, the clinical case manager and Mr. Bowen made a meal plan for the week, comprising foods that Mr. Bowen had on hand in his home.

Before leaving Mr. Bowen's home, the case manager spotted a basket full of medications on the kitchen counter. The medications were for Mrs. Bowen, and consisted of a variety of outdated antidepressants, pain medications, and antihypertensives, which she no longer required. Some of the medications were three years old. Together, Mr. Bowen and the clinical case manager reviewed the medications, and decided to discard them in order to prevent possible confusion between Mrs. Bowen's medications and those of Mr. Bowen. Because both Mr. and Mrs. Bowen suffered severe vision impairment and reported frequent problems in reading their medication labels, the case manager suggested they keep a magnifying glass in the basket of medications. The nurse also arranged for Mr. Bowen to receive a seven-day plastic medication box.

When visiting Mr. Bowen the next day, the case manager helped him arrange his medications appropriately. During this visit, Mr. Bowen reported relief from his constipation. He also reported having showered without difficulty, and his incentive spirometry volume had returned to baseline. Furthermore, his blood pressure was 140/78. The total time spent on the case manager's two visits to Mr. Bowen's home was one hour and ten minutes. These visits not only prevented potential injury related to electric shock from the pacemaker wires, but also eliminated the need for an additional office visit to the surgeon. Mr. Bowen's continued partnership with the clinical nurse case manager also enhanced his ability to follow his diet and medication regimens.

Following the two home visits, the clinical nurse case manager used the hospital transcription service to summarize her home-visit interventions. She forwarded copies of her summary to Mr. Bowen's surgeon, cardiologist, and primary care physician. She referred Mr. Bowen to a phase II cardiac rehab program in order to maximize his reconditioning and better prepare him for the physical demands of caring for his wife. Although continued follow-up by the clinical case manager was unnecessary for Mr. Bowen, a referral for community case management follow-up was made for Mrs. Bowen because of her chronic and debilitating condition. Mr. and Mrs. Bowen's continued relationship with a nurse partner should maximize their self-care skills and, hopefully, reduce the need for further hospitalization in the future. Because both Mr. and Mrs. Bowen belong to a capitated health care plan, reducing future hospitalizations is an important economic outcome.

Payer-Based Model

Payer-based case managers can be found working in insurance settings, clinical settings, and utilization management. A case manager working for a managed care organization is usually employed by an HMO, or other insurer, or by a specific medical group. The payer-based case manager's emphasis is on discharge planning, coordinating care, and ensuring that the level of care provided is appropriate for each patient. This type of case manager often serves as a gatekeeper, ensuring that resources are used in a cost-effective manner through effective discharge planning and utilization management. Payer-based case managers make decisions regarding the appropriateness of care and services based on a set of predetermined criteria or guidelines. These case managers are primarily accountable to the managed care system. They ensure that utilization of health care services is appropriate during each hospital episode and that an appropriate discharge plan is in place for each client.

One Payer-Based Case Manager

Mary, an associate degree nurse with several years of acute care experience, works for a large, managed care firm that is based in California and has branches in other western states. On an assigned floor in a Tucson, Arizona, hospital, Mary begins each day by reviewing the charts of all patients covered by her managed care organization. As part of her review, she compares each chart to utilization criteria to be sure that the patient meets the level of care required to remain in the hospital. When physicians order specialized and costly tests or invasive procedures that require the approval of the insurer, Mary is the person whom they must contact to obtain necessary authorization. Occasionally, Mary must enforce utilization guidelines and issue denial-of-care letters to patients and physicians.

If a patient who is otherwise ready for discharge is being retained in the hospital for nonmedical reasons, Mary facilitates the discharge by contacting the social worker or physician. Mary interviews patients to be certain they understand their plans of care. She collaborates with patients and their families to develop discharge plans. For noncomplex cases, Mary does the discharge planning herself, calling community agencies, arranging transfers to skilled nursing facilities, and making referrals to home health, hospice, or community nurse case management. For complex cases, Mary refers discharge planning to the social worker.

As part of the discharge planning team, Mary meets with hospital nurses, social workers, and home health liaisons during discharge planning rounds to review the status and discharge plans of patients. Any decision to transfer a patient to another level of care (e.g., from the hospital to a transitional care unit or home health care) requires that Mary obtain authorization. Thus, following rounds, Mary communicates the information she has gathered to the central office via computer linkages and spends the remainder of her time completing reports. For certain patients who had previously been identified as "at risk" for problems at home, Mary places follow-up calls to determine whether the transitions have gone smoothly.

Special Considerations. The preceding example makes clear that a payer-based case manager must be well organized and able to function independently. In addition, the role requires the ability to set priorities with regard to decisions and to communicate those decisions effectively to hospital staff, physicians, and patients and their families. Up-to-date knowledge regarding both acute nursing care and community resources is essential. Comfort with using technology—and, particularly, computer information systems—is also vital. This case management role is less likely than some to require a BSN or a master's degree. The nurse employed in this case management role must be able to derive satisfaction from a job that offers minimal direct contact with patients.

Program Model

Program case management, like clinical case management, involves working within an area of clinical specialty to establish and coordinate services, promote health, and reduce risks within a targeted population. The emphasis in program case management, however, is on the aggregate population rather than the individual patient. The extent of the involvement of the program case manager with the client may be limited by the payer or by the duration of health status changes (e.g., the term of a pregnancy or of recovery from a work-related injury). Like the clinical case manager, the program case manager must demonstrate outcomes of the program, frequently to external regulatory agencies.

On a daily basis, the program case manager may perform a variety of functions including assessing patients, planning patient care, planning programs, analyzing data, working with groups, writing grants, and evaluating outcomes of care. More than any other type of case manager, the program case manager is likely to be influenced by legislative changes. For example, recent legislation mandated that high-risk pediatric patients receive regular nursing follow-up. Health care arenas where the program case management model is often found include occupational health, diabetes care, and perinatal case management of high-risk mothers and infants.

Pediatric and Perinatal Populations. Some of the most rapidly expanding arenas for nurse case management are the pediatric and perinatal realms. Programs similar to the following may exist in your state, providing opportunities for the nurse interested in program case management.

Pediatric Early Intervention Program

Changes in federal law encouraged states to develop comprehensive, multidisciplinary early intervention systems to identify and service infants and toddlers who either are at risk for developmental delays or have been diagnosed as having significant developmental delays (Part H of Pubic Law 99-547). The title *case manager* was renamed *service coordinator* by this law. The philosophy and the role itself, however, remain the same. The functions of the service coordinator role are specified by law and include coordinating the performance of evaluations and assessment; facilitating the development of Individual Family Service Plans; assisting families in identifying providers; coordinating services and provision of medical care; and facilitating the development of a transition plan to preschool services, if appropriate (Carter, Lorber, & Carty, 1992).

The requirements for employment as a service coordinator vary and depend on available resources in the community. Nurse case managers generally are adequately prepared to be service coordinators. Additional training may be required, however, in order to be in compliance with federal mandates.

Newborn Intensive Care Program

Another example of program case management in the perinatal and pediatric arenas is the Newborn Intensive Care Program (NICP), which was founded in 1967 to better serve infants in the state of Arizona. This program was originally created to provide regionalized, tertiary care for high-risk pregnant women and acutely ill neonates following birth. A system of state transport was developed to bring these at-risk patients to tertiary centers where they could receive the medical and technological support needed to improve their health outcomes. The program is available to both rural and metropolitan families. A community health nurse functions as a program case manager to provide follow-up services for infants, including assessment, intervention, coordination of care for families, and collection of data for statewide evaluation of the program.

High-risk Prenatal Programs

Similar programs target pregnant women (Combs & Rusch, 1990). Some such programs use nurse case managers to provide outreach, identifying women who need prenatal care and managing them after they enter into a medical care system. Nurse case management services often continue after delivery to support the family's transition. Grant funding supports many such programs sponsored through state and/or county health departments. Existing and pending legislation impacting prenatal care can serve as a guide to locating such programs and projects.

Carondelet's Programs

The pediatric and perinatal nurse case management positions at Carondelet Health Services are contracted for one of the Arizona Health Care Cost Containment Service (AHCCCS) plans. AHCCCS is the State of Arizona's Medicaid program. Referrals for pediatric case management are made for infants and children who either have chronic health care needs or are recovering from acute episodes of illness and who require additional support in the home. Referrals for perinatal nurse case management are made for pregnant women with specific health conditions such as diabetes, hypertension, toxemia, substance abuse, preterm labor, or other medical concerns. The role of the nurse case manager is to provide nursing assessment to determine the level of health and functioning of the client and family; develop a plan with the family and medical providers that encourages independent functioning by identifying support needs; intervene through education and referrals to appropriate community and medical resources; advocate for clients and families; evaluate service provision and case management activities; and, finally, disengage nurse case management services when appropriate.

The AHCCCS contract is based on a medical model, resulting in the philosophy that when the client's medical issues have stabilized or appropriate other resources are in place, the case manager withdraws from involvement with the family. There is the provision for re-referral, however, in the event of an exacerbation or new illness. These nurse case managers serve families living in a variety of community settings including urban and rural environments.

A Study in Pediatric/Perinatal Program Case Management

The story of Michael illustrates differences in case managers' roles across agencies and the resulting need for collaboration when case managers of various agencies are involved with the family. Michael's story demonstrates how these services can be provided without overwhelming the family or duplicating services.

After a diagnosis of gastroschisis, Michael was delivered at thirty-eight weeks gestation by Cesarean section. He was admitted to the neonatal intensive care unit for small gestational age, respiratory distress, atrial septal defect, positive congenital cytomegalovirus studies, and gastroschisis repair. The repair was successful, and he was discharged home to the family at six weeks of age. The family lived in a rural area approximately an hour-and-one-half drive from the city.

Because Michael received care in the neonatal intensive care unit, he was eligible for and was enrolled in NICP. Michael and his family received periodic nursing visits from the NICP community health nurse while residing in the rural area. During that time, Michael had difficulties with chronic regurgitation and poor weight gain.

When he was approximately three months of age, Michael's family moved to the metropolitan area. The family consisted of both parents, who were unmarried and who lived together only intermittently, Michael, and his eighteen-month-old sibling. The maternal grandparents lived in the city and were supportive to the family. Shortly after the move, Michael began vomiting and losing weight. He was admitted to the hospital. Because of the family's limited income, the children received medical follow-up through one of the AHCCCS plans.

During Michael's hospitalization, a referral to nurse case management was made to monitor his nutritional intake and weight gain. Also during Michael's hospitalization, the hospital social worker expressed concern regarding his mother's parenting capabilities, including her method of setting limits with the eighteen-month-old. A Child Protective Services (CPS) referral was made to investigate the family and home situation. The nurse case manager made contact with the mother and Michael during hospitalization, at which time the mother was evasive and made limited eye contact with the case manager. The nurse case manager continued phone contact with the mother, the social worker, the CPS contact, and the various medical providers involved in Michael's care.

Three weeks after the nurse case management referral, Michael was transferred to a community medical care home because of continued feeding intolerance. Two weeks after Michael's transfer, a referral was made to the Arizona Early Intervention Program (the name of the program serving Part H of Public Law 99-457 in Arizona), and a service coordinator with a child development background was assigned. The nurse case manager began communications with the service coordinator to ensure continuity of care between the agencies. At the same time, the nurse case manager recognized that the family would need to be transferred to NICP community health nurses because the family had moved to another county. A new NICP nurse was thus assigned to and included in the communications about the case. The mother, service coordinator, and two nurses reached a mutual decision that the NICP nurse would begin home visits after the case manager was no longer involved with the family.

Approximately two weeks later, Michael was discharged home with nurse case management follow-up planned for three visits per week. These visits were supplemented by service coordinator visits. Weight gain continued to be inadequate, however, and Michael developed a respiratory infection requiring rehospitalization two weeks after discharge from the medical home. He was stabilized at the hospital and then transferred back to the same community medical care home.

The nurse case manager visited the home three to four times per week to check Michael's weight, provide information and support, and continue assessment and monitoring. The mother was compliant with medical appointments and began to contact the nurse case manager frequently with questions, and concerns, and to obtain support.

The nurse case manager alerted the mother to the existence of multiple other community resources such as parent aid, a toy lending library, and parenting groups. The family continued to remain a closed system with respect to involving other agencies, however. Thus, the service coordinator, nurse case manager, and mother communicated frequently to coordinate visits, scheduling them to supply the family with the most frequent contact possible. On occasion, combined visits occurred and were received well. The home environment was chaotic with multiple family members moving in and out of the home. Despite this chaos, however, Michael began to slowly and steadily gain weight, and his regurgitation decreased in frequency.

Relatives soon became involved in the educational and support process. When the nurse case manager assessed the mother and family members, she found them to have some learning limitations. She determined that discussion and modeling would therefore be the most effective teaching methods in this situation. The approach proved successful. On the next visit, the nurse case manager observed the mother and family members performing some of the discussed and modeled behaviors. The nurse case manager also identified multiple issues surrounding the older sibling, particularly with regard to setting limits. The service coordinator provided and taught the family appropriate developmental activities for both children.

As Michael's weight continued to increase and his regurgitation episodes continued to decrease, the nurse case manager began to visit less often, while the service coordinator continued her visiting regime. When the nurse case manager was notified by the AHCCCS plan that Michael was considered stabilized and that the nurse case manager visits were therefore to be discontinued, she held an informal discussion with the mother and the service coordinator. It was decided that the role of nurse was still needed and that this was the opportune time for the NICP nurse to begin visiting. This nurse made one home visit with the nurse case manager to meet the family. The nurse case manager spent time discussing the change in service providers with the mother, reassuring her that the service coordinator would continue to be actively involved with the family. The mother was encouraged to view the change as an important sign of success, indicating that Michael was doing well. Open communication between the agencies and the family led to a successful transition of service providers with minimal distress to the family.

Special Considerations. Coordination of services is especially important when working with the pediatric/perinatal population—not only to prevent duplication, but also to avoid overwhelming the family. Many providers may be involved with each family. The nurse case manager may work in conjunction with service providers such as physical, occupational, feeding, or speech therapists; nutritionists; mental health professionals; durable-medical-equipment providers; transportation providers; school personnel; substance abuse counselors; and traditional healers such as the Native American medicine woman or the Hispanic manor curandera (Attneave, 1982).

It is equally important for the nurse case manager working in this type of program to know that discharge of a family has gone well and that necessary resources continue to be provided for them. Working together as an interdisciplinary team provides mentorship and support for all providers. The nurse case manager works autonomously, yet collaborates closely with other team members, clients and families. Working interdependently and collaboratively with families and other service providers can be empowering for all.

Pediatric/perinatal program case management programs offer the nurse opportunities to operationalize a personal philosophy of family-centered care and replace a four-walled environment with an open-air atmosphere. Along with this leap to the "great outdoors" this nurse must be willing to accept a shift of control to the family—to be willing to accept the family without expecting to be the ultimate decision maker. For the nurse who is willing and able to make these concessions, an exciting career as a pediatric/perinatal program case manager may await.

Occupational Health. Similarities in the program case management model exist whether the target population is perinatal/pediatric or adults. Another growing application of case management is in the occupational health setting. In fact, the American Association of Occupational Health Nurses advocates for nurse case managers as the ideal professionals to coordinate clients' health care services from the onset of illness and injury to the safe return to work (American Association of Occupational Health Nurses, 1994).

Just as costs have risen in the acute care setting, costs of Workers' Compensation claims have steadily escalated. Thus, employers are seeking ways to control costs by minimizing injuries to workers; and employers increasingly are finding that nursing professionals can make valuable contributions to these efforts. The occupational health nurse case manager may be employed by industry, or rehabilitative-medicine practices, or may work as an independent case manager contracting services to multiple employers. The program nurse case manager employed in an occupational health setting is responsible for improving the overall health and safety of all employees in the work environment. Those employees at high risk for injury or illness in the workplace or those workers who have sustained illness or injury require a higher level of attention and intervention from the nurse case manager. The challenge for the occupational health case manager is to use the fewest possible allocated program dollars to achieve the maximum impact on health and safety in the workplace.

A Study in Occupational Health Program Case Management

Charlene worked as a patient-care transporter in a hospital setting. She had a forty-year history of diabetes, and had undergone cardiac bypass surgery two years ago. On several occasions, she had suffered episodes of disorientation and confusion on the job and was rushed to the occupational health office for evaluation by the occupational health nurse case manager. On one such occasion, Charlene required immediate transfer to the emergency department (ED) because she had become unresponsive. In addition to making an independent initial assessment and determining appropriate referral and follow-up, the occupational health nurse case manager also was responsible for ensuring that it was safe for Charlene to continue in her position as patient transporter.

The occupational health nurse case manager initiated communication with Charlene's supervisor. Together, they confirmed that there was a potentially serious threat to patients should Charlene experience another sudden hypoglycemic episode on the job. The ability to transport patients safely was considered an essential element of Charlene's job.

Regular visits to the occupational health office were scheduled for Charlene. During one such visit, Charlene reluctantly reported to the occupational nurse case manager that she had been experiencing problems with foot pain. Examination of the foot by the case manager revealed an ulceration that may have been contributing to fluctuations in blood sugar. The occupational health nurse case manager made an appointment for Charlene with the occupational health physician. Charlene was placed off duty until her blood sugars were under control and her own personal physician released her to return to work.

Despite these interventions, Charlene experienced another severe hypoglycemic episode while off duty. She had a one-car motor vehicle accident and sustained contusions and abrasions. The occupational health nurse case manager obtained Charlene's ED records with appropriate consent to release information. The reports revealed life-threatening hypoglycemia on admission to the ED.

Because Charlene was protected under the Americans with Disabilities Act for her permanent, physically disabling condition, it was the responsibility of the occupational health nurse case manager to collaborate with the occupational health physician, human resources department, and departmental director to determine whether Charlene could continue in her position without posing a direct threat to patients or to herself.

This interdisciplinary group developed a collaborative plan of care that enabled Charlene to take a short-term disability leave of absence from the workplace. The case manager arranged a referral to the diabetes program (also a program model of care delivery) for intensive diet and exercise education and careful monitoring of blood sugars. With

Charlene's permission, information about her progress in the program was shared with the occupational health nurse case manager and the physician. When Charlene had demonstrated stable blood sugars for two weeks, she was returned to the work environment.

Throughout this period, there was constant communication between Charlene, the case manager, the diabetes specialist, the supervisor, and the occupational health physician. The occupational health nurse case manager also kept the short-term-disability payer informed of Charlene's work status.

An individualized plan for snacks, glucose monitoring during the work day, and ongoing follow-up was communicated to Charlene, the departmental director, and the charge nurses. Charlene was able to return to work for approximately one month.

When another severe incident of hypoglycemia occurred, induced by the exercise demand of transporting, the case manager initiated a care conference with Charlene present. Charlene's options were identified and included taking a long-term disability leave, initiating application for Social Security Disability, or applying for transfer within the institution to a position that would not involve the exercise demand of patient transporting. The occupational health case manager facilitated an appointment with a human resources specialist to assist Charlene in developing a new résumé and completing a job application. Charlene applied for and secured a position in another department of the hospital.

Special Considerations. In Charlene's story, the program nurse case manager oversaw the worker and the workplace. Although the worker's condition was not caused in the workplace, the occupational nurse case manager intervened to prevent potential accidents and injury in the workplace. Managing Charlene's situation required a good amount of interdisciplinary communication and coordination, as well as constant sensitivity to the employee's dignity and confidentiality. The nurse case manager served as the primary contact for the employee. She responded to questions and interpreted the employee's condition for the short-term disability insurer and the departmental director. Through this ongoing relationship, Charlene felt supported during a difficult time of transition and loss of function due to a chronic illness.

During the process, Charlene reported that she had never really understood her diabetic condition in the forty years she had been coping with the disease. The program nurse case manager intervened to educate Charlene in becoming a more knowledgeable consumer of care. The education provided by program nurse case managers increases the self-care capabilities of individuals and reduces their requirements for hospitalization and other costly services. In

Charlene's story, the nurse case manager protected the workplace through early and continuous intervention. The worker did not sustain further injuries on the job, and federal legislative guidelines (the Americans with Disabilities Act) were enforced. While working with Charlene, the occupational health program case manager was also responsible for the health and safety of 1,100 other employees with varying needs.

The occupational health program case manager must continually set priorities with regard to workload in order to both provide health promotion teaching and manage occurrences of illness and injury. In this generalist role, the case manager must have broad assessment skills, in relation to both the individual patient and the workplace. The skill of assessing the workplace for hazards and threats to safety is equally as important as patient-based assessment skills. In addition, knowledge of the complex regulatory factors that impact the workplace is essential. As is the case with other program nurse case managers, the occupational health case manager must be comfortable with independent decision making and making appropriate referrals. He or she must also function effectively in interdisciplinary groups.

Community Model

In 1985, one model of community nurse case management was implemented at Carondelet St. Mary's in response to the DRG reimbursement system. At the time that DRGs were implemented, 65% of the individuals hospitalized at Carondelet St. Mary's in Tucson, Arizona, were on Medicare. Nurses became concerned about the resulting shortened hospital stays. These elderly clients were being discharged sicker and weaker, and readmission rates were climbing. Nurses felt that many of the readmissions might have been prevented had the elders been visited at home by a nurse shortly after hospital discharge.

Although home health nurses were available, these elders frequently did not qualify for their services. And whenever a chronically ill senior did qualify for home health visits, the visits were discontinued as soon as the patient's physical condition stabilized. Several months later, however, the patient would often be readmitted to the hospital, once again displaying signs of the same chronic illness. Nurses believed a different type of nursing service was needed to enable high-risk, chronically ill seniors to manage their health care concerns more effectively. They devised nurse case management as a strategy to assist in the care management of this population (Ethridge & Lamb, 1989). Under this community-based model, an individual identified as having deficient self-care abilities is targeted to receive nurse case management in the home for as long as the nurse and client feel these services are indicated.

The community nurse case manager's responsibilities when working with these clients are to monitor them; help them access the health care system when needed; teach them skills that allow them to manage their illnesses more effectively; connect them to community services for which they are eligible; obtain equipment needed to enhance their self-care abilities; familiarize them with their options in terms of both treatment and lifestyle; and advocate for them within the health care arena (Michaels, 1992).

Using a holistic approach, the community nurse case manager may work with a client for weeks, months, or years, depending on the self-care abilities of the client or caregivers, the amount of support available to the client, the severity of the client's disease, and whether the client is emotionally or cognitively challenged.

 One Patient's Community Nurse Case Manager

Mr. Perez is a typical elderly case-managed individual. He met his community nurse case manager when he was hospitalized with an exacerbation of his chronic obstructive airway disease (COPD). Mr. Perez had a history of taking his medications erratically, eating poorly, and continuing to smoke. He also waited until his exacerbations became severe before seeking medical attention. Although this had always been his pattern of self-care, the pattern became even worse after the death of his wife.

When the nurse case manager first visited Mr. Perez the day after his discharge, she found that he had not filled any of his prescriptions because he "had no way to pick them up." She also discovered that he was skipping meals because he was too short of breath to go grocery shopping. After arranging for short-term help in the home and for home-delivered meals, the community nurse case manager advocated with Mr. Perez's insurance company for a motorized scooter, which would allow him to both move around his apartment with ease and go to the shopping center two blocks from his home. He was delighted when the request was approved.

Over the next two years, Mr. Perez's nurse case manager visited regularly, assessing his respiratory status, teaching self-care strategies, and obtaining oxygen when his saturation levels indicated the need for it. Hospitalizations were averted on several occasions when upper respiratory infections were detected early and Mr. Perez was given prompt antibiotic therapy. Mr. Perez's hospital admissions went from three to four per year to one in two years. When he was hospitalized, he was visited by his nurse case manager, who took part in the discharge planning. Gradually, Mr. Perez's attitude toward his illness changed, as did his self-care abilities.

When interviewed two years after he first began receiving nurse case management, he described the change in these words: "I'm finally doing something right for myself. Before [nurse case manager], I stayed very much to myself. I never mixed or stuff like this. If she wasn't coming, I don't think I'd be doing all the things I've been doing. I don't think I'd be on my breathing machine. I wouldn't care if I took my medicine or not. I quit smoking. I'm drinking water now—because she told me it was good for me" (Lamb & Stempel, 1994, p. 10). He went on to say the reason he had made these changes was because the nurse case manager had cared about him so much that "I began to care about myself".

Special Considerations. Elders, particularly those with little or no family or other support persons, often feel poorly motivated to practice the self-care skills necessary to successfully manage their chronic illnesses. Frequently, they have recently suffered the loss of family members, and the resulting grief together with their marginal physical status makes them vulnerable to multiple illnesses and frequent hospital admissions. As in Mr. Perez's case, a nurse case manager not only helps with the medical management of the chronic condition, but also provides emotional support and helps motivate the client to more effectively manage the illness.

Since the Carondelet model of community nurse case management was initiated in 1985, other health care systems have implemented similar programs. The demand for community nurse case managers is growing, especially in areas of the country where managed care companies are moving into the health care marketplace.

ATTRIBUTES OF THE NURSE CASE MANAGER

In order to identify the attributes of the differing types of nurse case managers thus far discussed in this chapter, it is necessary to examine the focus of the work performed by these nurses. In short, all nurse case managers must internalize the following as attributes: honoring client choices, assessing and monitoring, promoting continuity of care, minimizing time constraints, linking care-team members, maintaining a holistic focus, and impacting quality and cost.

Honoring Client Choices

In honoring client choices, the nurse case manager must be adept at assisting individuals to clarify their values and their belief systems, while at the same time being sensitive to potential cultural differences among clients.

Thus, the nurse case manager must be flexible, nonjudgmental, and supportive. Learning to work as a health care *partner* rather than a health care *expert* is vital to achieving success in this role. This means supporting a client's choices even when they do not appear to be in the best medical interests of the client. Providing this kind of support is often one of the nurse case manager's greatest challenges (Newman, Lamb, & Michaels, 1992).

The nurse case manager may experience criticism from colleagues, conflicts with physicians and other providers, and challenges from risk managers. It is thus important for the nurse case manager to identify sources of support. Those case managers who are more experienced often can provide support and courage. When working with other professionals, consistently placing emphasis on seeing the situation from the patient's point of view may prove helpful. The most sound interdisciplinary plan of care will prove only as effective as the patient's ability and willingness to comply. As the patient's and family's advocate, the nurse case manager occasionally must remind colleagues that unless the plan considers the patient's preferences and abilities, it is doomed to failure. Encourage colleagues to brainstorm ways to satisfy the most important criteria for patients and providers.

Assessing and Monitoring

As illustrated by the case studies in this chapter, good assessment skills related to the targeted population are essential. The ability to recognize changes in health status and to direct clients to the appropriate levels of medical care is a key component of effectively managing cost outcomes for targeted individuals. The nurse case manager is responsible for recognizing a deterioration, improvement, or stabilization in an individual's health status. If a client experiences an exacerbation of COPD, for example, the nurse case manger must first assess the severity of the exacerbation and then decide whether the client should be sent to the ED, physician's office, or urgent care—or whether adjusting the client's medical regimen at home and under the physician's direction would be sufficient. When a client improves, as in the case of an injured worker, the nurse case manager must be able to recognize when the worker is ready to return to the workplace. Nurse case managers must therefore be self reliant and comfortable with making independent judgments (Lancero & Gerber, 1995).

Assessing and monitoring social situations are also important aspects of the nurse case manager's job. The nurse case manager often must assist clients in obtaining services such as mobile meals, household assistance, help with personal care, or entitlements such as food stamps or disability. A thorough knowledge of community services and the eligibility requirements for each is therefore vital.

Although some agencies and health providers employ nurse case managers having associate degrees in nursing, the trend is toward employing nurse case managers who have earned a minimum of a bachelor's degree. Today, many nurses are advocating that nurse case management become an advanced practice role for nurses. Several universities now offer master's degree programs with a major in nurse case management. In many health care settings, the role is rapidly becoming one of a clinical nurse specialist.

Coursework and related experience that strengthen your background in important components of the nurse case management role can facilitate your movement into case management. Many schools of nursing and other providers of continuing education offer case management courses. Broadening your knowledge of fiscal management, health care financing, physical assessment, outcome measurement and evaluation, and community services will aid in preparing you for case management. Investigate the specific qualification requirements and preferences of your potential employer.

A certification examination is available for case managers. You can obtain information about this examination by contacting one of the certification organizations listed beginning on page 157 of this chapter.

Maintaining a Holistic Focus

Unlike many other health care providers who focus mainly on the client's physical status, nurse case managers often employ a holistic approach to care (Newman, Lamb, & Michaels, 1992). Knowing that exacerbations of chronic illness may be triggered by unresolved personal issues—such as emotional, family, spiritual concerns—nurse case managers often explore these areas with clients who are ready to discuss them. The case manager can then implement interventions that address these underlying issues. In the case study of the injured worker, Charlene was assisted not only with her job functions but also with her diabetes self-management skills. The nurse case manager thus must have good listening and counseling skills in order to respond effectively to clients' needs in these areas.

Promoting Continuity of Care

As a client moves from the acute care hospital to a skilled nursing facility; a family adjusts to life at home with a neonate; or an injured worker returns to the workplace, the nurse case manger must be able to communicate pertinent information to the individuals involved in each setting (e.g., client, physicians, supervisors, family caregivers). It is also vitally important that nurse case managers, especially those working as managed care case managers, identify clients' needs at the time of discharge. Ensuring that appropriate care and services are in place is essential if clients are to be successfully discharged and returned to optimum levels of independence and wellness.

Minimizing Time Constraints through Awareness

Knowledge of how the differing payers and health care systems work is essential in helping clients move smoothly from one care setting to the next—and in obtaining additional services and equipment after clients have returned home. In particular, knowledge of who can authorize services and of the criteria used by each insurer to determine whether a client is qualified to receive the service or equipment being requested can greatly expedite such requests.

Linking Care-Team Members

The nurse case manager often is responsible for updating each health care team member on how well a client and caregiver are managing the client's care and coping with the client's illness. The abilities to communicate this information and to listen to the concerns of health care providers, clients, and families are thus important. When conflicts occur between health care providers and clients or families, the nurse case manager often plays the key role of negotiator.

Impacting Quality and Cost

Nurse case managers are frequently asked to demonstrate their cost-effectiveness. The abilities to identify and implement cost-effective interventions for targeted individuals and groups are thus key to the nurse case manager's job. As illustrated by the discussion of the clinical case manager's role, analyzing cost savings and communicating this information in language readily understood by providers, insurers, and administrators are essential.

FINDING OR MARKETING CASE MANAGEMENT WORK

Case management is an exciting career path, and may be an option you wish to pursue. Several variables are important to consider when pursuing work as a case manager.

First, assess your educational background and experiences to determine in which case management roles you would be most satisfied and successful. Case management is increasingly being viewed as an advanced practice role. There are, however, some options that can be pursued by any RN.

Second, assess your community for opportunities in case management. Investigate where nurse case managers are being employed and the credentials required for entry into practice. Explore not only opportunities in traditional health care settings, but also grant opportunities for developing new roles. Organizations such as the Multiple Sclerosis Society, Diabetes Association, and Councils on Aging have contributed to projects that promote case management role development.

Third, if you are currently working in a setting where case management might be a strategy to achieve more cost-effective and/or higher-quality outcomes with some group of high-risk patients, be assertive. Draft a proposal outlining how a nurse case manager could measurably impact cost, quality, and client health status. Include not only a description of the nurse case management role you wish to develop, but also a plan for how you would evaluate the program to determine whether you are meeting your goals. Utilize the growing body of literature and models to create a unique case management model tailored to the proposed target population.

Fourth, consider alternate settings. Physician office practices are now employing case managers to manage certain chronically ill populations. For example, a cardiology group within a managed care organization may find it cost-effective to employ a nurse case manager to oversee a population of elderly congestive-heart-failure patients in order to prevent costly readmissions.

And, finally, think creatively about ways to deliver care. Stanford University Hospital in Palo Alto, California, designed an innovative program wherein patients diagnosed with congestive heart failure are given scales to monitor their weights. Case managers, primarily through phone contacts, encourage patients to stay on therapy. Medications, weight changes, and symptoms are monitored through phone calls. Reductions in readmissions have been dramatic. And the Carondelet "Beyond-the-Walls" model of nurse case management was the creative idea of nurses who wanted to extend nursing care beyond the hospital setting and to the discharged patient at home.

RESOURCES FOR FURTHER INFORMATION

Following is a listing of several organizations for nurse case managers and other health professionals who work in related areas.

American Association for Continuity of Care
1730 N. Lynn Street, Suite 502
Arlington, VA 22209
Phone: 703-525-1191
Fax: 703-276-8190
Professionals served: nurses, social workers, discharge planners

Association of Medical Case Managers
6101 Ball Road, Suite 102
Cypress, CA 90630-3964
Phone: 714-220-0815
Fax: 714-220-0539
Professionals served: nurses

Case Management Society of America
    1101 17th Street NW, Suite 1200
    Washington, DC 20036
    Phone: 202-296-9200
    Fax: 202-296-0023
    Professionals served: nurses, counselors, social workers

Center for Case Management
    6 Pleasant Street
    South Natick, MA 01760
    Phone: 508-651-2600
    Fax: 508-655-0858
    Professionals served: nurses

Certified Case Manager
    1835 Rohlwing Road, Suite E
    Rolling Meadows, IL 60008
    Phone: 847-818-0292
    Fax: 847-394-2172
    Professionals served: nurses, social workers, allied health
    professionals, counselors

Certified Insurance Rehabilitation Specialists Commission
    1835 Rohlwing Road, Suite E
    Rolling Meadows, IL 60008
    Phone: 847-394-2106
    Fax: 847-394-2172
    Professionals served: rehabilitation counselors, nurses,
    insurance professionals, vocational counselors

Individual Case Management Association
    10809 Executive Center Drive, Suite 105
    Little Rock, AR 72211-6020
    Phone: 501-227-5553
    Fax: 501-227-8362
    Professionals served: case managers, nurses
    insurance professionals, discharge planners,
    rehabilitation counselors, managed care executives,
    social workers

National Association for Private Geriatric Care Managers
    1604 North Country Club
    Tucson, AZ 85716
    Phone: 520-881-8008
    Fax: 520-325-7925
    Professionals served: social workers, nurses

SUMMARY

The impact of managed care on the health care system has provided the impetus for a new role for nurses—that of nurse case manager. Although nurse case managers work in very diverse areas and health care systems across the country, four basic models of nurse case management are emerging. These models are clinical nurse case management, managed care nurse case management, program case management, and community case management. This chapter described these models and used case studies to illustrate how a nurse case manager would likely perform in each model.

The attributes and educational background needed to perform as a nurse case manager were also discussed, as were ideas for finding or developing and marketing case management work. Finally, a list of organizations from which further information on case management can be obtained was provided.

REFERENCES

American Association of Occupational Health Nurses. (1994). *OHN Position Statement*. Atlanta, GA: Author.

Attneave, C. (1982). American Indians and Alaska native families: Emigrants in their own homeland. In M. McGoldrick, J. K. Pearce, & J. Giordano (Eds.), *Ethnicity and family therapy*, 55–83. New York: Guilford Press.

Carter, B., Lorber, M., & Carty, L. (1992). *Early intervention advocacy network notebook*. Washington, DC: Mental Health Law Project.

Cohen, E., & Cuesta, T. (1993). *Nursing case management: From concept to evaluation*. St. Louis: Mosby-Year Book, Inc.

Combs, J., & Rusch, S. C. (1990). Creating a healing environment. *Health Progress, 71*(4), 38–41.

Ethridge, P., & Lamb G. S. (1989). Professional nursing case management improves quality, access and costs. *Nursing Management, 20*(3), 30–35.

Koerner, J. E., Bunkers L., Nelson, B., & Santema, K. (1989). Implementing differentiated practice: The Sioux Valley Hospital experience. *Journal of Nursing Administration, 19*(2), 13–20.

Lamb, G., & Stempel, J. (1994). Nurse case management from the client's view: Growing as insider-expert. *Nursing Outlook, 42*, 7–13.

Lancero, A. W., & Gerber R. M. (1995). *Work satisfaction among nurse case managers: A comparison of two practice models*. Manuscript submitted for publication.

Cipe, B. (Ed.). (1995). Managing care by managing risk. *Cost & Quality, 7*(1), 4–5.

Mahn, V. (1993). Clinical case management: A service line approach. *Nursing Management, 24*(9), 48–50.

Mahn, V., & Heller, C. (1994). Critical pathways at Carondelet St. Joseph's. In P. Spath, (Ed.), *Clinical paths: Tools for outcomes management*. Chicago, IL: American Hospital Publishing.

Michaels, C. (1992). Carondelet St. Mary's nursing enterprise. *Nursing Clinics of North America, 27*(1), 77–85.

Newborn Intensive Care Program. (1992). *Annual Report*. Phoenix, AZ: Arizona Department of Health Services.

Newman, M. A., Lamb, G. S., & Michaels, C. (1992). Nursing case management: The coming together of theory and practice. *Nursing & Health Care, 12*(8), 404–408.

Zander, K. (1988). Managed care within acute care settings: Design and implementation via nursing case management. *Health Care Supervisor*, 6(2), 24–43.

Chapter Eight

The Nurse Practitioner, Nurse Anesthetist, and Nurse Midwife

Joyce Crutchfield

INTRODUCTION

Specialization in nursing practice through advanced educational preparation has been available to the professional nurse for many years (Bullough, 1992). Among the early advanced practice nurses recognized were the nurse anesthetists whose duties and scope of practice were considered delegated tasks under the direction and supervision of a physician. Later, nurse midwifery was acknowledged as a specialty focusing on the care of the pregnant woman through delivery and the postpartum period. In 1965, nurse practitioner (NP) programs were started with the intention of preparing " physician extenders" who could provide primary care to improve the health of children (Murphy, 1990). Although the NP role was originated to substitute for or extend physician care, the role is now viewed differently. Today's nurse practitioner practice emphasizes the nursing components of holistic, preventive care tailored to individual client and family needs. Today's concept is one of adding advanced skills to the nursing approach rather than simply substituting for the physician role.

This chapter explores the advanced practice roles of the NP, the nurse anesthetist (CRNA), and the nurse midwife (CNM), as well as the contributions of these professions to health care. The chapter also identifies issues related to these advanced practice roles. You will find this chapter helpful as you explore potential career options in any of these three dimensions of advanced practice nursing.

NURSE PRACTITIONERS

Since the origin of the NP role in pediatric care, other vulnerable populations (e.g., adults, women, and elderly) and other health care services (acute or oncology care) have been targeted for nurse practitioner practice. The categorizing of specialty practice by either the client population served or the type of services provided can be somewhat confusing. Nonetheless, each nurse practitioner specialty affords unique services in both traditional and nontraditional settings.

Like so many other aspects of professional nursing practice, it is difficult to describe the exact functions and boundaries of the NP role. According to official statements circulated by the American Academy of Nurse Practitioners (AANP) in 1993, NPs are primary health care providers who order, conduct, and interpret appropriate diagnostic and laboratory tests, and who prescribe medications and treatments. They also provide health teaching and counseling to individuals, families, and community groups. The role of the NP can be defined by the specific types of NP practices recognized nationally, including family nurse practitioners, adult nurse practitioners, pediatric nurse practitioners, and gerontological nurse practitioners. The most recent nursing specialty group to be credentialed are acute care practitioners, who perform the advanced practice role in the hospital setting (Richmond & Kean, 1992; Stamoulis, 1992).

Although the roles of NPs can and have been defined by the client populations served, the type of care provided can also be used to define an NP specialty. Examples of type of care provided include cardiac, oncologic, and sports medicine. In addition to serving specific populations or providing specialty services, NPs can also practice as generalists in ambulatory centers where people receive primary care. Managed care has increased the focus on ambulatory and well-person care, creating opportunities for NPs to practice in outpatient settings including hospital-based clinics, freestanding ambulatory centers, and nurse-run clinics.

Approximately 32,000 NPs practice in the United States today. Dr. Jan Tower, of AANP, states that approximately 15% of these NPs are men (Personal Communication, March 18, 1996), a considerably higher percentage than the 4% of all practicing nurses who are men.

The Family Nurse Practitioner

Family nurse practitioners (FNPs) provide health services to clients who span the age spectrum. They care for pregnant women, newborn infants, children, adolescents, adults, and the elderly. Because FNPs are prepared as generalists, most FNP educational programs are somewhat longer than other NP specialty programs. Courses on family development, pediatrics, and care of the pregnant woman (excluding delivery) are part of these programs. FNPs often work in family practice clinics or rural areas, where more than one family member needs to be seen by the provider during the visit.

The Adult Nurse Practitioner

Adult nurse practitioners (ANPs) are prepared to deliver nursing and medical services to adolescents and to adults of all ages. The scope of practice does not however, include, maternal-child care. Depending on their educational preparation in health and illness care, ANPs may chose careers in ambulatory care, acute care, or specialty care (e.g., critical care, cardiac care, or oncologic care). The ANP works both autonomously and in collaboration with physicians, osteopaths, and physician's assistants. Among the settings in which the ANP works are outpatient clinics, public health departments, emergency rooms, health maintenance organizations (HMOs), school-based clinics, and employee health departments.

Pediatric and Gerontological Nurse Practitioners

Nurses certified as pediatric nurse practitioners (PNPs) or gerontological nurse practitioners (GNPs) are specialists in addressing the health needs of children or the older adult, respectively. Their services are targeted to these groups who have special needs because of vulnerability, pressing health concerns, or ongoing illnesses. The educational programs for these two specialties each include course work in theories on maturation (growth and development), aging, and common patterns of illness among the respective targeted populations.

Educational Preparation

Educational programs for NPs build on a bachelor's degree in nursing. Most programs are two years in length and are offered by universities or colleges that award a master's degree in nursing. Some colleges have also established postmaster certificate programs for returning, master-prepared clinicians wanting to broaden their knowledge and skills in another dimension of health care (Geolot, 1987). Although educational preparation for NPs is at the master's degree level, there are NPs currently practicing who received their preparation in nondegree-granting certificate programs. However, the few nonmaster's degree certificate programs remaining are being phased out.

You can obtain information about types of programs and specific programs by contacting your local university, your state's nurses' association, or your state's board of nurse examiners. Browsing through library copies of the *Nurse Practitioner* journal can provide you with additional information. Precise listings of programs across the nation are included, rather than advertisements for selected programs.

Most nurse practitioners are prepared to perform activities within the roles of direct provider of care, teacher, counselor, program coordinator, and evaluator of care through applications of quality assessment and research. Most importantly, NPs are trained to apply advanced physical assessment techniques in diagnosing and managing common acute health problems and stable chronic illnesses among a specified population. The curriculum usually includes advanced pharmacology, pathophysiology, and client care management for health promotion, illness prevention, and selected health conditions.

After completing an NP program, certification as a NP can be attained by achieving a passing score on the appropriate national certification examination. These examinations are offered by the American Nurses Credentialing Center (ANCC) and the AANP at various locations. Results of one or both examinations should be acceptable documentation for meeting state requirements. For the NP certified by ANCC, renewal is necessary every five years, depending on specified practice hours and continuing-education requirements. The standards for renewing certification are usually more stringent than those required for licensure renewal to practice professional nursing.

It is important to note that nurses prepared as NPs are neither physician substitutes nor physician extenders, as labeled in earlier literature (Ford, 1995; Ford & Silver, 1965). Rather they represent unique care providers who synthesize the skills and knowledge of nursing with the diagnostic and treatment measures that only physicians provided in the past. This blend of talents and abilities allows the NP to fill a pressing need for sensitive primary care services.

Personal Requirements

If this career option is sounding attractive to you, you may next wonder which personal characteristics would be desirable in the nurse filling the NP role? The ability to adapt to uncertain health care needs—either expressed or not so by those seeking care—is perhaps the greatest challenge faced by the NP. In the ambulatory care setting, expertise in collecting, analyzing, and labeling health problems is required in order to predict and provide services required by the patient. Considerable risk-taking is sometimes required because of the uncertainty surrounding many presentations. No longer is there the comfort of having a physician provide a diagnostic label for an illness being treated. The NP is expected to consider differential diagnoses and use available data and a sound knowledge base to recognize and treat ailments. These aspects of primary care present major challenges for the NP and represent a departure from the staff nurse role. It might be helpful to ask an NP working in primary care practice to share strategies for helping to meet these challenges.

NPs work in a variety of settings and serve persons from all walks of life. In addition to primary care facilities, they often work in schools, addressing the basic health needs of students and providing instructions regarding health promotion and illness prevention. Industrial settings also offer opportunities for employment. NPs with special preparation in occupational health can work for companies, promoting workplace safety, managing routine health problems, performing physical examinations, and implementing preventive programs. More recently, contracted services for emergency room coverage have included groups of physicians and NPs who manage the ever-increasing numbers of evening or weekend primary care cases. Many other opportunities are opening as the public becomes more informed regarding the nature of the services offered by NPs, especially in women's health. Many hospitals are establishing women's health centers to both attract new patients and provide additional well-woman and outpatient services in response to managed care.

Working Relationships

On a day-to-day basis, NPs employed in clinic settings work with one or more physicians, laboratory and radiologic technicians, and office personnel. For those working in managed care settings, such as HMOs, or large medical practice groups, the health team may consist of physician's assistants, physical therapists, social workers, RNs, and, occasionally, pharmacists. Similar working groups exist in long-term care facilities. The diverse talents of each professional contribute to a high caliber of care offered to patients.

Employment Opportunities and Compensation

Current employment opportunities for NPs seem plentiful, depending on the location desired (Styles, 1990). Such opportunities are published in newspapers or professional journals. Employers typically specify the exact type of expertise desired, or identify that no particular specialty is required as long as the NP has satisfactory credentials. Physician's assistants and nurse practitioners are both considered "midlevel providers," and some position advertisements list either preparation as acceptable. Survey the employment advertisements in your regional newspapers to identify opportunities.

Enrollments in NP programs increased dramatically in the early 1990s. Continued growth in NP practice opportunities will depend on public acceptance, provisions of state nursing acts, reimbursement policies, and the extent of physicians' acceptance and physicians' willingness to retool themselves for primary care practice. If more physicians elect to provide primary care, NPs will find fewer opportunities.

According to Dr. Tower, annual salaries for NPs average in the high $40,000 to low $50,000 range (Personal Communication, March 20, 1996). Experienced NPs may earn $60,000 to $70,000 per year, which is comparable to the annual salaries of family practice physicians working in HMOs (Van, 1995). Earnings vary greatly and are related to regional demands and scope of responsibilities.

 One NP's Practice

Marlene, is an NP working with seven physicians, four other NPs, an office manager, and various technicians in an ambulatory care setting. As a primary care provider, she performs many of the same tasks as do the physicians. When patients require more complex management, however, Marlene either requests a physician consultation or refers the patient to a general or specialty physician. Likewise, physicians sometimes refer patients to her for physical examinations, screenings, and health education.

Information Sources

The AANP can supply further information about NP practice. The journal Nurse Practitioner can also provide insight into NP practice and issues.

THE NURSE ANESTHETIST

Nurse anesthesia is an advanced clinical nursing specialty that was established in the late 1800s and is recognized by statute in each state. Certified registered nurse anesthetists (CRNAs) provide care to patients before, during, and after surgery or delivery of a baby. Specific activities include physical assessment, preoperative teaching, and preparation, administration, and maintenance of anesthesia. As specialists in anesthesia, CRNAs administer more than 65% of the 26 million anesthetics given to patients in the United States each year (AANA, 1993). CRNAs provide care during the recovery period and as part of follow-up monitoring during the postoperative course.

Approximately twenty-six thousand CRNAs are practicing in the United States today, making CRNAs the largest group of the three advanced practice roles described in this chapter. Men compose 40% of practicing CRNAs, making CRNA practice the most popular career choice for men in nursing.

Educational Preparation

Educational preparation of nurse anesthetists consists of a nurse anesthesia educational program approved by the Council on Accreditation of Anesthesia Educational Programs. An applicant is required to have a Bachelor of Science in Nursing or another appropriate baccalaureate degree, a license to practice professional nursing, and a minimum of one year of acute care nursing experience. Educational programs may establish additional requirements, such as critical care nursing experience.

Programs that prepare nurse anesthetists follow a standardized curriculum administered by schools and departments of anesthesia at medical centers or hospitals in conjunction with colleges or universities. Graduate course work over twenty-four to twenty-seven months includes a classroom component and clinical experience using specific techniques to administer a variety of anesthetic agents. At present, many programs confer a master's degree in nursing, allied health, or biological and clinical sciences, rather than a certificate or bachelor's degree. Graduates of nurse anesthesia programs must pass a national certification examination to become CRNAs. The American Association of Nurse Anesthetists (AANA) has established a target date of January 1998 for all CRNA educational preparation to occur in master's degree programs.

Following original certification as a nurse anesthetist, a minimum of forty continuing education credits must be accumulated every two years. Attending seminars at professional meetings is an excellent way to gain these approved credits while keeping current regarding new trends and developments in the field.

Personal Requirements

CRNA practice requires significant psychomotor skill; pharmacologic knowledge; refined skills in assessing, interviewing and teaching patients; and comfort with technology. The CRNA also must be able to cope successfully with stress. The operating room can be a highly charged, stressful environment, and some CRNAs have witnessed volatile eruptions on the part of surgeons. Whether or not working with surgeons is more stressful than working with other health care team members, the strict requirements for asepsis, the delicate balance in proper administration of anesthesia, and the narrow margin for error in surgery can all create tension. The surgical experience is also stressful for patients and their families. If you are considering a career as a CRNA, arrange several visits to the operating room and talk with CRNAs to gain insight into the culture and unique stresses associated with the operating room.

Working Relationships

Nurse anesthetists have working relationships with physicians, including surgeons, obstetricians, gynecologists, and anesthesiologists. As members of the surgical team, they also work with scrub nurses, circulating nurses, and operating room technicians during surgical procedures. In teaching hospitals, CRNAs also work with students and participate in teaching medical, nursing, and allied health students and residents. They also collaborate with operating room personnel to ensure that safety precautions are followed, and that supplies and equipment are available as needed. In addition, CRNAs work along with nurses in client monitoring and care management in postanesthesia units and critical care areas.

Employment Opportunities and Compensation

According to a 1989 Congressionally mandated study, CRNAs will enjoy many employment opportunities during the next twenty years. Careers available for consideration can be found in both the private and public sectors. Among the many choices, working in a group or private practice setting with other anesthetists and anesthesiologists presents definite benefits with regard to not only scheduling, but also sharing the costs of financial management. Large university medical settings, the military, public health services, and Veterans' Administration hospitals also afford opportunities for employment. In addition, schools of anesthesia offer teaching opportunities for qualified instructors. Lastly, locum tenens offers the anesthetist many short-term or temporary work opportunities. Such work can be pursued through agencies offering a wide latitude in length of work assignment and type of health care settings, all on a contract basis (Barton & Woglom, 1992).

When the nurse anesthetist begins to look for employment, the advantages and limitations of each type of position should be carefully considered. For example, a group practice provides a consistent level of income as compared with independent private practice. In addition, on-call time is shared among the members, permitting a greater amount of undisturbed leisure time. For the teacher, particular rotations or assignments of on-site practice can be negotiated in contacts with the medical center. And, finally, professional liability coverage, which represents a major financial benefit to many nurse anesthetists, can be part of a job's attractiveness.

The average annual salary for CRNAs is reported at $80,900 (AANA, 1993). This high rate of compensation reflects both the high level of responsibility and the potential risk of liability incurred with CRNA practice.

 One CRNA's Viewpoint

Karen, an experienced CRNA, is clearly proud of her career choice. She enthusiastically describes the many dramatic changes in anesthesia, from drop ether for tonsillectomies to the computerized techniques used today in coronary bypass surgery. Despite the abundance of advanced technology however, Karen adamantly emphasizes the need for direct observation of the patient by the nurse anesthetist throughout the operative procedure. She contends that warning signs of undesired changes can be perceived by the experienced nurse even before the mechanical monitors provide numerical evidence. Calling on all of her nursing knowledge and skills to deliver safe anesthesia is the core of her job satisfaction; she believes she is able to integrate the art and science of nursing into caring for her patients.

Information Sources

For additional information regarding CRNAs and their work, you may want to read the AANA Journal. Listings of specific nurse anesthetists programs can be obtained by writing to the AANA (address provided on page 175).

THE NURSE MIDWIFE

Nurse midwives are considered to be the first recognized nurse specialists. Advanced training programs have prepared nurse midwives for their specialty since 1931. In 1995, the American College of Nurse Midwives (ACNM) reported that 5,973 certified nurse midwives (CNMs) were practicing in the United States and its territories (Slattery & Burst, 1995). As compared to other advanced practice roles, fewer men practice as CNMs; approximately 1% of CNMs are men. CNMs provide a full range of prenatal, labor, delivery, and postpartum care. They also offer family planning counseling and gynecological services. They practice in private practices, as partnerships and groups in maternity centers, and in association with physicians and hospitals.

Educational Preparation

The formal education of nurse midwives includes a baccalaureate degree in nursing plus course work leading to certification. Many CNMs, pursue a master's degree in nursing, with midwifery as an area of concentration. Of all practicing CNMs, 70% hold master's and higher degrees, and 5% hold doctoral (PhD) or higher degrees. However, not only is a master's degree not required, but the American College of Nurse Midwives (ACNM) does not support requiring a master's degree for entry into CNM practice. ACNM has identified core competencies and standards for CNM practice, and views the education necessary for CNM practice as competency-based education. Educational programs vary considerably in length. A nurse who has practiced as a midwife in another country, for instance, might master any additional required competencies in as short a period as nine months. In contrast, the nurse without advanced practice experience or who elects to pursue a master's degree program would spend two years in the educational program. Some universities offer postmaster programs that award certificates in midwifery. These programs must be accredited by the National Council on Nurse Midwifery (Slattery & Burst, 1995).

Required course work includes traditional content in master's programs (e.g., nursing theory, research, advanced practice roles) plus specific courses in advanced pathophysiology, pharmacology, and maternal and infant care. Upon completion of an educational program, a passing score on a national certification examination is required before states will grant approval for practice. In most states, nurse midwives may work as nurse practitioners in the arenas of women's health and family planning.

Following original certification, the nurse midwife must comply with state licensing requirements for professional nurses. In addition, criteria for recertification as a midwife must be met. Because regulations vary among states, you must contact the regulatory board in your state to obtain precise information.

Personal Requirements

CNMs participate with families in one of the most intimate and significant events in life. The CNM must therefore be sensitive to individual needs, preferences, cultural beliefs, and practices. Skills in establishing rapport and in communication are essential. CNMs must have refined assessment skills, self-confidence, and sound clinical judgment, particularly regarding when to seek intervention by an obstetrician. In addition to having advanced knowledge and expertise related to women's health, pregnancy, the birthing process, and newborn care, the CNM must be committed to holistic practice. Most women and families who seek the services of a nurse midwife do so because they want a holisitic approach in addition to technical knowledge and expertise.

Working Relationships

Nurse midwives work closely with physicians, including obstetricians, gynecologists, and anesthesiologists. Nurse midwives are granted practice privileges by hospital medical staffs , and are subject to peer reviews similar to those performed among physicians. Nurse midwives may share aspects of work in the labor and delivery room with the nursing staff. In clinic settings, clerical and office staff contribute to the practice of the nurse midwife. Key personnel in many clinics and hospital units are the interpreters, who help communicate with patients who speak languages other than English. Under special circumstances, the nurse midwife may be called on to collaborate with radiologists or imaging technicians when a patient's condition requires the expertise of these practitioners.

Employment Opportunities and Compensation

Originally, job opportunities for nurse midwives existed primarily in rural areas of Appalachia and in relation to the Frontier Nurses program. The mission of these nurse midwives was to improve the health of mothers and infants in that region, a mission achieved through considerable effort and dedication. As medical care became more accessible to rural populations, however, the maternity services provided by midwives were seen as less essential. Then, the consumer movement of the 1980s redefined childbirth as a natural event rather than a medical condition. The result was increased demand for women's health care—and, thus, increased employment opportunities for licensed nurse midwives. Clinics, often associated with specialty hospitals or large medical centers, frequently serve as sites of practice.

Barriers to practicing as a CNM include obtaining the following: agreements for medical consultations and referrals, awards of practice privileges by physician groups, and reimbursement. All must be arranged prior to engaging in the practice of nurse midwifery. Malpractice insurance also must be obtained. The threat of litigation acts as a deterrent to practice for some CNMs.

Salaries for CNMs vary widely because of differences in practice patterns and regional norms. In fact, the ACNM has found it difficult to collect reliable data about CNM salaries because of these variations. But Kimberly Patamia, of ACNM, reports that annual salaries range from $40,000 to $70,000 (Personal Communication, March 21, 1996). Patamia adds that some CNMs are "paid in quilts" by Amish families who do not pay money for health care services.

Client populations served by CNMs are as diverse as the sites where care is provided. Some clients are self referred, often seeking alternatives to current or previous care. For the most part, CNMs provide care to healthy, low-risk women in association with one or more obstetricians. If complications occur during pregnancy or delivery, the CNM consults with the physician or, in cases of severe problems, arranges for transfer of care.

With the exception of the labor experience, the nature of the health services provided to low-risk patients by physicians and the CNMs is very similar. During labor, however, the CNM stays with the patient to monitor the progression of labor and give direct care as needed. It is during this period that nursing skills are used to help the patient master relaxation techniques and achieve some degree of comfort throughout the birthing event. Assisting a woman into motherhood is a special privilege, and, thus, contributes to the job satisfaction of the CNM.

 ## One CNM's Practice

Lisa, a CNM in a large urban medical center, works with three other CNMs. Together, they delivered 125 babies last year. Much of the prenatal care they provide focuses on preparing their patients physically and mentally for labor and delivery. Lisa and her colleagues familiarize themselves with one another's primary patients. This way, regardless of who is CNM on call when a patient calls or comes to the hospital for delivery, the patient is guaranteed informed, personalized care. Approximately 50% of their practice is devoted to low-risk gynecology, or well-woman care. They spend thirty to forty-five minutes on each office visit, and provide client education on gynecological and breast health, skin care, diet, and exercise. In addition to providing gynecological screenings, they counsel patients concerning family planning, menopause, hormone replacement, and osteoporosis (*Today & Tomorrow*, 1994).

Information Sources

For further information regarding CNMs and their work, you may want to read the *Journal of Nurse-Midwifery*. The ACNM (address provided on page 175) can also provide further information. Inquire about women's health centers at regional hospitals to learn more about local opportunities.

CONTRIBUTIONS TO HEALTH CARE

As health care agencies strive to accommodate decreasing revenue from public and private sources, the contributions of advanced practice nurses as direct care providers will no doubt increase. Underlying rationale for this perspective includes documentation of the high quality of care provided by advanced practice nurses and the moderate salaries traditionally received by nurses (Callan, 1992). In primary care roles, NPs and CNMs not only increase access to health care, but also assist patients in developing healthier lifestyles.

ISSUES

Issues for advanced practice nurses include reimbursement, legalities, accreditation, and acceptance by other professionals and the public. The roles of CNM (certified nurse midwife) and CRNA (certified registered nurse anesthetist) have longer histories and are more specialized and standardized than the NP role. Many of these issues are thus more troublesome for NPs than for CNMs and CRNAs.

Reimbursement

Services provided by CNMs and CRNAs as defined by their scopes of practice are reimbursed by federal, state, and private payers. Reimbursement for services continues to be a critical issue for NP providers, however. Historically, NPs have been excluded from the lists of professionals authorized for reimbursement by third-party payers. Congressional action during the

1980s, however, resulted in federal legislation requiring reimbursement for authorized care provided both by NPs in rural clinics and by NPs employed by nursing homes (Mittelstadt, 1993). Remuneration for services was set as a percentage of the customary payments given to physicians (OBRA, 1990).

Although federal policies specify the circumstances for and nature of services that are reimbursable, each state differs in regulating the practices of NPs. These variations reflect multiple barriers to practice, and frequently decrease access to care for those most often in need. Precise statutory requirements, published annually in the *Nurse Practitioner*, provide excellent data for making comparisons across the United States.

On the practice side, a newly hired NP working in a rural clinic recently admitted to her colleagues that becoming familiar with the processes of reimbursement was a real challenge for her. For example, she found that she had to translate the care provided to the patient into the "common medical procedure" term used on a standardized form. In addition, she had to become familiar with identifying the severity of illness treated during the office visit. These aspects of revenue-generation and accounting practices had not been a part of her nursing background as a staff nurse.

Reimbursement regulations and guidelines are constantly changing. When considering a career in advanced practice, it is thus important to seek information about anticipated changes that will affect practice. The professional organizations listed on page 175 of this chapter can supply such information. Advanced practice nurses must continually update themselves on reimbursement regulations, and, depending on their practice situations, may have to learn selected accounting skills, as was true of the NP discussed in the preceding paragraph.

Legal Issues

The failure of health care reform did not come as good news to NPs. Pearson (1995) suggests that the underlying reason for the lack of effective legislation to change health care in the United States was the enormous pressure exerted by special interest groups. There are too many individuals and organizations receiving concentrated incomes, and this money provides a powerful incentive to maintain the current system. This perspective holds true at national, state, and local levels, as is evident whenever changes to health care are proposed (Safriet, 1992).

For example, efforts to revise statutes governing nursing frequently meet with strong opposition from organized lobbies. And with regard to NPs, state laws often control their practice by limiting both the scope of practice and the ability to be reimbursed under insurance policies for services provided. Restriction of prescription authority also remains a thorny issue in many states. Further, statutory definitions of advanced practice nursing by state legislatures sometimes reflect the political sentiments—whether liberal or conservative—of the citizens, rather than national standards of preparation and practice.

States also regulate the practices of CNMs and CRNAs; however there is far less variation among states in defining the scopes of practice for these advanced practice nurses than for NPs.

Accreditation

As noted in the educational preparation sections for CRNAs and CNMs, professional organizations have taken a strong role in standardizing credentialing for these advanced practice roles. One serious concern for the public, as well as for professional nursing, is the limited accreditation standards for both the educational program and the credentialing process for NPs. Members of national nursing organizations and regulatory boards are beginning to work together to help resolve this problem. Once the fundamental issues are resolved, statutory language and regulations should be more precise and standardized across the nation. Hopefully, the scope of practice written and approved by regulatory boards will reflect the highest degree of autonomy. Meanwhile, considerable effort will be required in political arenas to explain existing constraints and to lobby for proposals that are in touch with the valuable contributions to health that NPs can make.

Acceptance by Other Providers and the Public

In the professional community, more controversy surrounds NP practice than CNM or CRNA practice. Because the latter roles are more clearly defined, are more standardized across states, and have longer histories, they are better understood by physicians, other providers, and the public.

Nevertheless, physicians and other provider groups are beginning to recognize that NPs can add value to patient care—and in a cost-effective manner (Terry, 1993). Although the American Medical Association (AMA) has not supported expanded roles for NPs in primary care, practicing NPs enjoy positive, collegial relationships with physicians.

Patients and physicians alike perceive value added by the contributions of advanced practice nurses. CNMs note that they "get a lot of return business" and that most of their patients would not want to go through the childbirth experience any other way (*Today & Tomorrow*, 1994). NPs assist patients and their families to problem-solve and take more control in managing their health and medical treatment. This proactive approach can lead to better general health, better compliance with prescribed regimens, and lower treatment costs.

Recent Gallup polls have shown increasing public acceptance of the NP as primary care provider: 86% of consumers would be willing to go to an advanced practice nurse instead of an MD for basic health care (Paully-O'Neill & Andreola, 1994). Consumers who have received care from advanced practice nurses are enthusiastic regarding their satisfaction with the care provided. Yet, many in the general public remain poorly informed regarding the expertise and scope of practice of advanced practice nurses.

RESOURCES FOR FURTHER INFORMATION

American Academy of Nurse Practitioners
P. O. Box 12846
Austin, TX 78711
512-442-4262

American Association of Nurse Anesthetists
222 South Prospect Avenue
Park Ridge, IL 60068-4002
847-692-7050

American College of Nurse Midwives
818 Connecticut Avenue NW, Suite 900
Washington, DC 20006
1-800-753-2266

SUMMARY

This chapter provided information about the advanced nursing practice roles of nurse practitioner, nurse anesthetist, and nurse midwife. (The clinical nurse specialist role, also an advanced practice role, is discussed in Chapter 9). In general, each specialty has its own distinctive history, and an equally unique future is predicted for each of these specialties regardless of any anticipated changes in the health care system. And, there will undoubtedly continue to be a need for health care for underserved groups such as children, pregnant adolescents, the elderly, and the indigent.

Historically, NPs, CNMs, and CRNAs have ministered to all individuals without concern for remuneration procedures or costs of care. However, changes are already occurring in nurses' levels of sensitivity regarding not simply the financial aspects of care, but also the public's trust that nurses help to manage our limited resources wisely. Perhaps the greatest challenge for nurses as direct providers of care is to tailor care specifically to individuals while at the same time striving to follow established practice protocols and standards of care. By following these guidelines, nurses in advanced practice can apply their skills, knowledge, and judgment in promoting wellness and managing health conditions.

As you explore a career change, consider the nature of advanced practice nursing. In particular, think about the autonomy offered in the three roles discussed in this chapter. Consider both the rewards and the demands that accompany advancement in the field of professional nursing. In many ways, you are probably quite similar to other nurses who have decided to expand their clinical expertise and scopes of practice. When one post-master student was asked why she decided to become a nurse practitioner, she replied that "with all the reorganization in health care organizations, downsizing, and job insecurity, I figured that the more diverse my practice and the more expertise I possess, the better my chances of keeping my job or finding another one." With this attitude, she is more than likely to be among those valued by her employer. Being proactive rather than reactive will keep her attention focused and her energy expended in a constructive manner.

As you proceed with your personal career planning, remember that a positive attitude will serve you well. A positive attitude and a strong desire to advance your practice will help you face the challenges of continuing your education. Advanced education is prerequisite for these advanced practice roles. Once a nurse begins advanced practice, self-directed, continuing education is necessary to ensure continued competence. With a commitment to advancing your practice as a nurse, you can develop a stimulating and rewarding career in advanced practice.

REFERENCES

American Academy of Nurse Practitioners (AANP). (1993). Scope of practice for nurse practitioners. Washington, DC: Author.

American Association of Nurse Anesthetists (AANA). (1993). Questions and answers about a career in nurse anesthesia. Park Ridge, IL: AANA, Education and Research Department.

Barton, C. R. & Woglom, J. (1992). *Guidelines for seeking professional opportunities in the contemporary practice of nurse anesthesia.* West Orange, NJ: Organon Inc.

Billingsley, M. C., & Harper, D. (1982). The extinction of the nurse practitioner: Threat or reality? *Nurse Practitioner, 7*(9), 22–30.

Bullough, B. (1992). Alternative models for specialty nursing practice. *Nursing and Health Care, 13*(5), 254–259.

Burst, H. V. (1995). An update on the credentialing of midwives by the ACNM. *Journal of Nurse-Midwifery, 40*(3), 290–296.

Callan, M. E. (1992) Nurse practitioner management of hospital-affiliated primary care centers. *Nurse Practitioner, 17*(9), 71–73.

Ford, L. C. (1995). Nurse practitioners: Myths and misconceptions. *Journal of the New York State Nurses Association, 26*(1), 12–13.

Ford, L. C., & Silver, H. K. (1965). The expanded role of the nurse in child care. *Nursing Outlook, 15*(1), 43–45.

Geolot, D. H. (1987). NP education: Observations from a national perspective. *Nursing Outlook, 35*(3), 132-135.

Koch, L. W., Pazaki, S. H., & Campbell, J. D. (1992). The first 20 years of nurse practitioner literature: An evolution of joint practice issues. *Nurse Practitioner, 17*(2), 64–71.

Mittelstadt, P. C. (1993). Federal reimbursement of advanced practice nurses' services empowers the profession. *Nurse Practitioner, 18*(1), 43–49.

Murphy, M. A. (1990). A brief history of pediatric nurse practitioners and NAPNAP: 1964–1990. *Journal of Pediatric Health Care, 4*(6): 332–337.

Omnibus Budget Reconciliation Act (OBRA) of 1990, Public Law No. 100–509.

Paully-O'Neill, S., & Andreola, N. M. (1994, February 7). Breaking down the barriers: Advanced practice nurses. *The Nursing Spectrum, Greater Chicago/Northeast Illinois & Northwest Indiana Edition, 7*(3): 8.

Pearson, L. J. (1995). Annual update on how each state stands on legislative issues affecting advanced nursing practice. *Nurse Practitioner, 20*(1), 35–47.

Richmond, T., & Keane, A. (1992). The nurse practitioner in tertiary care. *Journal of Nursing Administration, 22*(11), 11–12.

Safriet, B. F. (1992). Health care dollars and regulatory sense: The role of advanced practice nursing. *Yale Journal on Regulation, 9*(2), 149–220.

Slattery, L. E. & Burst, H. V. (1995). ACNM accredited and preaccredited nurse-midwifery education programs: Program information. *Journal of Nurse-Midwifery, 40*(4), 349–365.

Stamoulis, S. (1992). Inpatient nurse practitioner: To be or not to be? *Nursing Management, 23*(5), 85–90.

Styles, M. M. (1990). Nurse practitioners creating new horizons for the 1990s. *Nurse Practitioner, 15*(2), 48, 53, 57.

Terry, K. (1993). How " physician extenders" can strengthen your practice. *Medical Economics, 70*(22), 57–58, 60, 65, 68, 72.

Today & Tomorrow. (Fall, 1994). Certified nurse-midwives: Giving women another option for OB-GYN care. Chicago, IL: Northwestern Medical Faculty Foundation, Inc.

Van, D. (1995, Fall/Winter). Nurse practitioners take caring to a new level. *Rush Record.* Chicago, IL: Rush-Presbyterian-St. Luke's Medical Center.

Chapter Nine

The Clinical Nurse Specialist

Audrey Klopp

INTRODUCTION

Since the creation of the clinical nurse specialist (CNS) role in the early 1960s, CNSs have been recognized "change agents." From the beginning, curricula preparing CNSs have included theoretical and practice foundations for managing change and, in fact, for creating it. Retrospectively, the CNS's unique preparation for recognizing, creating, and managing change may explain how the role itself has readily adapted over the past thirty-five years to the constant paradigm shifts that have characterized health care in the United States. The future promises that this trend will continue for CNSs.

Interestingly, and to the credit of the CNS role, many changes have been stimulated and managed by CNSs acting proactively in response to opportunities for improvement (Wolf, 1990). This concept of using change positively (i.e., proactively), as opposed to reacting to the current tide of change, sets the

CNS role apart from others and provides important clues to the important characteristics of individuals who choose the CNS role. There is no doubt that the nurse who can use change constructively will continue to be an important player in the coming years.

This chapter describes the CNS role, including components of the role, the maturation of the role and the individuals filling the role, and information to enable prospective CNSs to identify strengths already in place and to propose strategies to ensure successful transition and role implementation. Opportunities and potential challenges for role development are also considered. In addition, examples of various CNS practice models are presented, both to demonstrate the diverse opportunities available to creative CNSs and to enhance understanding of this complex, highly varied role.

AN OVERVIEW OF THE CNS ROLE

A CNS is a master's prepared, advanced practice nurse whose care focuses on a specific patient population defined either by clinical type or geographical grouping (e.g., medical, surgical, diabetic, cardiovascular, operating room, emergency room, critical care), or by the needs of a specific age group (e.g., geriatric, neonatal). Leherr and Gift (1990) identify the medical-surgical CNS role as the most commonly utilized, followed by psychiatric and oncology CNSs. In considering current and probable future trends, greater demand for critical care, long-term care, and geriatric CNSs will emerge.

The CNS role, created approximately thirty years ago, arose from the need for the nursing profession to have an advanced level nurse who could improve both the art and the science of nursing. This need coincided with an explosion of knowledge and technological advances, which challenged the practice of nursing as it existed.

In a 1962 *American Journal of Nursing* (AJN) editorial, Johnson envisioned a new role being derived from the currently unsatisfactory delivery of nursing care. In this new role the professional nurse would be more available for direct patient care (Johnson, 1962). These concerns are eerily reflective of today's focus on the redesign of patient-care delivery systems. There were also ambitious hopes, only partially realized, that the CNS role would produce much needed nursing research (Notter, 1971; Cason & Beck, 1982; Robichaud & Hamric, 1986).

Numbering approximately forty thousand in the United States, CNSs are the largest group of advanced practice nurses (Moore, 1993). According to results of a 1992 survey the average annual earning for a CNS was $41,226 (American Nurses Association [ANA], 1994). Although CNSs have traditionally practiced in hospitals and similar acute care settings, the potential diversity of practice settings for the CNS is limitless.

A review of employment opportunities today indicates a shift of opportunities to the following: (1) better-defined populations (e.g., oncology or cardiology versus med-surg), (2) areas where technology continues to act as a major factor in the need for a CNS, or (3) where dramatic changes in the overall provision of health care has further enhanced the need for efficiency as well as quality (e.g., managed care, "rightsizing"). Positions for obstetric, operating room, and geriatric CNSs currently head the list of available jobs. CNSs continue to be sought for highly specialized populations, such as those with diabetes or those in need of enterostomal therapy. In addition, more positions are being created outside the traditional acute care and hospital settings. The shift of care delivery to the outpatient arena and to long-term care is opening relatively uncharted territory for the CNS role. Logic also dictates that CNSs roles that focus on keeping individuals out of hospitals will flourish.

As physicians grapple with capitation and the need to expand caseloads in order to maintain current levels of income, their willingness to delegate or share responsibilities for patient education, coordination of care, and long-term support will also create opportunities for CNSs. As late as 1990, interestingly, physicians who were self-employed were less likely than otherwise employed physicians to favor the use of advanced practice nurses (Curtin, 1990).

CNS ROLES

Traditionally, the CNS role has been subdivided into five dimensions: the clinician (or practitioner), the educator, the consultant (or collaborator), the researcher (or scholar), and the manager (or administrative/organizational). A great deal has been written about the feasibility of successfully implementing such a multi-faceted role. A two-year study of twenty-eight CNSs conducted by Boyd et al. (1991), however, found that CNSs were able to "merge and implement" all subroles, although not equally so. According to the survey, 67% of the CNSs' time was spent in clinical practice, 25% in education, 10% on scholarly activities, and 8% in consulting. Following is an in-depth examination of each subrole in depth, including ways in which CNSs implement each.

The CNS as Clinician

In the role as clinician, a CNS applies experience and advanced theoretical knowledge to complex patient-care situations. Using the nursing process, the CNS strives to improve outcomes. The related clinical activities may be direct (i.e., providing care) or indirect (i.e., directing others in the provision of care). A hallmark of the CNS's clinical practice is the ability to recognize the need to deviate from the norm, or the established rules, for the sake of individualizing care. Benner (1984) ascribes the ability to choose an appropriate action without necessarily analyzing the situation to the level of expert. This ability among CNSs becomes even more enhanced than that of the expert staff level nurse as the CNS intensely focuses on a specific population or set of nursing needs over time.

Although CNSs use physical assessment as part of the overall assessment of a patient's condition, physical assessment may be limited to the CNS's particular area of specialty, e.g., respiratory or cardiovascular. This system-specific use of physical assessment is one often-recognized difference between this advanced practice nurse and others, such as nurse practitioners (NPs) whose physical assessment skills are more global.

The CNS's skills in assessment are typically used to examine the entire clinical situation, the patient's and family's response to it, and the staff's needs for assistance, coordination, and support in providing needed care. The ability to see the Gestalt (i.e., the whole as more than a collection of individual pieces) is one characteristic of the CNS's clinical practice that patients and families readily recognize and value. They often view the CNS as someone who can see the whole picture and help to coordinate and advocate for them. This practice function of the CNS is one means of humanizing the health care experience and lessening the sense of fragmentation that patients and families often find to be an intolerable aspect of coping with illness and injury.

Radical changes in health care finance have occurred in the past few years and will most certainly continue for the foreseeable future. These changes have accelerated the rate at which patients and families are expected to navigate the care-delivery system. These changes have also made it necessary for patients and families to seek needed care in additional settings. This situation highlights two emerging clinical applications of the CNS role. One is as case (or care) manager, which also implies a role as cost manager. The other is as systems expert who works to make the complex network of systems that patients and families must navigate more efficient and user friendly. According to Kirk (1992), being responsive to and meeting customer expectations is paramount in the success of any operation. Health care is no exception.

With the rapid expansion managed care and the focus on its primary goal of curtailing the spiraling cost of health care, has come increased recognition that CNSs are uniquely prepared to assume the role of case manager (Cronin & Maklebust, 1989; Schull, Tosch, & Wood, 1992; Meisler & Midyette, 1994). So as not to repeat information already presented in Chapter 7, comments here relate only to those capabilities of CNSs that make them excellent candidates for the role of case manager. Schull, Tosch, and Wood (1992) indicate that organizing and coordinating services and resources, along with controlling costs, are the important goals of case management. These authors stress that a patient-centered approach involves the patient as a participant in operationalizing case management.

Case management emerges as a viable method of producing desirable clinical outcomes at affordable prices. Focusing on this goal legitimizes and gives structure to that which CNSs have always viewed as their contribution but have had minimal success in making tangible. As one author says, "Much has been written about what the CNS does, but little about what she achieves" (Beyerman, 1989, p.36). The lack of documentation (i.e., proof in outcomes research) demonstrating that the expenditure related to having a CNS on staff results in positive clinical outcomes and positive financial outcomes is a long-recognized and long-lamented problem for CNSs (Papenhausen & Beecroft, 1990; Beecroft, 1991; Boyd et. al., 1991; Gift, 1992). Care maps, critical paths, and similar written plans include not only clinical outcomes but time frames for achievement of those outcomes. By focusing on time frames, they highlight and quantify the impact of paying attention to moving the patient efficiently through the necessary components and aspects of the system. Case management closely parallels what CNSs have previously called "carrying a caseload": managing and directing the care of a specific group of patients. Carrying a caseload has not always emphasized formal measures of cost containment and legitimate ability to impact other players on the health team to the extent that case management does, however.

Much of what the CNS does, whether in a case manager role or not, is directed at managing the complexity of the health care environment. Tonges and Madden (1993) refer to these complexities as the interdependencies that exist in systems. Wolf (1990) describes a shift in the focus of organizational priorities during the mid-1980s from quality to a quality-cost balance. This more resource-driven focus highlighted the need for better coordination and communication among systems. To address these changes while at the same time maintaining quality of care and advocacy for patients and families, CNSs began expanding their scopes of practice to include systems. They began solving problems in systems by recognizing and dealing with the interdependencies, rather than looking at the individual components of systems. Wolf (1990) calls these CNSs "second-generation" CNSs and even proposes that complex environments might benefit from two levels of CNS: one with the traditional, patient-staff focus and the other with a systems focus.

Clinical practice has been described as the cornerstone of the CNS role, that portion without which the CNS role does not exist (Sparacino, 1991). In fact, the ANA Council of Clinical Nurse Specialists requires a client-based practice for fulfillment of the CNS role. And Hamric (1989) goes as far as to say that unless the CNS maintains a clinical practice, the title "clinical nurse specialist" should not be used.

CNSs operationalize their practice roles in a wide variety of ways. Some are unit-based, spending the majority of their work time on the same unit or couple of units, seeing most of the patients on those units. This is a likely model in situations where like patients are clustered by disease or nursing-need type, such as oncology patients who are receiving chemotherapy. Other CNSs may find their caseloads of patients scattered throughout a facility, and, therefore, find themselves practicing in many arenas. In some specialties, the CNS's caseload may include patients of all ages (e.g., a neuroscience CNS, an orthopaedic CNS, an operating room or emergency room CNS). For CNSs whose practices focus on clinical issues (e.g., a psychiatric liaison, wound-care specialist), the practice arena may extend to many inpatient and outpatient settings. Many CNSs follow patients through the continuum of health care provision, and, therefore, see inpatients as well outpatients. Others, because of a variety of organizational variables, may limit their practices to either inpatients or outpatients. Among CNSs, it is understood that the enormous variance in practice patterns is merely a characteristic of the role. Indeed, it is the need of a CNS's specific population that dictates which shape that CNS's practice takes. Novice CNSs or CNSs who initiate roles where none have existed before often find that such loose or nonexistent boundaries are not only challenging to establish and manage, but also sometimes poorly understood by staff and management who are accustomed to more traditional work assignments.

Activities in which CNSs typically engage while carrying out their practice roles include rounding to see patients or families (either alone or with other nurses or members of the interdisciplinary team); providing hands-on care or patient/family education and/or counseling; and directing and evaluating the overall plan of care, conducting formal or informal care conferences to enhance the plan of care and coordinating the delivery of care by communicating with anyone who is (or needs to be) involved with the care of the patient. Patients may be seen daily, more that once a day, every other day, weekly, or however often the CNS's assessment of the situation dictates. This exercise of judgment is another variable that staff and management may need help in understanding. Finally, CNSs spend a significant portion of their time supporting the staff who provide the bulk of direct care and dealing with difficult professional issues, such as ethical concerns (Fenton, 1985). Schaefer (1991) investigated this province of the CNS and described "caring" as the basic process by which CNSs are involved in caring for the caregivers, by "providing emotional and situational support" (p. 273).

The CNS's clinical practice allows a synthesis of the CNS's many areas of expertise, showcased in a way that is apparent and meaningful not only to the patient and family, but also to many others. The CNS's practice role provides a role model of expert nursing practice for the staff as well as for other members of the health care team who may not fully understand nursing's unique contributions. The public, whose image of nursing remains underdeveloped, gains greater insight into nursing practice through contact with an effective CNS. Holders of the purse strings (e.g., administrators and managed care providers) are beginning to recognize nursing as a generally underutilized vehicle for care delivery, and the role of the CNS, specifically, as an avenue to cost effective, high-quality care.

The CNS as Educator

Second only to the role as expert clinician is the CNS's role as educator (Boyd et al, 1991). Using principles of adult education in the role as educator, the CNS utilizes formal and informal teaching methodologies to impart knowledge to others. Activities in which the CNS typically engages when acting as educator include family and patient education, nursing staff education, education for members of the interdisciplinary team outside of nursing, community education, and education for undergraduate and graduate nursing students. In the role as preceptor for graduate-level nursing students, the CNS often assumes the role of mentor.

CNSs may be involved in patient and family education relating to any aspect of the patient's illness, injury, or need for health maintenance. Assessment of timing, level of information, method of instruction, and need for repetition are important activities in which the CNS engages when meeting the educational needs of patients and families. Depending on the population served, CNSs may provide education in one-on-one setting, or group settings.

Development of patient education materials is another important aspect of the CNS's role as educator. CNSs prepare and use printed materials, audio-visual materials, and models. They also coordinate and facilitate interactions with other individuals from whom the patient and/or family may gain information, understanding, or support. For example, the CNS may facilitate the use of "Y-me?" volunteers for breast cancer patients, or lay ostomy volunteers for patients with new ostomies.

Nursing staff education—often the most visible, measurable educational work of the CNS—comprises formal presentations such as inservices or workshops. The CNS may also provide staff education spontaneously, as when sharing expertise with staff at the bedside of a patient, or discussing some aspect of a patient's care. In addition to sharing purely clinical information, the CNS often interprets and communicates current research-based information to the staff.

CNSs are frequently called on as educators for professionals and others outside of nursing. Depending on a CNS's area of practice, the CNS may be called on to recognize educational needs of and provide education for any care provider in any system that interacts with or influences the overall experience of patient care. For example, physicians, medical students and interns, various technologists, and physical, occupational, and speech therapists may all benefit from the CNS's specialized knowledge. It is interesting to note that CNSs view providing education for those outside of nursing as one of the least satisfying aspects of their educator role (Tarsitano, Brophy, & Snyder, 1986). However, these activities are likely to increase as delivery systems are redesigned and CNSs are increasingly called on to provide education and manage the changes inherent in redesign.

Community education is an important aspect of the CNS's role as educator. CNSs often speak to laygroups which contact professional organizations to obtain guest speakers. CNSs' work with particular populations of individuals may also lead to speaking engagements in the community. For example, an oncology CNS may receive invitations from "Y-me?," the lay support group for breast cancer survivors, or from women's groups. Often CNSs' patients who are members of such lay groups recommend the CNS as a guest speaker.

CNSs may also be involved in providing information to the media through press releases or participation in the radio or television media. One underutilized medium among CNSs is popular literature. Advanced practice nurses are uniquely qualified to present professional health-related information in a manner that can be readily understood by the public.

Participation in formal graduate and undergraduate nursing education is another important aspect of the CNS's role as educator. In fact, in several practice models, the CNS spends a portion of time in the role of faculty member in graduate or undergraduate nursing programs. The potential success of such models lies in the CNS's current clinical knowledge and ability to teach. However, there are also potential practical problems of implementation relating to time management and the need to be available to the clinical arena. The CNS is therefore most typically used as a clinical preceptor, and is available to nursing students while they are focusing on the clinical components of their educational programs. This is particularly true in relation to the CNS's involvement with graduate nursing students, who look to the CNS as role model and mentor. Because of the wide variance in role implementation among CNSs, it is essential for the graduate nursing student who is interested in a career as a CNS to see how the CNS role can be operationalized in many different ways. By working with a practicing CNS, the student can gain insight into the rationale for one avenue of role implementation versus another. Many CNSs hold adjunct faculty appointments as recognition for their contributions to the education of graduate and undergraduate students.

The CNS as Consultant

The consultant role of the CNS, typically one of the last subroles to emerge (Sneed, 1991), involves the utilization of the CNS's expertise when invited into the care provided to a patient by another nurse or member of the health care team. Chisholm (1991) describes consultation as "an interaction or interrelationship between two professionals: one who has knowledge or skills, and one who desires help with a problem or a goal" (p. 57). At least two authors warn that the CNS must always remember that the individual who requests the consultation retains a significant amount of power (i.e., to either not heed the advice of the consultant or not invite the consultant back). Both authors suggest that respect for the role and knowledge of the consultee is paramount in creating a relationship where the CNS's skills and expertise can best be utilized (Chisholm, 1991; Hotter, 1992).

In its most conceptual format, consultation really means empowering another individual to succeed. This is clearly a strategy that CNSs use to improve the outcomes of clinical practice. Additionally, many CNSs use consulting as a forum for hands-on education, and most certainly as an opportunity for modeling expert nursing practice. One study regarding the CNS's consultative role demonstrated that the consultative activities of critical care

CNSs resulted in prevention of complications and maintenance of care standards (Gurka, 1991).

CNSs may also provide consultation to nurse administrators (Eichelberger, Fiscus, & Talsky, 1995) and nurse educators (Shawler, Steppler, & Kinnaird, 1990). Finally, it is worth noting that second generation CNSs provide consultative services to systems so as to improve systems' outcomes. Regardless of the recipient of the CNS's consultation, it is important to remember that the CNS's clinical expertise is the basis for this role as consultant.

The CNS as Researcher (Scholar)

Characteristics of a productive clinical researcher include intellectual curiosity, conceptual ability to work in the abstract as well as practical domains, clinical expertise, and creativity within the realm of practicality (Scholfeldt, 1974). These are clearly characteristics common to CNSs. Yet, the researcher/scholar facet of the CNS role is the last to emerge and consumes the least amount of the CNS's time.

The CNS's role as scholar includes not only involvement in research and research-related activities, but also efforts to disseminate research-based information and to work with staff nurses in applying new information to improve patient care. In every available study of the CNS role, research and scholarly activities account for the least percentage of the CNS's time when compared to the activities associated with other CNS subroles. Yet, studies have also documented that nurse administrators, nursing faculty, and CNSs themselves value the researcher/scholar role for the CNS (Cason & Beck, 1982; Wyers, Grove, & Pastorino, 1985).

A 1990 survey of CNSs regarding their involvement in research, found that nearly every CNS job description contains expectations for involvement in research and/or scholarly activities (e.g., publication, presentation at local and national levels, advancement of nursing). But only 16% of the reporting CNSs said that they were held accountable (i.e., evaluated) for actually being involved in research or scholarly activities (Klopp, 1990). CNSs believe that they operationalize their researcher/scholar subrole by reading; evaluating research for applicability in the clinical arena; serving on editorial boards for specialty-specific journals; publishing research-related information; attending and/or presenting at specialty-related conferences where others with similar expertise gather; addressing practice issues that require change; serving on an institution's research review board; collaborating with others (e.g., nursing faculty, physicians, other health care professionals) on research projects; and facilitating the research of others. It is apparent that these CNSs describe activities related to both discovery of new knowledge and use of research-related information, but that use outweighs discovery in the CNS practice.

Although many CNSs have successfully integrated research into their roles, CNSs are not involved in research to the degree originally anticipated by the profession. As early as 1983, Hodgeman succinctly articulated the problems related to the research facet of the CNS role: "This fantasy consists of the notion that regardless of how much or how little the CNS has been taught about nursing research in graduate school, regardless of how much time is consumed by other practice expectations, and regardless of the specialist's own interests and natural abilities, every CNS should be conducting the equivalent of a doctoral dissertation on the job" (p. 78).

As noted by Hodgeman, a variety of factors contribute to the reality of how well the CNS is generally able to incorporate the research component into practice. First is the issue of preparation in the academic setting for conducting research. Graduate-level nursing course work regarding research is typically geared more toward teaching the novice CNS to utilize existing research rather than conduct studies. The level of preparation that enables a nurse researcher is far more typical of the doctoral level of nursing education. (Incidentally, many senior CNSs pursue doctoral degrees at some point in their careers, and, subsequently, make significant scientific contributions as the result of this level of study.) It is also important to note that few graduate nursing faculty have themselves practiced as CNSs. Faculty who have not practiced as CNSs or who have practiced only in limited ways or for brief periods of time can offer only theoretical guidance in helping the novice CNS integrate the subrole of researcher. In particular, their guidance may not adequately address the practical issues involved in juggling research with clinical decision making.

The other major issue affecting the integration of research into the CNS role is that of reward. Unlike the CNS's academic counterpart, scholarly activities are seldom tied to financial incentive, tenure, or career advancement. In fact, scholarly activities are sometimes perceived as distractions by staff, administration, or other less "scholarly" colleagues.

Growing acceptance of qualitative methodologies, including case studies, may provide an avenue to a more comfortable fit for the CNS interested in research. Qualitative methods should more easily enable CNSs to use their own rich practice fields as data sources. Qualitative methods may also prove more relevant in considering highly complex, multivariate phenomena that require research in the realm of nursing. Use of nursing diagnoses, focus on patient outcomes, the movement toward case management and managed care, and the need to justify CNS roles are trends that have stimulated CNSs toward more research-related activities.

Unfortunately, the concurrent trend of rightsizing and redesign have challenged CNSs' abilities to incorporate this complex subrole into their daily practices. In 1986, CNSs were spending a scant 2.2% of their time on research (Robichaud & Hamric, 1986). In 1991, Boyd et al. found that CNSs were spending approximately 10% of their time on research and scholarly endeavors. Major changes that have unsettled health care since that time have surely not improved this situation, as CNSs find themselves devoting more and more time to systems issues and redesign.

CNSs can lend their expertise to collaborative research projects with nursing faculty and researchers in other disciplines. Such collaboration may offer opportunities for CNSs to contribute research without detracting from the other components of their roles.

The CNS as Manager

From the beginning, the CNS role has traditionally been a staff role. This means that, for the most part, CNSs have been free of administrative responsibilities such as staffing, budgeting, and personnel issues. This does not mean, however, that the CNSs are exempt from managing aspects of their own practices. They manage their time and the educational or research programs for which they are responsible, and they contribute meaningfully to the overall administrative functioning of the departments to which they belong. (Although CNSs are usually employed by nursing departments, other clinical departments occasionally do employ CNSs. And with increasing frequency CNSs serve product lines rather than departments.)

Organizational/administrative functions often include committee work. CNSs frequently contribute to policy and procedure committees, committees that review and strive to improve quality of care or care delivery, and committees that evaluate products. These are hand-in-glove roles for CNSs, enabling them to inject clinically focused expertise into an institution's decision making bodies.

As delivery systems are redesigned to provide more patient-focused care, CNSs are being called on to chair or serve on redesign teams. The goals of these teams are to reduce boundaries and make access to care seamless for all involved. Patients, families, and managed care providers have lost patience with care delivery designed with the system's best interest as the driving force. Patient-focused care seeks to restore the patient's best interest as the core of care delivery. This work is a natural extension for the CNS, who has always engaged in humanizing the health care experience and helping patients and families navigate the loosely connected aspects of the health care system.

CNS roles are less likely that others to be bureaucratically defined, and CNSs thus use individualistic frameworks for practice. This renders the CNS well-suited and integral to the major redesign that is currently underway in health care. In 1994 *AJN* editorial, Lucille Joel encourages nurses to "lay claim to our intrapreneurial heritage and cultivate a climate of change from within" (p. 7). Joel goes on to encourage intrapreneurs to "play intelligent hunches, trust . . . intuition, and thrive on risky business" (p. 7).

Who is better equipped to lead this movement than the CNS? Several colleagues who have evolved into second-generation CNSs are quick to agree that the organizational/manager aspects of their roles have grown considerably during the past three to four years. There is little doubt that all CNS subroles will be similarly affected as the paradigms continue to shift in care delivery. The career opportunities abound for CNSs who are up to the challenge of shaping the future of how America's delivery systems look and feel. Only lack of perseverance of those individuals in the roles will limit the opportunities.

The next section of this chapter explores the characteristics of the CNS. To gain the deepest understanding from this section, think back over the CNS subroles of clinician, educator, consultant, researcher/scholar, and manager and imagine how the characteristics discussed apply to the successful enactment of each subrole.

CHARACTERISTICS OF THE CNS

Much of what is important about the characteristics of the CNS relates to the traditional placement of the CNS in the organization, the CNS's methods of interacting with staff, and the manner whereby the CNS provides leadership.

The CNS in a Staff Position

As previously stated, most CNSs are in staff positions. Strictly speaking, staff nurses are not obliged to heed the advice of the CNS because of rank. So why do they? Two decades ago, Peter Drucker observed that several personal qualities make for success in a staff position. These qualities are most applicable to CNSs. They include the desire to enable or empower others to achieve a mutually desirable outcome without needing to "get the credit", being able to distribute attention fairly; and being able to allow others time to achieve goals—in other words, being patient (Drucker, 1974). Holt (1992) likens the work of a CNS to being "the wind beneath (someone's) wings" (p. 27). By this, she implies that the CNS supports and cares for others as they achieve desired outcomes.

Using a constant comparative method and theory developed by Leininger, one author studied CNSs for one year to discover the basis for their practice (Schaefer, 1991). She concludes that caring in the basic psychological process involved in the way that CNSs interact, not only with patients and families, but also with the caretakers. Caring in further divided into humanistic caring and scientific caring. Investigating (assessing situations and dissecting clinical problems) and teaching are ways whereby CNSs demonstrate scientific caring. They demonstrate humanistic caring through interactions with caretakers that enable, support, or bolster the caretakers' abilities and confidence.

Humanistic caring is also evidenced by the ways the CNS alters the environment to facilitate the delivery of care. This is reflective of the CNS's ability to see the whole picture in which the caretaker practices, and again highlights the notion that CNSs are taking more active roles in redesigning the systems wherein patients are provided care and caretakers function. The CNS also sometimes demonstrates caring just by "being there," providing a break, or assisting with a tedious procedure. Taken as a composite, these activities communicate to caretakers that what they are doing is important; feeling validated and worthwhile, the caretakers are thus energized to continue. In addition to these manifestations of caring, CNSs also use principles of coaching, constantly striving to help caretakers reach new heights and improve practice. This is empowerment in its truest sense, and represents the most powerful strategy that CNSs can employ in achieving their overall mission.

Leadership and the CNS

A central characteristic of the successful CNS is leadership. Although not typically the formal leader of a unit, division, or department, the CNS is in a key position to provide leadership to the largest group of professional caregivers in the health care environment: the nursing staff. Further, clinical focus distinguishes the CNS from management and often affords the CNS the attention and the opportunity to earn the respect of the staff nurse. This attention and respect form the basis from which the CNS's leadership strategies can influence improvements in practice and patient outcomes. Leadership "in the trenches" is a collective of behaviors and use of self employed by the CNS. Leadership that communicates caring truly empowers staff nurses to do important, customer-oriented things that redesign and patient-focused care requires of them—and that they truly want to provide. This leadership is far removed from the unfortunate notion prevalent in many corporate cultures and among well-meaning administrators that empowerment can be afforded by issuing a memo. Empowerment is not simply giving power to someone. Empowerment is generated by shoulder-to-shoulder work coupled with in-depth understanding of and passion for the essence of the work to be performed. When caring is communicated to staff, and systems are corrected, the staff becomes empowered in the truest sense of the word. This is the essence of the CNS's practice. Hotter (1992) also points out that CNSs are themselves inherently rewarded when those whom they have empowered succeed.

Transformational leadership has been the focus of a great deal of attention in recent years, and is helpful in understanding the ways whereby CNSs achieve success in influencing others. Transformational leaders relate individually to employees, are perceived as charismatic, and, through intellectual stimulation, help employees see opportunities in challenge. Medley (1987) demonstrates that the higher the transformational scores of CNSs, the higher the job satisfaction among staff nurses who work with them.

The complexity of and wide variance in CNS role implementation, makes it desirable to examine "snapshots" of the work of several real CNSs to gain a clearer understanding of this advanced practice role. In the next section of this chapter, thus, several actual CNS practices are described; comments and analysis regarding the ways whereby each CNS implemented the CNS role are also provided.

CNS PRACTICE MODELS

The practices of the five CNSs highlighted in the following vignettes illustrate the richness and variety afforded by the CNS role.

 Second-Generation CNS in a Hospital Setting

Marie is an ANA-certified, medical-surgical CNS whose clinical background includes medical-surgical and oncology nursing, as well in experience in nursing faculty and nursing management positions. Because of her professional interests and the needs of the institution for which she works, Marie added a certificate in enterostomal therapy to her educational background.

Marie manages a busy caseload of approximately ten to fifteen patients in a large, urban, medical center setting. Managing this caseload means identifying those individuals who could benefit from her services. She accomplishes this through referrals from nurses, attending and resident house staff physicians, nurse managers, and, occasionally, risk management. Care of these patients and families includes assessing needs and providing direct care (e.g., hands-on management of ostomies, draining wounds, pressure ulcers, and other difficult wounds). She also works with the staff to develop plans of care, and then acts as a resource to them as they provide the direct care. Because of the nature of her client population, Marie's clinical role requires her to practice on medical-surgical units, pediatrics units, in neonatal care, in pediatric and adult critical care, in psychiatric care, and in the emergency room. The operating rooms and recovery room also occasionally require Marie's expertise. And call from the x-ray Department is not at all unusual.

Marie's practice also encompases a busy outpatient wound clinic, which grew directly out of the need to organize the delivery of care to a growing number of outpatients having open wounds. Marie's ability to recognize the need for such services, rally an interdisciplinary team, and coordinate the necessary components of beginning a clinic through hospital management are important aspects of her clinical practice.

While her specific area of clinical expertise is ostomies and wounds, Marie's ability to coordinate care and navigate the patient and family through the health care system also requires an understanding of and attention to the overall aspects of the patient's care as it interfaces with multiple systems in the hospital and outpatient setting.

Marie also uses her clinical expertise to evaluate products, carry out clinical trials, and contribute to a variety of committees that deal with clinical issues. Marie's role is characterized by a practice that covers much territory while at the same time focusing on a relatively well-defined set of clinical issues. Because her expertise is highly equipment- and product-dependent, a large portion of her time is spent providing hands-on care. The one-on-one nature of her interactions with patients and families provides excellent opportunities for informal staff education. In addition, Marie's leadership and involvement with committees and quality improvement teams provide important avenues for using her expertise to influence problem-solving at the systems level.

 ## Solving an Important Practice Problem

Carla's clinical specialty is hematology/oncology and bone marrow transplantation. Because her client population is geographically clustered, her practice tends to focus on the care of patients on a single unit. This is not to say, however, that Carla's influence regarding any patient with hematologic or oncologic needs—adult or pediatric, inpatient or outpatient—is limited to that unit. As a frequently used consultant to any unit in her large, urban medical center; as a member of various clinically-oriented committees; and as chairperson of an interdepartmental, problem-solving task force, the influence of Carla's clinical expertise is realized in exponential dimension. The ways whereby her leadership skills and clinical expertise combine beautifully to solve an important clinical problem are illustrated by an example involving timely delivery of blood and blood products to the nursing unit where needed.

Carla, along with a highly professional and clinically competent nursing staff, were long frustrated by the length of time it took for a unit of blood or other blood products to be delivered from the blood bank (which was relatively long distance—several blocks, in fact—from the unit). Carla was encouraged by the administrative and quality-improvement structures to figure out how best to solve this apparently simple but in actuality complex problem. Carla decided that to solve the problem, she needed to convene a group composed of *all* involved persons. Her group consisted of members of the nursing staff, transporters and their supervisors and dispatchers, blood bank employees, and unit clerical personnel.

When the team began work, it took an average of forty minutes from the time of a call for blood to its actual delivery to the unit. Several months and many meetings later, the average delivery time had dropped to twenty-three minutes—almost half of what it had previously been. Carla believes that the face-to-face approach involving all players fostered constructive relationships among the players—in short, it fostered a sense of teamwork. She feels that escorts now better understand the importance of prompt blood delivery as it relates to patients' well-being. Likewise, the nursing and clerical staff learned how their practices may have contributed to the problem when, for instance, an escort was unable to find the nurse to whom to hand the blood. Carla reports that the resultant changes in policy, procedure, and practice resulting from this teamwork have saved time, money, waste, and frustration. These outcomes are both measurable and valuable. The ability of the CNS to persevere toward systems improvements, as did Carla, is an invaluable commodity in a health care system struggling to improve efficiency and provide care in more customer-satisfying ways.

 A CNS Who Moved out of the Hospital

Sandra redesigned her own role when her position as a critical care CNS was eliminated. It was the second time she had lost a CNS position in this way. Sandra accepted a position working with a group of pulmonologists in an outpatient setting, and began developing a caseload of patients who primarily needed her services. That role has evolved so that she sees patients not only in the outpatient setting, but during hospitalizations as well.

How did she adapt her practice as she changed from critical care, the most acute inpatient setting, to an outpatient setting? Her primary focus in critical care was case management of patients having challenging respiratory needs; this is still the case. Her methods in critical care involved patient teaching and helping patients and families cope with health-related issues; she continues to use these methods. Her practice in critical care required a collaborative approach with other disciplines; her current practice does as well. Her experience as an inpatient critical care CNS enables her also to teach patients in the outpatient setting so that they are prepared for the experience of hospitalization.

Sandra's movement to a different practice setting illustrates that the CNS with a strong clinical foundation can identify opportunities and develop roles in previously unidentified settings. As more CNSs leave hospital settings, for whatever reasons, they will undoubtedly apply advanced practice nursing in numerous creative ways. They will continue to carve out practice settings where the public sector, other health providers, and payers will be more easily able to differentiate the advanced practice nurse from other nurses and health professionals. This trend is surely a step in the right direction for establishing the CNS as an autonomous practitioner of nursing.

A CNS Becomes an Independent Consultant

Laura practiced in an urban medical center setting as a surgical CNS and ran a busy enterostomal therapy service. Several successful years into this role, Laura found her services being requested more and more frequently outside the hospital setting and by a variety of "customers," including several long-term care facilities. Laura's expertise in preventing and managing pressure ulcers was a highly visible and highly valued clinical commodity. Upon agreeing to provide isolated services for individual facilities, however, Laura recognized that some facilities were in need of consultation designed to put long-term "fixes" in place. They needed policies, procedures, protocols, equipment and supply selections, ongoing nursing education, and clinical consultation. Laura gradually reduced her affiliation with the medical center, and her private consulting services now account for more than 80% of her work time. Laura is quick to point out, however, that while her consulting services are valued from a variety of perspectives, it is always her reputation for clinical expertise that opens doors and affords her the credibility required to function in the consultant role.

Performing Research as a CNS

Harriet has case managed a population of heart-failure patients for almost twenty years. Administratively, she is not part of the nursing structure in her facility. Rather, she works in a medical department. Her role has always included a significant research component, much of which has been undertaken collaboratively with other members of the health care team. At this writing, Harriet reports that her renown in the area of heart failure has led to an opportunity to participate in research evaluating the effectiveness of advanced practice nurse management of the heart-failure population as compared to traditional management of this population. This opportunity seems especially fitting given Harriet's involvement in structured efforts to strengthen the role of the CNS. Notably, Harriet was instrumental in creating the national ANA Council of Clinical Nurse Specialists, after nurturing her local chapter for several years. She remains extremely active in the advancement of advanced practice nurses, while at the same time continuing her clinical practice.

The Varied Practice Models

The preceding vignettes highlight the variance in CNS role implementation. Make no mistake, however, that the basis for each and every practice model—and for success—is the clinical expertise of each CNS. Remember also that these vignettes focus on only one aspect of each CNS's practice; each CNS also integrates all other CNS role components. Each expresses concern but at the same time recognizes that current changes in health care open a vast expanse of opportunity for nursing, in general, and for advanced practice nurses, in particular. They collectively agree that titles may change, arenas for practice are already changing, and that more change is certain to follow. But each believes that the current essence of CNS practice will continue to exist in some form, because clinical excellence is always valued. Indeed, the advancement of the profession of nursing will hinge on the recognition and value of that which the advanced practice nurse has to offer. The challenges for the short- and long-term future are to maintain high standards for clinical practice; demonstrate a fit between what Americans want from the health care system and what advanced practice nurses provide; and demand that nursing contributions be equitably rewarded.

LEARNING MORE ABOUT A CNS CAREER

Chances are that any nurse considering the CNS role as a career choice has had positive contact with one or more CNSs. Staff nurses who have experienced first-hand the powerful influence of a successful CNS have a head start in truly understanding that which a good CNS does and how a successful CNS operates. Prospective CNSs are advised to create opportunities for contact with CNSs in their personal areas of interest. Staff nurses working in facilities with CNSs should have little difficulty scheduling either interview time or time to spend with a CNS in practice. Pursuing several such opportunities would be the best way for a prospective CNS to see the widely varying ways of implementing CNS roles.

Local chapters of the ANA Council of Advanced Practice Nurses (formerly separate councils of CNSs and nurse practitioners (NPs)) are another resource for finding and learning about local CNSs. Also, because many CNSs choose certification as a means for professional recognition, prospective CNSs can either contact the certification board directly or consult The National Distinguished Service Registry in Nursing (ANA, 1988), which lists by locality and specialty certified nurses in advanced practice.

Graduate schools of nursing that offer CNS tracks are also excellent sources for identifying CNSs practicing in a prospective CNS's area of interest. Graduate schools also will have already arranged preceptorships for their CNS students and can thus cite practicing CNSs who can share information about their practices. Reviewing curricula and requesting syllabi from specific courses allows a prospective CNS to preview course content before enrolling, or helps the prospective CNS in selecting one program over another. Prospective CNSs today are likely to find changing curricula, as schools adjust to health care reform and the trend toward advanced practice preparation rather than separate preparation for CNSs and NPs. The final section of this chapter is directed toward evaluating the CNS role as a career choice.

CNS AS A CAREER CHOICE

The decision to choose the CNS role as a career is not as straight forward as it once might have been. During the 1970s and 1980s, nurses who desired advancement and preferred clinical practice to the management track chose the CNS role, and typically practiced in a hospital setting. Today, in an environment where every role will be involved in revamping the health care system in the United States, there are several variables to consider: (1) The shift of health care out of hospitals will affect the number of traditional CNS roles; (2) CNSs who remain in hospitals will spend increasing amounts of time and effort redesigning systems; (3) CNSs who develop practices in home health, collaborative practice, independent practice, or long-term care will discover uncharted aspects of the role; and (4) As CNS practice shifts out of hospitals, CNSs will face the challenge of working in isolation from one another. Although each CNS in a given setting is typically "one of a kind," there has thus far existed a kinship related to issues, as well as a basis for support and networking among CNSs working under one roof.

In terms of education, an advanced degree is a minimum requirement. Master's-degree programs in nursing vary widely. The prospective graduate student interested in the CNS role as a career choice is advised to "shop" available graduate programs. Along with the practical issues of scheduling, time, money, and location, select a program for one or more of the following four reasons: (1) The program will significantly enhance an area of interest in which the prospective CNS already has expertise; (2) The program will add an area of expertise that the prospective CNS (or a market niche) has identified as necessary for the development of a specialty role; (3) Members of the program faculty are recognized for expertise in an area of interest to the prospective CNS; and/or (4) The program affiliates with facilities that employ recognized clinical experts from whom the prospective CNS can anticipate preceptorship.

It is unrealistic and inadvisable to expect a graduate program alone to enable a complete change of focus. In other words, a nurse whose background includes only psychiatric clinical experience but who wants to become a pediatric CNS should not anticipate that a clinical rotation in pediatrics during her graduate education will be sufficient to make such a switch. This nurse would be well advised to work as a staff nurse in pediatrics for a minimum of one to two years. Although clinical experiences garnered during a graduate program enhance clinical knowledge, these experiences are more likely to be geared toward application of the prospective CNS's clinical knowledge and development of skills that will enable the prospective CNS to understand and practice the subroles of the clinical specialty.

The foundations of the CNS role as a career choice have not changed. A strong background in and commitment to clinical practice remains the most important, non-negotiable characteristic of anyone who is considering the CNS role. The nurse who is considering becoming a CNS would be wise to introspectively evaluate personal preferences. Unless a prospective CNS feels a passion for the clinical arena—whether in a med-surg unit, an operating room, an outpatient clinic, or a patient's home—that prospective CNS is doomed from the outset. In general, it seems that those who fail as CNSs are those for whom the CNS role seemed a "way out" of clinical practice, rather than an opportunity to savor it.

A fondness for and ability to share knowledge is also important. This is not to say that exquisite, formal teaching skills are required; but the willingness to share information as a method of interaction and accomplishment must be present. And for the CNS, patience is definitely a virtue. Recognizing that each patient, each family member, and each nurse requires an individual teaching plan will spare the CNS much frustration. Furthermore, the "students" in the clinical classroom keep changing. The CNS is further advised to remember that the teaching role requires repeating the same information to new audiences of learners. For every caregiver or patient whom the CNS guides to a higher level of expertise, at least one new "student" comes forward needing basic information.

The ability to achieve satisfaction through the accomplishments of others is another characteristic inherent in the CNS role as a career choice. Cheerleaders rarely get carried off the field on the shoulders of the team, although their support and encouragement may have spurred the winning point. So it is with the CNS, whose "behind the scenes" work may go unrecognized by many.

A healthy respect for change and how others feel about change is also important. Not only will future CNSs be involved in managing extrinsic change (such as change related to mergers and reimbursement issues) they will also continue to strategically create change for the sake of implementing research-based knowledge and improving patient-care outcomes. Ironically, this means that CNSs will increasingly redesign their own roles.

Creativity is another desirable attribute in the CNS. It is important to remember that creativity can be developed (von Oech, 1990). Creativity is often little more than a matter of looking at a situation from a different perspective, or applying a simple idea in an unusual way. Brainstorming, using humor in problem-solving, and thinking "what if?" are strategies suggested by von Oech in his creativity primer *A Whack on the Side of the Head.*

Additionally, any nurse contemplating the CNS role as a career choice would be wise to consider both personal and professional needs for support and reward. By design, the CNS role can lead to a feeling of isolation. Because there will typically be only one critical care CNS, and only one med-surg CNS in a given setting, for example, no two CNSs will be doing exactly the same job in any given setting. Peer relationships therefore are limited unless one's personal and professional attitudes are amenable to networking and making use of collegial support, the CNS role can feel very lonely indeed.

Finally, the prospective CNS would be wise to reflect on the type of leadership that he or she personally requires in order to feel supported. Remember that the CNS is often in the unique position of reporting to someone who may be less knowledgeable about fundamental aspects of nursing than is the CNS. This scenario presents a potential challenge for many CNSs, particularly novice CNSs who are establishing and defining roles while being managed and evaluated by less knowledgeable supervisors.

A nurse who is willing to take risks—to do things differently, to suggest the "we-tried-that-once-and-it-didn't-work" approach just one more time, to be sentimental, to break some rules—and, more importantly, to live through the inevitable challenges and potential the failures associated with the CNS role) possesses important characteristics for succeeding as a CNS. After all, the successful CNS lives for the consult that begins, "We've tried everything . . .."

SUMMARY

The CNS role, like other nursing roles, has changed along with the health care environment. Clinical expertise, knowledge regarding creating and managing change, and a desire to continually improve processes and systems characterize the CNS role today . The CNS role remains an excellent career choice for the clinically excellent nurse who wants to both positively influence one-on-one patient-care situations and improve the processes that compose health care systems.

REFERENCES

American Nurses Association (ANA). (1988). *The national distinguished service registry in nursing, incorporating the national registry of certified nurses in advanced practice.* Kansas City, MO: Author.

American Nurses Association (ANA). (1994). *Today's registered nurse—numbers and demographics.* Washington, DC: Author.

Beecroft, P. C. (1991). *Measuring clinical nurse specialist effectiveness. Clinical Nurse Specialist, 5*(4), 179.

Benner, P. (1984). *From novice to expert: Excellence and power in clinical nursing practice.* Menlo Park, CA: Addison-Wesley.

Beyerman, K. (1989). Making a difference: The gerontologic CNS. *Journal of Gerontological Nursing, 15*(5), 36–41.

Boyd, N. J., Stasiowski, S. A., Catoe, P. T., Wells, P. R., Stabl, B. M., Judson, E., Hartman, A. L., & Lander, J. H. (1991). The merit and significance of clinical nurse specialists. *Journal of Nursing Administration, 21*(9), 35–43.

Cason, C. L., & Beck, C. M. (1982). Clinical nurse specialist role development. *Nursing and Health Care, 3*, 25–38.

Chisholm, M. (1991). Use and abuse of power. *Clinical Nurse Specialist, 5*(1), 57.

Cronin, C., & Maklebust, J. (1989). Case-managed care: Capitalizing on the CNS. *Nursing Management, 20*(1), 39–47.

Curtin, L. L. (1990). From captain to quarterback. *Nursing Management, 21*(1), 7–8.

Drucker, P. (1974). *Management: Tasks, responsibilities, practices.* New York: Harper and Row.

Eichelberger, K. M., Fiscus, J., & Talsky, J. (1995). Nurse manager and CNS: One collaborative role. *Nursing Management, 26*(1), 56–57.

Fenton, M. (1985). Identifying competencies of clinical nurse specialists. *Journal of Nursing Administration, 15*, 31–37.

Gift, A. G. (1992). Determining CNS cost effectiveness. *Clinical Nurse Specialist, 6*(2), 89.

Gurka, A. M. (1991). Process and outcome components of clinical nurse specialist consultation. *Dimensions in Critical Care Nursing, 10*, 169–175.

Hamric, A. B. (1989). History and overview of the CNS role. In A. Hamric & J. Spross (Eds.). *The clinical nurse specialist in theory and practice* (pp. 1–18). Philadelphia: Saunders.

Hodgeman, E. (1983). The CNS as researcher. In A. Hamric & J. Spross (Eds.), *The clinical nurse specialist in theory and practice* (pp. 1–18). Philadelphia: Saunders.

Holt, F. M. (1992). Invisible leadership. *Clinical Nurse Specialist, 6*(1), 27.

Hotter, A. (1992). The clinical nurse specialist and empowerment: Say goodbye to the fairy godmother. *Nursing Administration Quarterly, 16*, 11–15.

Joel, L. A. (1994). New changes from within. *American Journal of Nursing, 94*(1), 7.

Johnson, D. (1962). Consequences for patients and personnel. *American Journal of Nursing, 5*, 96–100.

Kirk, R. (1992). Total quality management and continuous quality improvement. *Journal of Nursing Administration, 22*(4), 24–31.

Klopp, A. L. (1990, April). The clinical nurse specialist and research: Putting research into your daily practice. Symposium for clinical nurse specialists, sponsored by the Cook County Graduate School of Medicine, Chicago, Illinois.

Leherr, M. A., & Gift, A. G. (1990). Utilization pattern of clinical nurse specialists in the Baltimore-Washington area. *Clinical Nurse Specialist, 4*(4), 196–199.

Medley, F. (1987). Transformational leaders and job satisfaction of staff nurses. *Florida Nursing Review, 18*, 33–34.

Meisler, N., & Midyette, P. (1994). CNS to case manager: Broadening the scope. *Nursing Management, 25*(11), 44–46.

Moore, S. (1993). Promoting advanced nursing practice. *AACN Clinical Issues in Critical Care Nursing, 4*, 603–608.

Notter, L. (1971). Empirical research in nursing. *Nursing Research, 20*, 79.

Papenhausen, J. L., & Beecroft, P. C. (1990). Specialization vis-a-vis the clinical nurse specialist. *Clinical Nurse Specialist, 4*(2), 61.

Robichaud, A. M., & Hamric, A. (1986). Time documentation of clinical nurse specialist activities. *Journal of Nursing Administration, 16*, 31–36.

Schaefer, K. M. (1991). Taking care of the caretakers: A partial examination of clinical nurse specialist practice. *Journal of Advanced Nursing, 16*, 270–276.

Scholfeldt, R. (1974). Cooperative nursing investigations: A role for everyone. *Nursing Research, 23*, 452–456.

Schull, D. E., Tosch, P., & Wood, M. (1992). Clinical nurse specialists as collaborative care managers. *Nursing Management, 23*(3), 30–33.

Shawler, C., Steppler, H., & Kinnaird, S. W. (1990). Model for integration of CNS with nursing management and staff development. *Clinical Nurse Specialist, 4*(2), 98–102.

Sneed, N. V. (1991). Power: Its use and potential for misuse by nurse consultants. *Clinical Nurse Specialist, 5*(4), 58–62.

Sparacino, P. S. (1991). Expert clinical practice: The cornerstone of CNS practice. *Clinical Nurse Specialist, 5*(1), 11.

Tarsitano, B. J., Brophy, E. B., & Snyder, D. J. (1986). A demystification of the clinical nurse specialist role: Perceptions of clinical nurse specialists and nurse administrators. *Journal of Nursing Education, 25*(1), 4–9.

Tonges, M. C., & Madden, M. J. (1993). Running the vicious cycle backward and other solutions to nursing problems. *Journal of Nursing Administration, 23*, 39–44.

von Oech, R. (1990). *A whack on the side of the head: How you can be more creative.* New York: Warner Books.

Wyers, M. E., Grove, S. K., & Pasterino, C. (1985). Clinical nurse specialist: In search of the right role. *Nursing and Health Care, 4*, 203–207.

Wolf, G. A. (1990). Clinical nurse specialists: The second generation. *Journal of Nursing Administration, 20*(5), 7–8.

Chapter Ten

The Nurse-Manager-to-Executive Track

Elizabeth J. Falter

INTRODUCTION

As the coordinator of the Institute for Nurse Executives for the Lienhard School of Nursing at Pace University in New York for ten consecutive years, this author can make you a promise: nurses who pursue the executive track will have unprecedented opportunities to influence the direction of health care and set the course for health care provider organizations in the future. This is definitely not a mission for the faint of heart or for those who want "nursing only." Rather, it is about embracing change, thriving on chaos, and committing to a vision. It is about possessing the desire to lead all health care professionals to high-quality, fully integrated health care systems.

Today, American institutions of all kinds are undergoing change on a scale never before seen. Evidence of such change can be found in virtually every hospital in the United States. Managed care is forcing hospitals and other health care institutions to become as effective and efficient as possible. If this has not already affected your institution and your career, it will very soon. If you are a nurse manager contemplating a management career and the executive track, pursuing this goal will not only alter your current expectations, but will dramatically change your future as well. For some, it will be a difficult experience. For others, it will be an opportunity to move further and faster along the executive track than ever imagined.

Before proceeding, it is important to clarify two key terms: nurse management and executive track. These terms represent a continuum rather than two alternatives. Those who pursue the executive track very likely will have a succession of management positions, beginning with assistant head nurse moving through director of nursing and to vice president for nursing. The executive track should not be viewed as an alternative to nursing; it is not pursued "instead of nursing." Rather, it involves exercising authority and accepting responsibility for activities beyond nursing and at the highest levels in the health care organization.

Barriers that have long existed are fast disappearing. Growing numbers of nurse executives are breaking the "glass ceiling" described by Jolene Tornabeni, herself an RN, Administrator of Fairfax Hospital, and Senior Vice President of Inova Health System (Tornabeni, 1995, p. 30). Some nurses are becoming chief executive officers, chief operating officers, vice presidents for patient care services, and, even, Vice President for National and International Health Care practice in a large consulting firm. Some of the most notable successes in the health care industry have been spearheaded by executives who are nurses. Why? Because nursing still remains the art and science most closely tied to the core competency of health care: patient care.

Are you a staff nurse who is considering or presently working in your first management position? Are you a student who enjoys seeing "the big picture" of health care and the way that nursing fits into that picture? Do you enjoy organizing and leading groups? Do you feel challenged and exhilarated by change? Do you get pleasure out of helping someone else succeed? Do you enjoy working with nurses and other professionals as much as with your patients? Do you thrive on chaos? If so, management and the new "empowerment" may be the track for you.

This chapter outlines three subjects related to the pursuit of a career in management:

- changes in management competencies
- self-assessment for the management track
- seven tips to a successful management career

CHANGES IN MANAGEMENT COMPETENCIES

Like many other industries in the United States, the health care industry has experienced profound change in the way business is conducted.

Traditional approaches have proven inadequate in an environment of new structures requiring new core competencies. Entirely new skills are necessary to function effectively in this new environment.

Traditional Management Practices in Health Care Industry

What are termed *traditional management practices* in the health care industry are not significantly different from those in large, private-sector firms. Over an extended period of time, management practices that were successful in private industries were gradually adopted by their counterparts in health care, notably hospitals. In many small communities, the local hospital very often had a role in the economic life of the community very similar to that of a private corporation. It was the largest institution and the largest employer. Even in large urban centers, hospitals are frequently among the top two or three employers. By virtue of their size and complexity, hospitals have, with the support of their trustees, tended to adopt for their use the tried-and-true management structures of private industry.

It is not surprising, then, that the traditional management structure of a hospital resembles very closely that of the traditional corporation. Devised in the 1950s and 1960s, managerial authority (or, as some then called it, "power") had the following characteristics: (1) administrative, (2) conformist, (3) hierarchical (i.e., chain of command), (4) stable, (5) introspective, and (6) apprenticeship (Dilenschneider, 1992). These characteristics were evident throughout the hospital and particularly in nursing departments, serving as clear reflection of the environment in which hospitals found themselves. The culture of the entire country, in fact, reflected stability, conformity, and introspection. Authority was respected throughout. All careers began on the bottom rung and in the form of an apprenticeship. The key to success was to learn from your supervisor and pass it along to those who would apprentice to you.

During the post World War II years, technology as we currently understand it was in its infancy. Compared to their present-day counterparts, the hospitals of the 1950s were low on technology. The focus was hands-on patient care. It was a labor-intensive environment and, like many other occupational settings dominated by women, it was a low-wage environment. Hospitals in the 1950s were able to provide consistently high-quality care at low cost, due principally to the large number of professional, dedicated RNs. The responsibility of the nurse manager in this environment was to focus entirely on the unit and the welfare of the patient.

With few exceptions, this basic management structure has remained in place until the present, although significant modifications have been made to accommodate the changing hospital environment. Reflecting the increased numbers of college-educated BSNs entering the workforce, management practices have been modified in a positive direction. Apprenticeship, for example, has given way to mentoring. Rather than requiring a rigid and highly detailed indoctrination in patient-care practices on the unit, the focus has shifted to developing a more open, supportive, and consultative role between manager and subordinate. Greater attention is given to guidance, and individual initiative is viewed favorably.

As increasing numbers of nurse managers secured advanced degrees, their ranges of activities and interests increased beyond the purely administrative. Reevaluating internal procedures, initiating quality-improvement activities, and developing the talents of their nurses became increasingly important. What had been administrative authority, thus, became management authority. Policies and procedures were still to be followed, but they were also to be reevaluated. Yet, the basic management structure remained in place because there was no apparent fundamental shift in what society demanded from its health care system or in the costs associated with that system.

The Realities of the Reengineered Environment

It has become increasingly clear that many of the traditional concepts of management and management structure operate at cross purposes to the current needs of health care institutions. Where there was once stability and introspection, there is now radical change accompanied by the need to look outside the bounds of individual responsibility. The pace of technological advance is accelerating and with it, the cost of acquiring that technology. Identifying that which must change is the very antithesis of conformity. True change initiatives cannot survive the hierarchical management structure. There are too many impediments to success. The change process requires more than most managers themselves can provide. Change requires leadership. A leader must possess vision and the ability to step outside the current boundaries and visualize an entirely new and different process that goes to the heart of the cost/quality issue.

In one sense, methods of communication highlight the deficiencies in the traditional management model. Traditional management communication practice may be best characterized by the passing of a physical document—e.g., a report—from hand to hand. This represented the accomplishment of administrative tasks, whether or not a tangible outcome was achieved. The passing of the document through the hierarchy rather than the purpose for which the document or report was originally written tended to become the focus of concern. The process itself was slow and cumbersome, as befitted the document.

Contrast that with information technology, in which there is no document and no limit to the number of individuals who can simultaneously receive the information. The document itself may not be tangible, but may instead reside only in computers. Finally, the document can be altered or deleted entirely with a single key stroke. The document is no longer the focus of the process.

Rather, its content and the desired results are the focus. There are no limits or boundaries to what information in this form can do. Modern information technology, then, will play a key role in the evolution of the new management skills and practices required to meet the current challenges to the health care system.

The New Core Management Competencies

Reengineering is the most dramatic expression of the total-quality movement. The goal of the process in almost every case is to create a more customer-responsive organization. Fewer layers and further-empowered management teams reduce response time and increase customer satisfaction. Whatever you call the process, the underlying principles will dramatically change how things are done. To date, successful efforts have been led by nurses and physicians, resulting in the establishment of core competencies in health care. Current position titles are being changed and new ones created based on these core competencies. The title "nurse executive," for example, has been challenged and replaced by the broader and more functionally descriptive "vice president for patient-care services." More significantly, new and expanded career paths are emerging for nurse practitioners (NPs), case managers, and nurse midwives (CNMs). The broader perspectives of these new careers, coupled with advanced degrees in business administration or public health, are clearly preparation for the executive track.

At a recent presentation to the Institute for Nurse Executives, Katherine Vestal (1995), Vice President for Health Care Practice for the Hay Group, identified twelve important management competencies for the future:

- analytical thinking
- achievement orientation
- self-confidence
- interpersonal sensitivity
- initiative
- strategic innovation
- facilitation of others
- group management
- influence strategy utilization
- direct persuasion
- development of others
- fiscal responsibility

Success in the new environment will require the ability to look outward, beyond the boundaries of one's own experience and to the experiences of others. More than ever before, a new set of management competencies will be required to work effectively in a team environment. The manager as team leader will see personal skills and attributes become core managerial competencies. Analytical thinking, combined with initiative and an achievement orientation will provide the framework in which the team will operate. The direction will be determined by strategic innovation, which may come from any member of the team but which the manager must recognize and make his or her own.

Not only will more be asked of the nurse manager in terms of output, but the complexity of the health care organization will very likely increase significantly. Nurse managers will have to manage an increasingly broader array of technically skilled RNs, as well as a greater proportion of less skilled staff. Further, they will rely more heavily on other areas of the institution (e.g., pharmacy and rehabilitation) to provide a significant share of patient care. Instilling a sense of cooperation and team focus will be critical to achieving overall success and will require greater reliance on group skills such as facilitation and influence strategies. Nurse managers will become coaches to the team, addressing each member as an individual and working with each to achieve the greatest possible output and personal growth.

As noted earlier, the executive track is an extension of the management track. All of the managerial competencies previously described continue to apply. What differs is the scope and scale of activities at the executive level. It is an environment where the impact of every decision is magnified by the number of individuals who will have to execute it. The big picture, or larger view, must always be kept in mind. The short-term and long-term implications must be reconciled. Strategic planning becomes a paramount concern, whether the subject is new services, facilities, or personnel assignments. Authority increases, but so, too, does personal responsibility and visibility. Those to whom executives are personally responsible include not only senior management, but also trustees and regulators. Interpersonal skills of the highest order are required to negotiate the crosscurrents of opinions. Ultimately, the most challenging task may well be communication—communicating your vision to those who work for you and to those whose support you need in order to succeed.

Acquiring the Necessary Skills

The dramatic changes thus far discussed will be disconcerting to many who either currently hold, or aspire to hold, nurse management positions. For many others, however, new organizational structures, responsibilities, and skill requirements will offer something very significant. For perhaps the first time ever, nurses will be able to consider pursuing more than one career path. By virtue of the traditional management organization and the "glass ceiling," nurses have historically been confined to a narrow, well-defined career path. The only way up was through the well-worn path of unit nurse, charge nurse, evening supervisor, day supervisor, assistant head nurse, head nurse, multiple levels of assistant director, and vice president. Because professional options were for the most part limited, career advancement depended less on individual abilities than on seniority. Positions generally were available only upon the retirement of incumbents. Given the general lack of mobility among nursing staffs, it was typically years before individuals could hope to achieve their goals. Education acquired early in a career was very often lost, and the criteria for advancement was familiarity with existing procedures. Traditional management structures and attitudes were constantly reinforced. Professional focus was on twenty-four-hour patient care in a hospital setting.

Three Opportunities for Professional Growth

One by-product of the review and overhaul of the health care delivery system is a dramatic expansion of the career options for nurses. Opportunities exist not only in the traditional hospital environment, but in many outside settings as well. Michael J. Hammer, author of best-sellers on reengineering the corporation, sees three separate career paths emerging in the new, reengineered environment. One such path is designed as a transitional role for managers who have progressed through traditional management positions (Hammer, 1994).

The first of these paths, the transitional role for traditional managers, involves taking on new responsibility as a coach. Hammer suggests that this "means taking a group of professionals, mentoring them, advising them, coaching them, educating them and developing them." It entails passing on one's own expertise to others so as to accelerate the change process.

The second emerging career path is for managers who become completely involved in the reengineering process on a continuing basis. These managers will be responsible for change in the health care organization.

The third path is that of specialist. It will be populated not only by traditional managers reverting back to their technical competency bases, but also by those who elect to build their careers around clinical specialties.

SELF-ASSESSMENT FOR THE MANAGEMENT TRACK

How do you know whether you want to pursue a management career path? First of all, the decision is not made day one on the unit. The decision to follow a path toward management evolves over time and should be based on a thorough and honest evaluation of personal strengths and weaknesses. Success in the new environment will depend on possessing core competencies, in terms both of personal and interpersonal skills.

The foundation for success in management will lie in the development of key individual competencies. Technical competency and the ability to understand and perform detailed analyses will remain critical, particularly in the health care field. In fact, Professor Stephen M. Shortell recently criticized health care executives as not having a "sufficient understanding of clinical processes" (Shortell, 1994, p. 12). Although the nurse typically has sufficient knowledge of clinical processes, the nurse executive will require knowledge beyond that related to nursing. The issue that each nurse must address in contemplating a career is the choice between a technical path (e.g., NP, Clinical Nurse Specialist (CNS), etc.) and a managerial one. It is important to emphasize that the executive track is knowledge based, just as is the technical path.

The future will be process-oriented and will thus require personal skills of a high order. Proficiency will demand not only a broad base of knowledge, but also critical- and conceptual-thinking skills—and all in a process-oriented environment. The focus will be on the way tasks are accomplished rather than on the qualities of the individual asked to do the job or the particular organizational structure within which the individual operates. This is a dynamic process and quite different from the static structure characteristic of traditional management approaches. Process analysis is the only means of overcoming the limitations of organizations and individual players. Process analysis, therefore, attaches greater value to individual initiative, to flexibility, and to self-control.

Before deciding to pursue a management career path, it is thus important to engage in a critical assessment of both your personal and interpersonal skills. To do so, you must first engage in a conversation with yourself and then seek the advice and counsel of others. Examine your career to date, and specifically, those experiences that will give you an indication of your future potential as a manager. Have you performed any duties or assumed any responsibilities that give you insight into your managerial potential? Along personal lines, you must to evaluate what excites and motivates you in pursuing your career. What do you like doing? Do you prefer playing on the field or coaching the team? Are you willing to coach a quarterback who makes more money than you do? (Some clinical specialists make more money than do some managers.) Have you ever wanted to come to work and reorganize everything on Monday morning? Do you like being in charge? Do you like to manage projects? Do you like politics? Do you like to step back and say, "what are we all about? What should we be all about?" The answers to such questions help define who you are and what motivates you to pursue your career and succeed as a manager.

There are, however, another group of questions you must ask yourself with respect to working with others. Do you gain pleasure from helping colleagues succeed? Do you enjoy other people? Do you enjoy going to a meeting to negotiate? Do you value communicating with others? Do you like bringing others together? Are you open and flexible in your approach to others? These and similar questions, are those that you must ask yourself in evaluating your potential as a manager.

The Educational Process

The educational process comes only after a thorough self-assessment of core competencies—those required skills that you possess and those that you must acquire. The self-assessment of core competencies should drive your decision regarding pursuit of an advanced degree. This is the same decision process being made by neophyte managers in the corporate world. For example, should I secure an advanced technical degree—say in computer science or mechanical engineering? Or should I pursue a nontechnical, advanced degree—say a Master of Business Administration or a Master of Public Health or Administration? Or should I pursue a combination of both? This may be the biggest decision you will make.

Furthermore, there is considerable disagreement among nurse leaders on this very issue. For now, you should look at trends in both your community and the places where you want to work. The traditional advice has been to focus exclusively on advanced nursing degrees, both at the master and doctoral levels. For a career that will include a significant academic commitment, doctoral preparation is a requirement for advancement. In fact, the professional practice models require a leader who is a doctorally prepared nurse.

If you know that you want to pursue a career in a health care institution, it would be wise to give serious consideration to an increasingly common alternative; the MBA/MPA. This combination of a master's degree in business administration and a master's degree in public administration, being offered by more and more graduate nursing programs as a joint degree, is intended to focus attention on a broader range of management issues. One-half of the degree program focuses on management practices common to the private sector, which are more closely attuned to the quality/cost issue by virtue of the profit orientation of this sector. It is important to note, however, that a literal application of these ideas and principles to the public and nonprofit sectors is impossible, because services offered by hospitals, foundations, and other similar organizations are bound by responsibilities beyond the profit motive. What is required, and what these programs seek to accomplish, is a broad synthesis of the two—the cost effectiveness of for-profit organizations and the public-service orientation of not-for-profit institutions. Some schools instead offer a combination MSN/MBA with a public health focus.

Joint MBA/MPA programs are still in the development phase. Not surprisingly, you may find that the curriculum itself varies among institutions. Of one thing you can be quite certain, however; the number of courses focusing entirely on nursing and nursing-related issues will account for less than one-half of the program, and may account for as little as one-quarter. For example, Harriet R. Feldman, RN, PhD, and Dean of Lienhard School of Nursing at Pace University, suggests that an MPA/MBA with a concentration in nursing management might including the following requirements:

- organization theory
- management of public and nonprofit organizations
- budgeting and financial management
- public policy analysis and formulation
- human resources management

- quantitative methods in decision making
- management information systems
- strategic management in health-delivery systems
- fiscal management of the nursing organization
- ethical and legal issues in nursing management
- managing change in nursing service
- the culture of nursing management

Of the twelve courses in a program of this type, only four refer to nursing in their titles; thus a full 75% of the courses focus on areas other than nursing. That is not to say that these courses are not relevant to nurse managers, however. These courses address the issues of organizations, management theory, finance, information systems, and decision making from a perspective that applies to all forms of organizations, both corporate and public. Even those courses that refer to nursing issues in their titles are very likely to have a broader focus in a joint curricula. The broader perspective required of nurse mangers in the current environment is clearly reinforced in such joint programs.

Becoming familiar, and even comfortable, with ideas and approaches associated with other interests in our society—whether those interests be for-profit or not-for-profit—will obviously have a positive impact on an individual's approach to resolving problems and issues upon return to the hospital or other institutional setting. Furthermore, personal contacts made while attending classes common to the MBA and MPA/MBA programs will provide a network of resources for the future.

What is learned and the way in which it is learned must reflect the reality of the daily work environment, which is becoming increasingly complex and interdisciplinary. Everything done on behalf of patients involves many other areas besides nursing. In order to do their jobs, nurse managers must thus understand not only what others do, but also the constraints under which others operate. Education for the future must take the same approach. An interdisciplinary approach to education reflects the reality of a managerial career. Health care reform is forcing administrators to be much more business focused. An interdisciplinary approach offers not only exposure to other perspectives regarding day-to-day issues, but also preparation for that point in the future when, as a senior executive of an institution, you will have the opportunity to work closely with others who may hold their own perspectives, as trustees or fund-raisers. The sooner in your career that you can establish a rapport with the broadest possible spectrum of managers in other areas, the sooner you will be able to develop innovative solutions to the issues you will confront as a manager.

SEVEN TIPS FOR A SUCCESSFUL MANAGEMENT CAREER

The change train is in the station, and it is up to each individual to make the decision whether or not to get on. The conductor has made the last call, and further delay is not possible. No matter where you are in your career, there are things you can do and steps you can take to make sure you are on your preferred car. Although the specific steps you take depend on where your are in your personal life and your career, there are actions that you—and everyone—can take now to prepare for the future. Following are seven steps that nurses can take to advance themselves after they have completed their self-assessments.

Familiarize Yourself with Career Opportunities

Make it a part of your weekly routine to survey the health care sections of your local newspapers and survey professional magazines for employment opportunities. Do not look for jobs resembling your current position, but for those that might be your next position and maybe the position after that—in other words, jobs that could compose your desired career. Where are the management positions? What are the related requirements, experience, education, are the skills required related just to nursing, or do they reflect a mix? If a mix of skills is required, how will you go about acquiring the needed skills? Pay particular attention to health care providers in managed care networks. Who are they hiring? What skills are they seeking? This is the most innovative edge of the health care industry, particularly of the private component. Managed care providers will be looking for the nurse managers with the most advanced form of academic credentialing, the joint MPA/MBA or the PhD.

If you are already on the management track in your institution, you still must inquire. Is there succession management planning, a process that identifies high-potential individuals and tracks their careers? If so, investigate getting on the list or determine which positions are included in succession planning.

Love Learning and Ask the Right Questions

It is a widely accepted theory that most people will have several major course corrections during their careers. Prepare for that likelihood by becoming an enthusiastic learner. Engage in self-learning as broadly as possible. Periodicals like the *Journal of Nursing Administration* and *Nurse Manager* are valuable guides to management practices. You can write to the American Organization of Nurse Executives (AONE) about joining their Association for Nurse Managers. The address is 840 North Lake Shore Drive, Chicago, Illinois, 60611. Also read the *Wall Street Journal* or *Fortune* magazine.

Investigate the graduate programs in your area. What programs have been added or are growing rapidly? Is the program near you increasing its NP program while decreasing its other administrative programs? That should signal something to you. Does your local graduate program offer the joint MPA/MBA degree? If so, you may want to inquire about not only the requirements and curriculum, but also who is hiring the graduates. The best way to determine whether you like something is try it on for size. A management career is no exception. There are any number of opportunities to take management courses while deciding whether to make a commitment to the management track.

Most professional conferences have one or more sessions on management issues and practices. Make sure you attend at least one such session. Determine which supervisory and management courses are offered by your training department. Finally, see what is available at local colleges and universities. If you can gain admission to a management course in the business school, so much the better. Not only will you gain immediate benefits from the experience, including an expanded network of contacts, you will also gain insight into your future.

Variety in experience will give you much more than knowledge. No one individual can ever possess all of the knowledge required to do one's own job, let along everyone else's. And at the very top levels of management, in fact, just the opposite often is necessary. As Jolene Tornabeni notes, "The real key to my success, I believe, has been not in coming up with all the answers, but in asking the right questions. By asking questions, an executive is able to identify the problem, then envision a process by which to move the organization toward the desired outcomes" (Tornabeni, 1995, p. 34). The goal should always be to ask the right questions.

Coach Someone

As noted earlier, coaching will be a desirable management skill in the reengineered workplace (Hammer, 1994). Whether you are currently in or aspire a management position to, you can get a head start by going out of your way to help your peers. Competition is out, and teamwork is in. As mentioned previously, the current environment requires the accomplishment of more while using less. This means that all players must contribute to their maximum abilities, a goal that simply cannot be accomplished in a traditional environment characterized by control, both of individuals and information.

The alternative is empowerment. Empowerment means giving others the authority and required information so that others can do the job. The result invariably is of a higher quality and may even be innovative and cost efficient, as well. People are empowered by coaches, not cops. Coaches impart information and instructions and then leave it to the individual to perform the task. The sharing of knowledge and offering of assistance can occur at all levels and among all personnel.

Seek Out a Mentor

In the traditional environment, where career opportunities for nurses were fewer and the career path was well defined and well-trodden, the view of the horizon was quite clear. It was quite easy to see where you were headed, and you knew that you had plenty of time to navigate your way. In the current environment, however, career options are greater as well as more fluid. Looking at an organization from the bottom up, it is difficult to comprehend the range of opportunities that might be available now, within the next year, or within the next five years. What is needed is perspective. A mentor can provide not only perspective, but, very often, a road map as well. A mentor, quite simply, is an individual who is interested in you and your career and is willing and able to help you. As Jolene Tornabeni observes, "I was fortunate . . . to have such a mentor, who demonstrated the qualities of leadership I most admired, who recognized my potential, and who encouraged (at times even coerced) me to stretch beyond what I thought were my capabilities" (Tornabeni, 1995, p. 31). For this reason, it is unlikely that your boss will double as your mentor.

Finding a mentor is not easy, partly because the relationship requires personal chemistry. Quite often, a mentor is not a part of your organization. Having a mentor is not a substitute for performance as you proceed along your career path. Rather, a mentor provides advice and counsel, and helps you avoid fruitless effort and dead-end positions. In a constantly changing environment, both of these things can happen with discomforting frequency. It is important to remember that the idea of mentoring is well established in the corporate world. Individuals with whom you have a close personal relationship and who are in a position to provide perspective and guidance will generally be happy to do so. It is up to you to ask them.

Practice Being a Leader

The best time to start practicing being a leader is at the first opportunity that presents itself. The earlier the better. Management *concepts* are learned from a book; management *skills* are learned on the job. At every opportunity, volunteer to participate on or, better yet, lead a team. If you are a participant, make sure that you are visible. Make a solid contribution at every meeting. There are many opportunities for taking a leadership position: as a charge nurse, as a team leader on a task force, or when leading a team such as patient care, professional practice, quality improvement, or rewards and recognition. The best teams are those that are multidisciplinary. You will learn by doing and be well-prepared to handle increasing responsibilities as those opportunities arise.

People too often overlook opportunities to develop skills in risk-free environments—their own communities. There are any number of opportunities to volunteer in a community whether for a church, school, or civic organization. This kind of volunteer work affords a way of testing and developing your management skills and more importantly, of determining whether or not you like management—whether or not it is "for" you. Being active in a professional organization also can expand your knowledge, as well as your network of personal contacts.

Interview the Vice President of Human Resources

Management has to do—first and last—with people. Talk to your human resources staff about their jobs and their perspectives on the organization. These perspectives will most certainly differ from your own. Learn about the technical side of human resources: job descriptions, hiring practices, and benefit plans. Perhaps your organization uses assessment tools in the hiring and skills-evaluation processes. You can investigate tests such as the Strong Inventory, Myers-Briggs, and Stress Endurance. Compare the competencies noted in the job description for a manager to those noted in job descriptions for staff. Better yet, ask whether you can have a copy of an assessment tool—and ask your friends/peers for feedback on yourself!

Understand Yourself First

Understanding yourself ties into the self-assessment process described earlier. In his book *The Seven Habits of Highly Effective People*, Steven Covey (1990) talks about understanding ourselves. He observes that before we can enter the public arena, we must prepare ourselves with "private victories" (p. 63). The most important principle of personal management, he says, is to "put first things first" (Covey, 1990, p. 145). Ordering our priorities is so important, in fact, that Covey was compelled to write another book, entitled *First Things First* (1994). Both books are worth your time. What is most important to you? Consider the kind of balance you want in your life. Although many executives have families, management careers are very demanding in terms of time and other sacrifices. Management is not a 9:00-to-5:00 responsibility. Your work week may be upwards of 50 to 60 hours on a regular basis. Is this something you are willing to do?

Perhaps the greatest challenge that confronts managers amidst change is coming to terms with their own limitations and getting beyond those limitations. How can you prepare yourself to handle situations that you have never before confronted, and to do so with energy and confidence? Some people prepare on the athletic field. There are other similar means of developing not only the physical stamina, but also the mental and emotional stamina required to survive the chaos of change. Do something that you have never done before and that will challenge all of your senses: climb a mountain, learn to scuba dive, ride a horse, run a marathon, ride the rapids in a kayak, participate in an Outward Bound program, sing in public, or remodel a house. What you do is less important than that it be challenging and unrelated to nursing. While there is much to be gained from any such experience, Jay Conger suggests one benefit associated in particular with outdoor-adventure activities: "They . . . empower participants through experiences that teach them to take responsibility for their situations—rather than blame problems on the job or outside influences or events" (Conger, 1992, p. 46). Is there any more useful attitude in surviving change?

And, one last recommendation: have fun! Until you are in the throes of change, you will never truly learn the therapeutic value of a sense of humor. Quite often, it is humor that breaks down the barriers that seem impervious to logic.

SUMMARY

If you think you can make a difference in health care by leading, and if you are willing to invest the required time, effort, and commitment, you are definitely needed in management. Nursing will play a major role in the health care systems of the future. It is not enough, however, to like management and nursing. You must also be interested in leading, motivating, and influencing. As a nurse, you have already successfully dealt with the challenges of technology and human nature within the confines of delivering patient care. As a manager pursuing the executive track, you will be asked to do the same for the entire organization. You will bring a unique set of skills and experiences to the senior management team in your organization. The most valuable of these will be humaneness. You must not forget—and must not allow anyone else to forget—that the focus of health care is the patient. Humaneness, incorporated in management's philosophy at the highest level, will become a true mark of excellence in the health care environment of the twenty-first century.

REFERENCES

Conger, J. A. (1992). *Learning to lead*. San Francisco: Jossey-Bass Publishers.

Covey, S. R. (1990). *The seven habits of highly effective people*. New York: Simon & Schuster, Inc.

Covey, S. R. (1994). *First things first*. New York: Simon & Schuster, Inc.

Dent, H. (1995). *Job shock*. New York: St. Martin's Press.

Dilenshneider, R. L. (1992). *A briefing for leaders*. New York: Harper Collins Publishers.

Feldman, H. R. (1994). *Preparing the nurse executive of the future*. Presentation to the Ninth Annual Institute for Nurse Executives, White Plains, New York.

Hammer, M. (1994, Fall) Reengineering . . . blasting away the old rules of business and work—an interview. *Wyatt Communicator*. Washington, DC

Shortell, S. M. (1994, August 5). Are today's hospital CEOs prepared to lead networks? *Hospitals & Health Networks, 68*(15), 12–15.

Tornabeni, J. (1995) Shake the kaleidoscope: One woman's response to gender-related barriers in health care management. *Nursing Administration Quarterly, 19*(2), 30–34.

Vestal, Katherine. (1995) *Towards a new definition of leadership: executive competencies for the year 2000*. Presentation to the Tenth Annual Institute for Nurse Executives, White Plains, New York.

Chapter Eleven

Home Health Care

Benne Druckenmiller and Margaret Hadley

INTRODUCTION

Ten years ago, this chapter would not have been included in a book about new opportunities for nurses. But, much has changed in that time period. Specifically, the home health care market has grown—and continues to grow—rapidly. The current home care market is estimated at $20 billion, up from $3 to $5 billion in 1986. Growth estimates for the next decade range from 10% to 12% annually. This growth can be seen in all segments of the home health care market. Medicare, for instance, which pays for the health insurance of the fastest-increasing segment of our population, has seen an increase of 135% in the number of visits made to Medicare recipients from 1986 to 1992. The number of Medicare-certified home health agencies has grown from 4,258 in 1983 to over 6,000 today. (Lerman & Linne, 1993). Ten years ago, home health expenditures accounted for approximately 5% of the Medicare budget; today, that figure is closer to 12%.

THE GROWTH OF HOME HEALTH CARE

Continuing growth in home health care will result in many opportunities for nurses. You can take greater advantage of these opportunities if you understand the trends influencing this growth. The growth in home health care can be attributed to several factors, particularly, changes in Medicare, technological advances, payer and patient satisfaction, managed care, and continuity of care.

Changes in Medicare

The Medicare Prospective Payment System was instituted in the mid-1980s as a cost containment tool. It dramatically reduced the average length of stay in acute care hospitals—not only for Medicare patients, but also for those covered by other third-party payers—and has kept hospital-based costs from increasing as rapidly as they might otherwise have. Although patients were staying in the hospital for shorter and shorter periods of time (average length of stay is now fewer than seven days), however, the need for care did not change. The program thus merely shifted the burden of care to the patient, family members, and/or other paid caregivers. Home health care's growth was a natural response to the change in acute care reimbursement and to cost containment efforts.

Technological Developments

New, computer age technology has also been a factor in the growth of home health care. Miniaturization and computerization have made possible the administration of many high-tech procedures at home. Patients who used to stay in an acute care hospital for several weeks for intravenous antibiotics or chemotherapy, for instance, can now be treated safely at home. Sophisticated fetal monitors, Kangaroo pumps, peritoneal and hemodialysis machines, ventilators, and cardiac monitoring systems have all made it more feasible for certain patients to be treated at home for conditions that would otherwise have required hospitalization.

Payer and Patient Satisfaction

Third-party providers and consumers alike are highly satisfied with home health care. Providers are able to demonstrate cost savings. While consumers of home health care have traditionally been extremely satisfied with home health services, patients in acute care hospitals or skilled nursing facilities have often complained about those environments. Unappealing food, noisy hallways, sleepless nights, and seemingly long waits for answers to call bells are just a few of the irritations that can be avoided when a patient is provided care for at home. Other sometimes more serious problems are minimized as well. For example, nosocomial infections and, medication and treatment errors can occur when a number of patients occupy one nursing unit. These "adverse side effects" of institutionalization can be avoided in the home setting. Furthermore, patients and families are often more relaxed, feel more in control, and participate more in care when that care is provided at home. Finally, client and family teaching and learning can take place in an atmosphere and at a rate most appropriate for the situation. Rather than having to transfer learning to the home environment, patients and families learn needed skills and information in the setting where they will use that learning. Not all disease conditions and recuperative periods can be managed in the home environment. But home health care permits many patients to enjoy the advantages of the home setting.

Managed Care

Insurance benefit packages and managed care have made expanded home health care coverage available to a larger segment of the nonMedicare market at the same time that the absolute number of Medicare-eligible recipients is growing. That segment of the population that is 65 years of age or older has increased in the last ten years and will continue to increase well into the next century and as the baby boomer generation ages. Thus, just when more services and procedures are able to be provided in the home, there are more patients in need of those services and procedures.

Continuity of Care

As medical care has become more sophisticated, it has also become more fragmented. One patient may be seen by several physicians, and in several different care settings. This has led to a need for ensuring continuity of care and to an emphasis on home health care as a means of integrating hospital and community-based care, concepts incorporated into both the *Medicare Conditions of Participation* (the regulations under which Medicare-certified agencies operate) and the *Joint Commission for Accreditation of Health care Organizations (JCAHO) Standards for Home Health Care Accreditation.* These will continue to be important components of any care system, putting home health care at the center rather than the periphery of such systems. And home health care nurses have traditionally been the agents of continuity of care.

The preceding trends have led to the explosive growth in home health care over the last ten years. At the same time that home health has grown, the need for acute care beds has decreased. For the first time in over thirty years, hospitals are closing units and downsizing. Nurses are thus finding themselves without the wide array of hospital-based job choices available just a short time ago. In fact, new nursing graduates are finding it difficult to find jobs in some hospitals. Home health care is an attractive alternative for many nurses. Certainly, as the field has grown, so has the need for highly skilled, talented employees who can function in an ever-expanding range of roles.

DIFFERENCES BETWEEN HOSPITAL AND HOME CARE NURSING

Every aspect of nursing offers certain attractions to professionals wanting to work in specialty areas. Why would a nurse choose home health care, and what are some of the fundamental differences between home health care and other settings? Nurses who choose home health care do so because they enjoy working in the community instead of an institution. There is more community involvement and socialization. For example, shift report may be given at the dining room table, where the patient and caregivers are waiting to learn how to carry out the plan of care until the next nursing visit. Home health nurses get to know community members from neighborhood pharmacists to clergy, and are resourceful in finding the only podiatrist or dentist in town who makes house calls. These nurses understand the intimacy of a family's home, functioning as invited guests rather than as gatekeepers in the unfamiliar setting of a hospital.

The Home Environment

A former ER nurse was initially attracted to home care for its flexibility. She soon recognized, however, that she was a guest in the patient's home. "I had less control, more of a need to establish rapport. So much of my work revolves around teaching, especially as patients are coming home sooner from the hospital, and so much more sick."

Armed with the latest technology and gadgets—from beepers, car phones, and laptop computers to glucometers and pulse oximeters—these nurses brave the inclement weather, rough neighborhoods, traffic, and snarling dogs to make a difference in the lives of the patients and caregivers depending on them. There is thus a greater sense of autonomy, as well as of self-direction, among these nurses.

The aroma of a favorite stew simmering on the stove in a patient's home, contrasts pleasantly with the odors of a hospital. The whoosh of an oxygen concentrator competes with, but does not eliminate, the familiar sounds of home. The home care nurse in the living room is able to make the patient the center of attention for as long as the nurse is there. The nurse is free from interruption by other call buttons, loudspeakers, and room pagers, not to mention the patient in the next bed who has a problem at the same time.

Assessment and Improvisation

Home health care nurses are masters at assessment. They often must quickly pick up on subtle changes in a patient's health status in order to avoid a major crisis, and they often must do so without the benefit of a stat x-ray, telemetry units, or the assistance of other nurses and health care workers on-site. They troubleshoot when IV settings are askew, keep current regarding the latest skin care products, and know where to purchase food thickeners for people with swallowing difficulties. They improvise catheter clamps, crush pills with rolling pins, and use egg cartons to organize medications. They make sure circuits are not overloaded when the latest in medical technology is plugged in at home. They also help determine which other disciplines can benefit the patient's recovery and help hasten desired outcomes. Home care nurses thus operate under a broader definition of health care than do their colleagues in the hospital. And they face the need to improvise more frequently. One staff nurse who made the transition to home health after twelve years in hospital nursing puts it this way: "The biggest difference that I have noticed in home care is that the routine is gone. The supplies you have to work with are whatever you happen to have brought in your car. I have used a bag of frozen vegetables for a cold pack" (Healy, 1995, p. 6).

Work Schedule

The closer-to-normal working hours offered by home health care can be drawing cards for nurses looking to escape sometimes exacting hospital schedules. Usual hours are on weekdays, with occasional on-call, weekend, and holiday hours. With the demand for home health care ever-increasing, however, flexibility within that framework is the rule. A staff nurse who works with hospice home health, for example, explains, "Home care is a commitment—it doesn't recognize time frames like 7:00 to 3:00 or 3:00 to 11:00. You can expect calls at any time, and you may need to quickly modify your schedule to visit a patient with unexpected concerns or problems. Quick turnaround can divert ER visits and hospitalizations. The nurse's visit is often the determining factor when the physician changes medications or starts a PCA (patient-controlled analgesia) pump. It's a lot of responsibility, but it's also gratifying to know you have made a difference in that patient's quality of life and that you can be there when they need you." Thus, while these nurses have more independence with regard to time management, they is also must be flexible when it comes to their work schedules.

Technology

Although improvisation and adaptability remain cornerstones in home health care nursing, there have been significant advances in the level of sophistication reached by the industry. The home care nurse is driven to keep up with the technology; if it came out yesterday, it can probably be used in the home today. Today, patients can receive care at home that at one time could be provided only in the hospital. For example, home phototherapy units now allow jaundiced newborns to be discharged along with their mothers. Related education is provided by home care nurses, and babies no longer have to be re-hospitalized for high bilirubin levels. And feeding pumps are now widely used in the home for gastrostomy tube feedings. Other services that can now be offered in the home include apnea monitoring, respiratory care, IV therapy (such as for hydration), chemotherapy, antibiotic therapy, and pain management. As technology continues to improve, more services will be added to this already broad array. High-tech services indeed constitute an integral part of home care.

One RN who is an IV infusion specialist recalls a case involving TPN (total parenteral nutrition) infusion, where adaptability met high tech in the home: "The family needed to be taught how to administer TPN through a central line—all in the home. Nobody in the family had a high school education. They were lovely but unsophisticated people. We had to translate verbiage from high-tech to simple, everyday language that anybody in the home could read. I also taped instructions for those who learned more easily by listening. Then it dawned on me that there were teenagers in the house. I incorporated the use of the teenage grandchildren. In five minutes, they were able to demonstrate to me and to the family how to program and use the feeding pump. Unknowingly, they acted as interpreters. That is the beauty of home health" (Healy, 1995, p. 5).

Interdisciplinary Collaboration

There are many other challenges for nurses in home health care. In particular, multidisciplinary interactions are integral to the delivery of care in the home setting. Nurses thus not only must be self-directed, but they also must be able to collaborate with physicians and multidisciplinary team members. Home health care offers a wide array of services ranging from skilled nursing to assistance with activities of daily living as provided by a home health aide to physical, occupational, and speech therapy. The nurse must identify what the patient needs based on functional limitations in such areas as feeding, grooming, dressing, bathing and toileting. The nurse also must determine when interventions can be safely and effectively performed only by a therapist. Is the patient's mobility at risk, as evidenced by decreased strength, pain and contractures, need for assistive devices, or difficulties in coordination? Are there communication deficits such as swallowing difficulty and expressive or receptive aphasia? Are there safety concerns such as frequent falling, impaired balance, environmental hazards, loss of sensation, or infection? The home care nurse may either coordinate with members of other required disciplines at the initiation of service or first discuss with the physician why the patient will benefit from multidisciplinary intervention. Medical social services also are often needed. Many patients experience social problems (i.e., economic, marital, environmental, and other difficulties) that are or are expected to be impediments to effective treatment. The medical social worker is essential in providing direct interventions to assist in patient adjustment, including referring the patient to community resources.

Communication

The best home health care nurses are those who can communicate well, partly because the patient, physician, and home health agency are separated by distance. Home health nurses must thus maintain open communication channels to effect the plan of care and coordinate the services of the multidisciplinary team. Home health care nurses also find themselves working with people who have unique convictions and ways of doing things. Good communication fosters effective working relationships with patients and caregivers despite differences.

Because it is less expensive for the patient to receive multiple services in the home, hospital stays are now shorter. At times, discharge occurs even before it can be determined whether a new medication or treatment modality will help the patient. Patients and caregivers receive less preparation regarding how to best function upon returning home. In the patient's home, the home care nurse can observe and actively address any aspects of the patient's home environment that may have initially contributed to the patient's problems, rather than relying solely on the patient's description of the home setting and situation.

Autonomy and Flexibility

Leaving the institutional setting to work in the patient's home affords certain freedoms in practice. Although the physician is just a phone call away, the plan of care and number of visits are frequently adjusted by the home health nurse. These nurses set up their own daily and weekly schedules, adding patients to their caseloads as requested and adjusting their schedules accordingly. As indicated previously, improvisation with regard to supplies, equipment, or therapies in the home setting is necessary and requires flexibility and creative problem-solving. Home health care does not take place in a controlled environment.

Documentation

The focus of documentation in home health care is influenced by Medicare guidelines and is quite different from that in the institutional setting. Accurate, precise documentation reflects the quality of patient care, validates the need for services rendered, and serves as a basis for reimbursement by Medicare and other insurers. Home care nurses are often concerned about getting insurance companies to approve continued visits when a patient has just started on a new medication or has an unexpected change in condition.

The nurse's understanding of insurance regulations, thus, affects patient care. Home care nurses assume a major part of the responsibility for understanding insurance reimbursement.

Ongoing Learning

The role of the home health care nurse comprises elements that are clearly outside those of the traditional nursing role. Confidence and competence are essential in order for the home care nurse to work well in a variety of home environments. Because home health nurses function with a high degree of independence, their influence over the quality of patient care is significant. Patients in home care are viewed in the context of their households. Home care nurses thus assess not only the patient's health care needs, but also the social, economic, and environmental factors that may affect care.

Because home care is so different from traditional nursing, a good orientation program for new home care nurses is essential. It is important that you receive an adequate orientation for a long enough period of time. Be sure the agency is committed to the orientation process. The agency should also have standardized policies and procedures, including protocols for teaching and a documentation philosophy based on regulations and grounded in the process of care delivery. Continuous quality improvement (CQI) should be an ongoing policy grounded in the viewpoint that no matter what you're doing, you can always do it better. Finally, the agency should encourage ongoing inservice training or education beyond minimal requirements.

ROLES AND VARIATIONS IN HOME HEALTH NURSING

What is it like for nurses to work in home health care? The answer to this question depends on several factors, including the size and location of the agency, whether the agency is for-profit or not-for-profit, and which roles are available to nurses within the agency.

Agency Size

Home health care agencies range in size from those managing several thousand visits per year to those managing hundreds of thousands of visits per year. Working in a small agency offers some advantages to the nurse just starting in home care. For example, because many smaller agencies do not have the budgets to support a wide variety of workers, the majority of nurses employed by these agencies often perform many different tasks or see many different types of patients. Such experience can be extremely valuable. For instance, an agency that is too small to hire its own enterostomal therapy (ET) nurse will expect all of its nurses to become proficient in ostomy and wound care. Any nurse who has the initiative can become that agency's "expert" in wound care. This can, in turn, lead to educational, consultative, and even speaking opportunities that might not be available in a larger organization, where roles often are already highly differentiated. Supervisory and management experience can also be obtained in smaller agencies. An agency that is too small to have a quality improvement department, for example, will expect its entire staff to participate in quality improvement activities. Or the smaller agency may have no intake nurse, in which case anyone answering the phone will be expected to help out. If you enjoy public relations, you may be asked to promote a smaller agency by speaking before a local church group or dropping off some brochures when visiting your own doctor. For a nurse interested in learning many different aspects of the home health care business and willing to take some initiative, then, the lack of highly structured, differentiated organization characteristic of a small agency can provide many opportunities for training, professional growth, and development.

On the other hand, for those who prefer and excel in a structured environment, larger agencies have much to offer. Larger agencies are more likely to offer a broader range of benefits to staff, such as educational materials and opportunities, clinical expertise, supervisory expertise, role models, greater specialization, and better benefit packages. Furthermore, large agencies often have different branches, corporate offices, or other sites of business, which may offer an advantage in regard to moving up the career ladder.

Nature of the Community

Home health care, of course, grew out of community nursing; and the type of community in which a home health care agency is located will affect the experience of any nurse working for that agency. Nurses who work in rural agencies, for example, do much more driving than do those who work in urban areas. (They are also more likely to provide care to relations, acquaintances, or acquaintances of acquaintances!) Working in an urban setting makes it easier for a nurse to maintain the required productivity because of the shorter driving times associated with caring for several patients in a small geographic area. For instance, one nurse may have several patients in a high-rise for senior citizens. Safety, however, has become an issue for some nurses working in urban areas. Most home health agencies have addressed the realities of urban life by sending nurses in teams or with escorts, when deemed necessary. The rewards of caring for often very needy, inner-city residents can be great, however.

Ownership of the Agency

Although not often factored into career-path decisions, the ownership of a home health agency does sometimes influence the nursing practice of the agency. Although it is difficult to generalize, several observations might be useful to consider. Following are brief overviews of the major ownership categories of home health agencies as categorized by the National Association of Home Care (NAHC).

Visiting Nurse Associations (VNAs). VNAs are freestanding, voluntary, non-profit organizations, each governed by a board of directors and usually financed by tax-deductible contributions in addition to earnings. Contributions and grants often allow VNAs to provide care to indigent populations and to provide services that are not always covered by third-party reimbursement. Recently, however, many large VNAs have been bought by national companies and managed like any large business. During a job interview with any VNA, therefore, ask questions to clarify ownership of the agency.

Public. Public agencies are government agencies operated by a state, county, city, or other unit of local government and have a major responsibility for preventing disease and providing community health education. Although such agencies provide care for which the costs are reimbursable by third-party payers, the focus of care is that of the more traditional community health model. Many of these agencies are in rural areas, where they are the only providers of home health services in the area.

Proprietary. Proprietary agencies are freestanding, for-profit businesses. Some of them have very high standards of care and are leaders in the field, however, their emphasis is business. They tend to be in urban and suburban areas having population densities high enough to support many agencies within the given area. These agencies can provide wonderful opportunities for nurses who are interested in both learning more about managing a business and becoming more entrepreneurial in their approaches providing care. It should be noted, however, that charity care is minimal.

Private, Not-for-Profit. Private, not-for-profit agencies are freestanding and privately developed, governed, and owned. As not-for-profit agencies they offer charity care, develop programs funded by grants, and often contract with local governmental agencies to provide services to specified needy populations. They also provide care under third-party reimbursement mechanisms.

Hospital-Based. Hospital-based agencies are operating units or departments of hospitals. Most are not-for-profit. Hospital-based agencies often provide desirable benefit packages in addition to the other advantages generally associated with being part of a larger organization. However, the management structure of the hospital is often cumbersome to the home health agency. Hospital-based home health care agencies traditionally have had a difficult time because hospital administrators traditionally have known little about home care. This may be changing, however, as home care agencies become more important to the viability of the hospitals that own them. Nature of the community, ownership of the hospital and size of the agency will also affect the corporate culture of an agency. It is important for nurses to understand that these factors can influence the work, experience, and opportunities available to them in home health care.

Home health care also offers a vast array of roles for nurses. As home health has grown, so have the opportunities for professional growth.

The Expert Generalist Skill Set

Traditionally, home health nurses have been expert generalists, meaning they are expert at treating a wide range of conditions and diagnoses. Within the scope of this role, caseloads often are based more on scheduling or geographic considerations than on the type of care needed. Many home health nurses still function this way. These nurses are particularly adept at long-term decubitus ulcer treatment, use of Foley catheters, care of bedbound patients, and care of patients with multiple medication needs or multiple diagnoses. They are comfortable with providing care to patients who will get better as well as those who will not. They may see a patient to change a dressing and at the same time teach diabetic care to that patient. Another patient may need to have pain medications titrated.

As the marketplace changes, the need for more nurses with special training is emerging. Patients are being seen sooner in the course of their illnesses, at the more acute stages. Indeed, some patients never make it to a hospital at all, and are, instead, referred to home care in lieu of hospitalization. Home health agencies are finding it advantageous, therefore, to hire or train nurses who are specialists in different areas of nursing. In the last few years, many new niches in home health care have become available for specialists, including rehabilitation, cardiac, psychiatric, infusion therapy, maternal/child, pediatric, hospice, and wound care, to name just a few. Specialty nurses typically function in several ways. They may be case managers for a group of patients who are predominately in need of specialized care and/or may act as consultants to other staff members on particularly difficult cases. They may also serve as community educators. Agencies have found that specialized programs are important to customers and referral sources alike—that is, that it is both clinically imperative and good business to develop specialized clinical programs within the home health agency.

Roles Other than Direct Care

Many other roles besides direct patient care are available to nurses in home health care. Some of these are discussed following.

Community Education. Most home health agencies of medium to large size have found it useful to employ nurses to provide information about home health care to doctors, discharge planners, and other referral sources. A general lack of understanding regarding home health care exists among many other health care professionals, as well as the general public. Educating the

Community allows agencies to market to the public as well as provide needed information to those in positions to make referrals to agencies.

Hospital Liaison Nurses/Admission Planning. Because many patients are referred to home health care after hospitalization, home care nurses often are responsible for helping the patient make the transition from hospital to home. They thus work with the discharge planning departments of hospitals to ensure that patients are referred appropriately to home care. They also provide information to patients regarding the services offered by the home care agency. Further, they work to obtain in a timely manner get whatever durable medical equipment, supplies, and/or supplementary help will be needed in the home and they make sure that agency nurses have the medical information required to provide the needed continuity of care. Finally, they also work with physicians to develop initial treatment plans for patients referred to home care.

Intake Coordination. Intake coordinator nurses usually work in offices, where they provide the same type of services to patients over the telephone as hospital liaison nurses provide to patients leaving a hospital. They verify that the patient meets home care criteria, and has insurance coverage for the needed services, and they work with the physician to develop an initial treatment plan. This role requires an in-depth understanding of nursing, home care, and business.

Quality Improvement, Risk Management, Utilization Review, and Staff Development. Most nurses are familiar with the functions of quality improvement, risk management, utilization review, and staff development in the hospital setting. Each of these is also needed in the home health agency. Some large agencies have separate staff who function in these roles. Smaller agencies may combine these roles or make these roles part of other job positions.

Information Resources. As home health agencies increasingly turn to the computer for help with the overwhelming amount of documentation required of them, they are finding the need to employ people who understand computers and computer systems. Several highly sophisticated home health care software packages on the market today integrate the various functions needed by all home health agencies (i.e., financial, credit and collections, accounts receivable, payroll) with clinical information, and often provide detailed statistical reporting capability as well. Because of their very complexity, however, these software packages are not always "user friendly." Yet, computers are becoming more important to the industry. Thus, most agencies can no longer function without employing people who have skills in computer systems and programming.

Management and Supervision. Agency management structure is often determined by size, but all agencies need nurses with management and supervisory skills. But one note of caution: it is often impossible to tell from a job title alone exactly what the job will entail. When interviewing for a management or supervisory position, therefore, make sure you obtain a copy of the job description and ask questions to clarify the tasks and responsibilities associated with the job. Also, make sure you understand the authority and responsibility that goes with the job. Because most home health agencies do not follow one general pattern in terms of management structure, job titles used in the industry can be misleading.

THE NURSING PROCESS IN HOME CARE

What is the nursing process in home care? It starts with an initial visit, which encompasses functional, physical, psycho-social, and environmental assessments. Patients typically visited in the home require nursing intervention related to one or more of the following: chronic obstructive pulmonary disease (COPD), congestive heart failure (CHF), autoimmune deficiency syndrome (AIDS), bladder dysfunction, cerebrovascular accidents (CVAs), wound care, cancer, diabetes, or other chronic illnesses. Managing patient care at home thus demands a scientific as well as a caring approach.

Before the first visit, the home care nurse reviews the information on the physician's referral to determine the purpose of the visit. The information collected on the initial visit is used to develop the nursing care plan and provide the physician with further guidelines for the medical plan of treatment. The physical assessment is a major source of information and provides a baseline for future comparison and evaluation. Documentation of the data is standardized. On later visits, it may be necessary to assess only specific problem areas. Information about all prescription and nonprescription medications is gathered as well. The nurse reviews the patient's health history and assesses the patient's and family's capabilities and limitations to manage the care plan at home (e.g., level of knowledge, resources, and functional limitations). The home care nurse also assesses the abilities of the patient and caregiver to meet basic requirements (e.g., rest, elimination, nutrition, and activity) as well as requirements specific to the illness (e.g., diet, dressings, or colostomy care). The nurse must consider questions such as "Is home care the appropriate setting for this patient's treatment?"; "Can necessary procedures be done at home?"; and "What are the patient's problems, needs, requirements, and knowledge deficits?" Other factors influencing home management include age, culture, and psycho-social, socio-economic, and environmental factors. Once the assessment is complete, the nurse develops a nursing diagnosis, nursing plan of care, and medical plan of treatment.

The nursing diagnosis generally identifies specific problems and needs, such as "impaired skin integrity on abdomen due to postop wound infection." A nursing care plan is established that reflects goals and interventions of the home care nurse and other home care professionals. The nurse establishes priorities. She discusses approaches to meet those priorities with the patient, family, and other caregivers. Priorities change as the patient's condition changes. Goals are based on the nursing diagnosis, take into account the patient's perspective, and must be attainable and realistic, for example, "Patient or caregiver will demonstrate correct understanding of universal precautions by next RN visit" or "Will demonstrate good aseptic technique in wound care in two weeks."

After goals are established, the home care nurse works with the patient to identify those interventions, actions, and therapies that will help the patient achieve the goals. The care plan is then implemented. Implementation involves referrals, coordination of services, ongoing assessment, education, and direct care. It is important that the nurse makes sure the patient and caregivers understand the purposes of any other involved disciplines. Specifically, the nurse identifies who will do what and when, for example, "RN to do wound care daily and teach wife procedure"; "Complete bed bath, personal care by home health aide 3x/week"; or "Physical therapy 1-3x/week to improve strength and ensure safe ambulation with walker." The nurse informs the physician of significant assessment findings, makes plans to achieve goals, and obtains the physician's approval for the plan. Client education is fundamental to home care nursing because it is the only way to ensure continuous care after the nurse has left. The patient and caregivers are considered active participants and are thus taught how to recognize problems or changes that need to be reported to the nurse or physician. Careful attention is also paid to documentation. Accurate documentation reflects high-quality client care, validates the need for services, and serves as a basis for reimbursement.

The final step in the nursing process is the evaluation of care, which involves the patient, caregivers, physician, nurse, and multidisciplinary team. The patient's progress, or lack thereof, is evaluated on each visit. Is the plan meeting all of the patient's needs? Is the plan helping the patient reach and maintain his or her highest level of functioning? When goals are met or the patient no longer requires home care, discharge occurs, and the process of home care delivery is complete.

QUALIFICATIONS

As you have probably already concluded, home health care nursing requires special preparation and knowledge. Nurses usually should be educated at the baccalaureate level or have extensive experience in a variety of hospital units including medical-surgical. Home care nursing requires management and organizational skills with an emphasis on critical thinking and decision making. The home care nurse should possess intuitive and advanced assessment skills. Home care requires a high level of technical competence on the part of the generalist as well as the specialist; in short, sound clinical skills are a must. The home care nurse also must be willing to assume responsibility and accountability. Finally, effective communication skills, sound judgment, flexibility, creative problem-solving, and self-direction are additional qualities required in a good home care nurse.

RESOURCES FOR FURTHER INFORMATION

Information about home health care is available from many sources. The National Association for Home Care (NAHC) is one of the largest home care associations. It produces several publications including *Caring* magazine and *Report*, a weekly update on issues related to home care. *Report* also has an employment section, which lists opportunities available throughout the country. NAHC is located at 519 C Street NE, Washington, DC 20002-5809, telephone 202-547-7424. NAHC also offers a national directory of home care agencies.

The Hospice Association of America and the National Hospice Organization (NHO) are both good sources of information about hospice care. The Hospice Association of America is located at the same address as NAHC. NHO is located at 1901 North Moore Street, Arlington, VA 22209, telephone 703-243-5900.

Home Health Care Nurse is a bi-monthly journal focusing on clinical management of home care patients. It is the official journal of the Home Health Care Nurses Association.

Other publications of interest include:

Home Health Care Services Quarterly

Hospital Home Health

Journal of Community Health

Public Health Nursing

American Journal of Nursing

American Journal of Public Health

Finally, a *Statement of the Scope of Home Health Nursing Practice* is available from the ANA at 600 Maryland Avenue, SW, Washington, DC 20024.

SUMMARY

The home health nurse will continue to play an important role in educating and informing members of the community regarding how to effectively manage their health care needs. As home health care continues to evolve, the home health nurse will have a wonderful opportunity to influence and contribute to nursing of the future.

REFERENCES

Healy, K. M. (1995, June 12) Taking home health nursing into the 21st century. *The Nursing Spectrum, 8*(13), 5–7.

Lerman, D., & Linne, E. (1993). *Hospital home care strategic management for integrated care delivery.* Chicago: American Hospital Association.

Chapter Twelve

Occupational Health Nursing, Employee Health Nursing, and Case Management in the Workplace

Dennis Ondrejka

INTRODUCTION

Recent changes in the practice of nursing within the community have introduced new challenges in categorizing the various nursing subspecialties. The concept of practicing in the community as compared to the hospital setting is the first level of differentiation. The nursing specialties discussed in this chapter collectively compose a portion of the group that falls under the community nursing domain: occupational health nursing (OHN), employee health nursing (EHN), and case management (CM). CM, which was discussed in Chapter 7, has historically been a part of the practices of the OHN and EHN. Today, however, CM has become a subspecialty in its own right.

This chapter examines OHN, EHN, and CM for their similarities and differences by exploring the clients they serve, regulatory issues, clinical practice, and administrative structures. The chapter also examines how these subspecialties interrelate, and describes some of the unique skills required in and opportunities afforded by these subspecialties.

TRACING THE SUBSPECIALTIES

The literature and professional organizations supporting these subspecialties can be consulted to begin the process of differentiating the subspecialties. As recently as 1991, for example, the *Journal of the American Association of Occupational Health Nursing*, or *AAOHN Journal*, incorporated employee health services administration in its assessment guide for occupational health nurses (Manchester, Summers, Newell, Gaughran, & DeCourcey-Spitler, 1991). In addition the entire April 1991 issue of the *AAOHN Journal* was dedicated to EHNs working in hospitals. It might be somewhat frustrating for EHNs at this time to be considered as within the domain of the OHN subspecialty because EHNs are well on their way to creating a separate specialization group. The progress toward separation continues despite few differences between the roles of the OHN and the EHN as we know them today. Distinctions are clarified in this chapter as they present themselves.

Both OHN and EHN are within the community health nursing domain, which includes several subspecialties and can be described in terms of practice using the traditional, three-tiered method of primary, secondary, and tertiary clinical levels. CM continues to be part of the OHN and EHN roles, but CM also is becoming a specialty in its own right. Nursing, thus, seems ready to proliferate into subspecialty domains of practice, affording nurses opportunities to explore more practice options, but also demanding more expertise from nurses.

As is evident from Table 12.1, the major feature differentiating community health nursing practices is the clientele served. (This chapter does not address the community health subspecialties of parish nursing, home health care nursing, school nursing, and public health nursing.)

As table 12.1 shows, there is some overlap among the subspecialties with regard to clientele served. This overlap brings some of these subspecialties closer together, which can create challenges when trying to categorize a nurse in one subspecialty versus another. It is very likely that nurses serve in more than one capacity and, thus, can be categorized under two or more subspecialties.

PROFESSIONAL AND CERTIFICATION ASSOCIATIONS

A client-based classification system reveals areas of overlap with regard to the populations served by the community nursing subspecialties, as well as some distinctions between the subspecialties. A powerful influence in creating

Table 12.1 **Domains of Community Health Nursing**

Subspecialty	Client/Clientele Served
Occupational Health Nursing	Blue- and white-collar work forces, specialty clinics focusing on work-related injuries, corporate businesses, industry, some hospital employees
Employee Health Nursing	Hospital and medical-research employees
Case Management	Insurance groups; occupational medicine clinics that treat work-related injuries; specialized private contracting CM groups; internal business insurance departments; all OHN and EHN locations
Parish Nursing	Specific church groups and their congregations
School Nursing	K–12 schools (with an emphasis on students)
Home Care Nursing	Client within the home and needing special nursing care (e.g., continued acute care, rehabilitation, hospice)
Public Health Nursing	One or more members of a family

any subspecialty group is the professional association that constructs standards of practice and, sometimes, certification processes to test the basic knowledge of professionals in that subspecialty. Although some community health subspecialties are very similar in mission as well as population served, a division has recently occurred, with EHNs and CMs creating their own subspecialty organizations. They have done so in order to build collegial relationships and specialization.

The OH Nurse

The professional association for OHNs is called the American Association of Occupational Health Nurses (AAOHN). AAOHN has developed standards of practice, an ethical code, continuing education, and many educational tools for nurses in this field. It preceded the other groups discussed in this chapter and laid much of the foundation for EHNs and CMs.

The AAOHN has its roots in the early 1900s, when the National Organization of Public Health Nursing (NOPHN) established an industrial nursing section in 1920 (Cahall, 1981). Rogers (1994) describes the formation of the American Association of Industrial Nurses (AAIN) around 1922, which involved several factory nursing groups coming together in the United States and Canada.

The AAIN continued to expand in numbers and purpose by adopting bylaws in 1943 and developing a core curriculum outline for various schools by 1944. In the 1950s, AAIN, the American Nurses Association (ANA), the National League of Nursing (NLN), and the Public Health Service (PHS) examined a host of activities related to curriculum and definition of practice. This resulted in assigning the specialty a broader name: "occupational health nursing." In 1977, the AAIN changed its name to AAOHN to reflect this broadening of scope. AAOHN currently has approximately twelve thousand members.

In 1972, AAOHN developed a certification body, the American Board of Occupational Health Nursing, Inc. (ABOHN). ABOHN offers a one-day examination to measure basic competency of any nurse who meets the criteria to take the examination.

The EH Nurse

EHN continues to evolve as a subspecialty. The distinct features of this subspecialty were more formalized in 1982, with the formation of the Association of Hospital Employee Health Professionals (AHEHP). The goals established by the AHEHP centered primarily around communicable infections within the hospital setting and the goals of employee health services (EHS) in hospitals reflect this focus. Hamory (1991) states that the EHS goals are to "reduce the risk of exposure to contagious diseases, reduce work-related injuries, and decrease exposure to toxic exposures such as antineoplastics and asbestos" (p. 5). Harmony goes on to describe the realm of EHS as "preplacement screening, immunizations, annual screenings, evaluation of communicable diseases, and postexposure prophylaxis" (p. 5).

In 1994, the AHEHP changed its name to the Association of Occupational Health Professionals (AOHP), reflecting a broader dimension and direction for EHNs within the hospital and medical-research settings. Current national membership is approximately fifteen hundred, according to an interview with the Colorado chapter president Colleen Casaceli (Personal Communication, March 15, 1995). However, because many nurses who work in the EHN subspecialty do not join AOHP, this number does not accurately reflect the number of nurses actually working in this subspecialty.

Massante (1995, p. 24) reclarifies the primary goals of EHS as:
- preventing and treating work-related diseases and injuries,
- promoting health,
- creating and ensuring a safe work environment, and
- providing CM to control costs of injuries and illnesses.

Massante thus suggests a broader definition of EHN that blurs the line between this subspecialty and that of OHN. The very first conference of EHNs was held in Atlanta, Georgia, in 1982 and was documented by

American Health Consultants (1982) in a collection of program manuscripts. The features differentiating the EHN role from the traditional OHN role become clearer when examining the content of the program. The program included topics on accidental chemical exposure to anesthetic gases and ethylene oxide, as well as on a host of infectious agents including the tuberculosis bacteria, HIV, and nosocomial viruses.

At the conference, Dr. William Valenti emphasized the need for effective employee health programs by affirming: (a) the need for a safe working environment, (b) the need to address the challenges of Workers' Compensation, (c) the need to support the entire work group toward being a productive workforce, and (d) the need to ensure compliance with regulatory demands (American Health Consultants, 1982). By describing such similar goals between the two groups, Dr. Valenti provides another reason to continue considering OHN and EHN as one specialty group.

There is no certification body for the EHNs. The certified occupational health nurse (COHN) certification process established by ABOHN is at present considered the best assessment for this subspecialty of nursing practice. The AOHP is currently exploring the boundaries of EHN practice, including where EHN overlaps with OHN and when it exhibits uniqueness.

The CM

CM was organized in the late 1980s by what is known today as the Case Management Society of America (CMSA), which currently boasts 3,500 members. The process allowing nurses to become certified case managers (CCMs) began in 1992. The CMSA offers a historical perspective of CM tracing back to the turn of the century. Clinicians of that era tried to coordinate the best services for the patient. The CMSA suggests that the current practice of CM was formalized in the early 1970s as a response to Medicaid and Medicare initiatives. Early CMs were little different from any clinicians who provided the best possible services to their clients. When insurance companies and businesses started to capitalize on the nurse's knowledge and understanding of services available, however, CM began to be viewed as a distinct specialty.

The scope of practice and the boundaries of CM extend into a host of settings. Only recently, however, has there been in-depth discussion, development and marketing of CM as a separate nursing specialty.

HISTORICAL INTERRELATIONSHIPS AMONG OHN, EHN, AND CM

A look at the historical development of these three nursing subspecialties provides perspective on their similarities, as well as the differences that led to their establishment as separate specialties.

The Beginning of Industrial Medicine

OHNs trace their history back the farthest of the three subspecialties, to the beginning of industrial medicine in around 400 B.C. Hunter (1978) provides a progressive account of occupational health issues as they developed throughout the world. The adverse affects of lead exposure on miners were first recorded by Hypocrites in 400 B.C. However, it wasn't until the first century A.D. that personal protective equipment was recommended and used. In *Encyclopedia of Natural Science,* Pliny the Elder referred to the use of bladders by "mining refiners" who were trying to protect themselves from breathing cinnabar dust, which contained mercury sulfide. It took another 1,400 years before descriptive assessments were conducted for occupational exposures, however. In 1473, Ulrich Ellenbog recognized the dangers associated with certain metal vapors. He described symptoms of industrial lead and mercury poisoning and suggested preventive measures.

Hunter cites the father of industrial medicine as being Bernardino Ramazzini (1633–1714), giving Ramazzini this honor because he wrote the book *The Diseases of Workmen.* This text discussed one hundred different occupations and their associated hazards through the use of case studies. The question developed by Ramazzini and still used today by all occupational health specialists is, "Of what trade are you?" (Hunter, 1978, p. 37). This question thus marks the start of the diversion of occupational health specialists from other health care clinicians. Rogers describes Ramazzini's work as focusing on the "significance of faulty posture, want of ventilation, unsuitable temperatures, personal cleanliness, and protective clothing" (Rogers, 1994, p. 18). Such insights and concerns now constitute the special realm of industrial hygienists, ergonomists, occupational physicians, safety specialists, and occupational health nurses.

The Beginning of Industrial (Occupational Health) Nursing

Phillipa Flowerdaye has been described as the first industrial, or occupational health nurse. She began her work for the Jeremiah Coleman Company in Norwich, England, in 1878. The company manufactured mustard. The socially conscious wife of Mr. Coleman asked Ms. Flowerdaye to work in the plant from 9:00 a.m. to 12:00 p.m. and then make home visits to the workers to assist with family illnesses and injuries (Hunter, 1978; Rogers, 1994).

Cahall (1981) and Rogers (1994) trace the beginning of OHN in the United States to Betty Moulder who worked with Pennsylvania coal miners in 1888. More is written, however, about Ada Mayo Stewart, who began working for the Vermont Marble Company in 1895. She typically used her bicycle and occasionally used the company horse and buggy to visit the sick and injured in their homes. She provided a variety of nursing care including emergency care, education regarding healthier ways of living, obstetrical care, and pediatric care. Ms. Stewart's records identify few visits for industrial accident treatment and follow-up, however. Her work was therefore more characteristic of public health nursing, but was a service provided by an employer. The true beginnings of OHN may thus be found among the first self-insured benefit programs for workers and their families, which were based on the nurse's roles and practice.

The Beginning of Nurse CM

OHNs have functioned in many industries including hospital settings and have provided CM for decades as a part of their usual practice. The August 1994 *AAOHN Journal*, in fact, was dedicated to the issues and demands of CMs who see themselves as OHNs, thus illustrating the interrelatedness of these two subspecialties.

In the early 1980s, the emerging need to control health care costs caused a dramatic shift in the practice of OHNs who were working for large corporations. Nearly every on-site OHN was providing some level of CM by the mid-1980s, but the CM aspect of the OHN role was poorly defined in terms of special skills and was only one of many subroles played by the OHN. Benefit managers historically were not nurses. In the 1980s, however, a slow influx of nurses to this arena began. Nurses also witnessed a shift in terms of businesses providing more reward and recognition for managing benefits than for providing employee advocacy and client care. Nurses were well prepared to play a greater role in controlling the benefit costs of an organization by virtue of their knowledge regarding benefit plans, employee needs, community resources (those that worked and those that didn't), alternative care strategies, and potential abuse of the system.

Nurses became more notable players in CM because of their increasing role in providing utilization review (UR) and prehospital certification cost-containment strategies. The insurance companies hired nurses as well as physicians for the express purpose of CM. The insurers sought clinicians' expertise in defining the need for hospital admissions and in suggesting alternative treatment strategies and lengths of inpatient stays. This opened the door to case managing any lost-time injury or illness, even when hospitalization did not occur. CM as a nursing subspecialty was born out of the complexity of keeping abreast of clinicians and dealing with treatment plans, lost-time, system abuse, and problems communicating with patients regarding actual care and treatment options.

As evidence of this transition and the formation of new standards of care, consider how the treatments for alcohol addiction and childbirth have changed, specifically with regard to length of stay. In the mid 1970s, the standard alcohol treatment plan called for an inpatient stay of thirty days. Five years later, Case Managers were using fifteen days of inpatient care as a maximum, followed by transfer to outpatient care. The 1990s have seen the standard decrease to three to four days of inpatient detoxification followed by outpatient care. Likewise, the length of stay for vaginal childbirth went from three to four days to twenty-three hours during this same time period. CMs originated these changes, which, in turn became the standards of care as defined by insurance companies. Most utilization standards for inpatient services are automatic, and costs for hospital stays exceeding the standards will not be reimbursed.

The first area of focus for occupational health CMs was Workers' Compensation, especially as companies became self-insured and found they could significantly control costs through CM. Today, however, every illness or injury is case managed by either the actual employer or the insurance company that oversees health benefits for the employer. To facilitate their work, CMs have developed collegial relationships and training conferences that now use broader strategies to reduce costs by preventing and treating illness and injury more generally. Industry and insurance companies also demanded efficient prevention and treatment programs to keep employees safe on the job. These demands have led to the subspecialty of CM as we know it today.

Conflicting priorities greatly challenged nurses who tried to remain clinicians and patient advocates as they continued to develop skills in CM. The CMSA views the CM as the intermediary between the providers of care and the payer. Others are more inclined to view the CM as an advocate for business and cost-containment, and clinicians such as OHNs and EHNs as advocates for the employee. Advocacy can be viewed on a sliding scale and is different for every setting. Within any given setting, however, advocacy can be identified and measured for each specific role. The scale can be used by consultants to determine whether there is desirable division of roles and where conflict might arise when trying to perform multiple roles.

OHN AND EHN

In order to gain a deeper understanding of the OHN and EHN subspecialties, both the similarities and the differences between these subspecialties must be closely examined.

Setting and Program Influences

Both subspecialties involve assessing newly hired employees, a process requiring a variety of skills. A new-hire assessment can include preparing the patient for a physical examination, performing screenings, and performing the actual physical examination. OHN and EHN nurses are expected to understand the current legal implications of these assessments. Most nurses practice in one- or two-nurse units and have a host of job responsibilities. Their practice can be a full blend of medicine and nursing practice and, therefore, often requires using standing orders.

Special Skill Requirements

Simple treatment of a headache can be demanding in terms of one's beliefs about nursing practice and medicine. Such beliefs impact the boundaries of OHN and EHN practice. A typical client visit to an EHN or OHN in either an industrial or hospital setting can provide insight into the special skills needed to practice in these subspecialties.

A Tool and Die Maker Complains of Headache

Jerry is a fifty-four year-old male who works in a plant as a tool and die maker. On one occasion, he visits the plant nurse, complaining of a frontal headache. Jerry states that the pain starts every morning and typically lasts all day, but sometimes goes away at night. Before performing an actual assessment or treating the headache, the nurse first asks Jerry more about the workplace and his work.

Jerry states that his group started a new job four days ago. They had some problems with the degreasing process and had to get some new material to degrease the dies. The nurse, knowing that every new chemical must have a Material Safety Data Sheet (MSDS), calls Jerry's supervisor to obtain the MSDS for the new degreasing material. The nurse then checks Jerry's vital signs, performs a quick eye assessment, and asks some questions about neurological status, such as whether Jerry was experiencing numbness or tingling in the hands or in other parts of his body.

When the MSDS arrives, the nurse reviews the medical section, which states that the degreaser must be used in a well-ventilated area and that it can cause headaches and neurological intoxication symptoms. Recommended treatments are fresh air and elimination of exposure. The nurse makes note of this causation and treatment information, so as to both treat Jerry and protect all other employees at risk.

Jerry's vital signs are blood pressure 150/90, pulse 90, and respirations 20. Jerry states that he usually gets good results with acetaminophen. The nurse gives him 1,000 mg of acetaminophen along with dosage-information for the rest of the day (including to self-administer every 4 to 6 hours, as needed). The nurse then tells Jerry to come back the next day for follow-up. Next, the nurse notifies the safety department and ask Jerry's supervisor to work with the safety department to ensure safe use of the new degreasing chemical in the plant. The nurse also asks Jerry's supervisor to refer any other employees who may be feeling ill. Finally, knowing this to be a mandated Occupational Safety and Health Administration (OSHA) log entry requiring an incident report and investigation documenting what is going on in the work area, the nurse initiates these processes.

Knowledge of potential work etiology and skill in interviewing are critical aspects of the OHN and EHN subspecialties. The language used and knowledge required in gathering needed information is unique to these professionals. For example, these nurses ask clients questions such as, "What is your profession?"; "What do you specifically do?"; and "What do you work with?" Some questions that are likely to challenge the average nurse but that serve to illustrate some of the terminology and knowledge required to function in the OHN or EHN role include, "Do you know what an MSDS is and how to use it?"; "What is a 'First Report of Injury,' and is it the same as an incident report?"; "What needs to be reported on the OSHA 200 log and why?"; "When is an OSHA 101 form needed?"; "What would you do if a safety specialist were unavailable?"; "Do you have general knowledge of toxicology so as to make useful physical assessments related to the use of certain chemicals?"; and "When was the last time you performed reflex assessments and measured pupillary responses for a client with a headache?"

The OHN or EHN nurse is also challenged to practice as an independent practitioner. In the preceding scenario, how much medicine was practiced, according to your own definition of medicine? How confident would you be in providing the care and actions of the nurse in the scenario without the aid of a medical opinion or sophisticated hospital testing? Are you practicing medicine when you dispense over-the-counter (OTC) medications? If not, when does practice move beyond the realm of nursing practice and into the practice of medicine?

EHNs and OHNs must have a host of first-line assessment skills and treatment strategies to be effective in the areas of cost control and early intervention for the employer and workforce. Physicians are becoming less available in the actual workplace, often working instead in centralized clinics or being available for only short periods of time. Standing protocols that straddle the nursing/medicine boundary must be clarified within the directives.

OHN and EHN specialist work entails providing care for foreign bodies in the eyes, chemicals in the eyes and on the skin, second-degree burns, early repetitive-motion injuries, trauma, back sprains, nail hematomas, toxic exposures, needlesticks, viral infections, tuberculosis contamination, and sudden death. When a nurse is not available to provide early intervention, define treatment strategies, and establish prevention programs, the first responder to the incident performs these functions and refers anything that is beyond first aid to the local hospital or clinic. First responders who lack a nurse's judgment skills, however, may make decisions resulting in danger to the employee and/or increased cost of care. Judgment is key to the practice of OHNs and EHNs, as Rogers describes, "the challenging role of the occupational health nurse [places] emphasis on autonomous decision making, independent functioning, health promotion, prevention, analytical and investigative skills, and management of health care services" (Rogers, 1994, p. 34).

For the EHN functioning in the hospital setting, the decision to provide care or refer is compounded because there usually are emergency departments (EDs) or triage areas nearby. The ED's primary mission, however, is to serve the community, and if the ED treats employees, the ED is challenged to comply with regulatory requirements and return-to-work restrictions.

Brown states, "the primary goal of occupational health nursing (employee health nursing) is to assist the worker to attain and maintain optimal physical and psychological functioning" (Brown, 1981, p. 4). Rogers provides a philosophy of occupational health nursing service, stating, "The occupational health service (employee health service) contributes to the safe and healthful work environment through programs aimed at reducing and eliminating work-related hazards and enhancing health promotion. Occupational health services are provided to individual workers and the collective workforce within an environment that considers and meets the needs of a diverse workforce" (Rogers, 1994, p. 34). She further cites the integration of the worker into the family and community. Rogers emphasizes that everyone is a part of the same interconnected system and, therefore, that each part influences the others. The OHN and EHN are also concerned with protecting the worker's ethical and legal rights and with creating communication to enhance the health of all workers and their access to excellent care in the community.

Legal and Regulatory Responsibilities

The EHN and OHN share the same legal and regulatory concerns, for the most part. Both must comply with OSHA requirements. Because the EHN serves employees in a hospital setting, the EHN must also comply with Joint Commission on Accreditation of Health Care Organizations (JCAHO) and state health department requirements. Although complying with OSHA regulations also serves to fulfill JCAHO requirements, the EHN must prepare different documentation for each agency.

Nurses in these subspecialties must know the regulations in order to protect their employers, safeguard the rights of the employees, and prevent costly litigation related to violations. In some cases, the nurse is not the clinician responsible for the actual implementation of these requirements. This creates the additional demand on the nurse to educate management, other clinicians, and risk managers regarding their responsibilities and risks in these areas. Unfortunately in many work settings the nurse is neither placed at a sufficient level of management nor on the right committees to impact this issue directly, making the process even more difficult. Nurses in such settings thus must have both high self-confidence and political savvy to create awareness and change.

Federal compliance concerns fall under four areas and two major federal departments, which are as follows:

1. Equal Employment Opportunity Commission (EEOC)
   1.1. Americans With Disabilities Act (ADA)
   1.2. Title VII Civil Rights Act of 1964 with the amendment of 1972
   1.3. Section 503, Rehabilitation Act of 1973
2. Department of Labor (DOL)
   2.1. OSHA

EEOC. For more than twenty years, the EEOC has been an influential force in the areas of antidiscrimination and affirmative action. Since 1972, the EEOC has been allowed to file class action suits against any employer who discriminates on the basis of race, color, religion, sex, or national origin under Title VII.

In 1973, section 503 of the Rehabilitation Act mandated that most employers include handicapped persons in affirmative action. In 1990, this mandate was expanded and redefined as the ADA. Title I of the ADA prohibits entities from discriminating against a qualified but disabled individual in all aspects of employment. Discrimination as defined under the ADA takes any of the following forms:

1. Limiting, segregating, or classifying a job applicant or employee in a way that adversely affects employment opportunities for the applicant or employee because of his or her disability.

2. Participating in a contractual or other arrangement or relationship that subjects a qualified applicant or employee having a disability to discrimination.

3. Denying employment opportunities to a qualified individual because she or he has a relationship or association with a person who has a disability.

4. Refusing to make reasonable accommodation for the known physical or mental limitations of a qualified applicant or employee with a disability, unless the accommodation would constitute an undue hardship on the business.

5. Using qualification standards, employment tests, or other selection criteria that screen out or tend to screen out individuals with disabilities, unless these measurement methods are job-related and necessary for the business.

6. Failing to use employment tests in the most effective manner to measure actual abilities. Tests must accurately reflect only the job skills and aptitude of an employee or applicant with a disability.

7. Discriminating against an individual because she or he has opposed an employment practice of the employer or filed a complaint, testified, or assisted or participated in an investigation, proceeding, or hearing to enforce provisions of the act (Rogers, 1994, p. 459–460).

The primary impact of the ADA on the practice of EHNs and OHNs relates to new-hire preplacement evaluations and to placement of restricted employees. Past practice was to perform a preemployment physical that tended to be used with bias, specifically, to screen out certain persons even when the potential risks to their successfully performing a job were minimal. Today, preemployment physicals are not acceptable under ADA; postoffer and preplacement examinations, however, are acceptable. After a person has been offered a position, the assessment for the position can be as extensive or as minimal as desired by the employer, as long as the assessment process is consistent. Additional testing or assessment can be performed depending on the various risks identified in the assessment. An offer of employment in a given position can be contingent on completing—as opposed to passing—the new-hire assessment process for that position. The only time a person can be denied employment in the position is when either there exists an eminent risk to health or the new-hire is unable to actually perform the job (EEOC, 1992).

Reasonable accommodation is an issue that applies to new hires as well as current employees. If an employee or new hire needs some job modification, assistive equipment, or relief from nonessential functions of the position, the employer is obligated to make such accommodations, unless doing so would create a hardship for the employer (EEOC, 1992). This is a very demanding issue for the employer, with case law and definitions of hardship based on the size and resources of the parent company both ever increasing.

OHNs and EHNs are equally involved in ensuring compliance with hiring regulations. Although external clinics often are used to perform new-hire examination, internal nursing personnel must monitor the process to ensure that no one is violating the regulations.

DOL. The DOL oversees OSHA, which has many compliance requirements relevant to OHNs and EHNs. For example, there are regulations regarding documenting injuries and illnesses on the OSHA 200 log. Documenting on the OSHA 200 log is accompanied by completing an OSHA 101 form. The OSHA 101 form tracks all work-related diseases and injuries that go beyond first aid or fall into automatic recording categories. In addition, the 29 CFR 1910 regulations cover a host of programs that are typically enacted in work environments. Programs pertinent to OHNs and EHNs include the following:

- hearing conservation programs
- bloodborne pathogen programs
- chemical exposure medical surveillance programs
- ergonomic general duty clause and requirements
- medical equipment management programs
- respirator medical clearance and fit testing programs
- medical resources needed and emergency response team programs
- employee access to medical and exposure records
- drug testing standards for Department of Transportation drivers

Most of these programs require expert understanding of federal regulations. In addition, compliance encompasses clinical practice, education, administrative controls, and engineering controls. Nurses must determine exactly what is expected of them in their respective work environments, because in any given work setting, the nurse may be responsible for only a portion or all of the OSHA-compliance issues. Furthermore, the nurse may be responsible for corporatewide compliance encompassing many locations, states, and countries. OSHA-compliance curriculums are not taught at the associate or baccalaureate nursing level. Thus, nurses usually learn the required skills either in the work environment, or when working at the advanced practice level as OHNs.

State guidelines for Workers' Compensation also impact EHN and OHN practice. Reports must be generated based on state guidelines and sometimes are generated on the same form used for the OSHA 101 compliance. Rules regarding Workers' Compensation vary among states. Some states pay all the costs, and employers pay into the Workers' Compensation fund based on their past records and types of jobs offered. Other states allow employers to be self insured. All programs use some type of CM to control costs and prevent abuse of the system. Employers who have their own OHNs or EHNs typically either require these nurses to integrate CM into their practices or locate CM in a separate department with which the nurses have periodic contact to discuss cases.

Special EHN Regulations. EHNs must address the specific concerns outlined by the JCAHO, state health department, and the United States Department of Health and Human Services (Rogers & Hayes, 1991). These concerns relate to identifying, tracking, and reporting communicable diseases such as tuberculosis, measles, HIV, and any infectious outbreaks. The tuberculosis program is an OSHA-mandated program that is also required by the JCAHO and local state health departments. Because the agencies may ask for differing information, it is necessary to maintain excellent surveillance databases for these programs, unless the nurse is willing to dedicate many hours each year to calculating correct numbers.

Roles and Responsibilities of OHNs and EHNs

Thus far, OHNs and EHNs have been described in terms of the environments in which they practice; priority setting based on the needs of their employers; their clientele; and regulatory concerns. A more in-depth examination of roles and responsibilities is required, however, in order to more fully understand these subspecialties. Both OHN and EHN offer a variety of practice modes depending on the needs and priorities of the employer and the qualifications of the individual nurse.

Diversity in Skills, Settings, and Roles. In general, OHNs and EHNs use the same clinical skills. Among individual nurses, however, clinical skills used on the job can vary greatly based on the nurse's clinical proficiency, academic preparation, certification and currency with regard to professional practice. Nurses in these subspecialties range from new graduates with no generalized experience and no academic training in the subspecialties, to master-prepared clinical nurse specialists who may also be certified nurse practitioners.

Working environments vary as well; from the single-nurse unit with minimal medical support and resources to the multinurse unit with extensive support staff including a full-time physician, x-ray technicians, and separate case managers to the external clinic providing occupational health services to a host of local businesses and employers. OHNs and EHNs may also travel to multiple facilities, taking care of the needs of several smaller sites within the same company; work as consultants for insurance companies; work as, independent consultants, providing services to a host of companies; or, finally, work as federal government occupational nurse specialists educating, regulating or investigating to determine needs and risks within the various work settings. Such diversity in work settings and resources can pose some unique challenges depending on the expertise of the nurse.

OHN and EHN Practice. The role of the nurse as described by Rogers (1994) can fall into one of five categories, and possibly, combinations of these. The first is the clinician/practitioner role, which is more clearly described as primary, secondary, and tertiary clinical practice. The second is administrator, a role that entails handling a host of issues relating to development, management, accountability, and evaluation of that which is being provided within the work environment. The third role is that of educator, a role that exists within the academic setting to provide nurses or nursing students with the knowledge and skills required to perform within these subspecialties. The fourth role is that of researcher, a role that is often tied to the academic setting and that can be pursued as either student or faculty. (Although there are practicing nurses who conduct independent research, this tends to be rare because of the time and skill necessary to perform research.) The fifth and final role is that of consultant. The consultant role demands a broad understanding of what has been, what is, what could be, and how to make a program match the needs of any particular working environment.

Leavell and Clark (1965) were the first to classify clinical care in terms of prevention levels, which are defined as follows: (a) primary prevention, which comprises the clinician's and client's actions to prevent an occurrence of a disease or injury and the use of protective strategies that act as internal or external barriers to a harmful agent; (b) secondary prevention, which comprises early diagnosis and prompt treatment designed to control and limit any disability; and (c) tertiary prevention, which comprises actions that allow for optimum rehabilitation and stabilization of the client at the highest possible level of functioning.

The Leavell and Clark classification method continues to serve as a practical model of subdividing clinical roles and functions within the OHN and EHN subspecialties. Many authors (Davidson, Widtfeldt, & Bey, 1992; Rogers, 1994; Massante, 1995) have discussed the clinical role of the OHN and the EHN. The role can be classified into three levels of prevention equivalent to those of the Leavall and Clark model.

Clinicians in Primary Care. Wellness and health promotion programs make use of health risk analysis (HRA) tools that allow workers to examine a host of health-related areas in which they may be personally at risk. Rogers (1994) identifies fifty-one different HRA tools that are currently used to evaluate personal health risks. After assessing health risks and needs, prevention and health promotion programs are tailored to the needs identified. Common programs include stress management, healthy eating, exercise and fitness, balanced lifestyle, smoking cessation, and parenting skill development.

OHNs and EHNs must also be involved in prevention and surveillance programs to determine potential risks to the workforce. More common in the industrial environment are hearing conservation, biological sample testing, and plant rounds programs. More common in the hospital setting are the tuberculosis screenings using purified protein derivative (PPD); rubella, rubeola, and varicella zoster screenings; and hepatitis B vaccination programs. Equally common in both settings are new-hire examinations, periodic examinations, work station ergonomic assessments, medical clearances for the use of respiratory protection, and provision of other personal protective equipment such as eye shields.

Clinicians in Secondary Care. Clinicians in secondary care provide first aid and advanced treatment for a host of work-related and nonwork-related illnesses and injuries. Common in such practice are steri stripping deep cuts, removing foreign bodies from eyes after straining the eyes, and performing assessments for cumulative trauma disorder. In addition, the typical clinician also must provide care for flu symptoms, colds, allergies, headaches, and chronic-disease maintenance.

Most care, including burn and wound care, is provided in a clean versus a sterile environment. Emergency showers and eye wash stations are used for immediate removal of chemicals. Patient-stabilization equipment and skills are used for serious injuries, including major burns, lacerations, amputations, projectile wounds, and scalping injuries resulting from hair being caught in machines. Stretchers, wheelchairs, oxygen, dressings, and burn blankets are items commonly used in initial treatment and while someone calls an emergency transport service. Rarely available to such clinicians are intravenous setups, advanced cardiac- and life-support equipment, and personnel trained to use such equipment. More commonly available are an EKG machine, trauma bag, and oxygen. An emergency response team is often available to help control the environment, call for an ambulance or paramedic support, and assist with CPR, when needed.

Clinicians in Tertiary Care. Sometimes, an employee is stabilized after a chronic illness or injury and returns to work. In such a case, most workplaces ask the attending physician to provide a release for the employee to return to work. In cases where injury was the disabling problem, workers may be returning with limitations or trying to resume their regular jobs even though they are incapable of performing the work. An inappropriately early return to work can thus be even more problematic than delayed recovery and prolonged time away from the job. It can also be dangerous.

The nurse must obtain medical specialty examinations so as to negate any potential discrepancies regarding the worker's ability to return to work. Such discrepancies may result from the attending physician's advocacy for the patient in conjunction with the patient's description of the work situation. The nurse cannot let the worker return to work without administration of a discriminating examination to measure return-to-work ability. The most significant challenge for the nurse is when the medical evidence differs from the worker's perceptions of personal ability. Some workers, in fact, require additional therapy or training to assist them in becoming more capable of performing their previous work. Effective rehabilitation is benefited by counseling and a supportive work environment.

Burgel and Gliniecki (Munday, Moore, Corey, and Mundy, 1994) suggest that disability behavior is actually prolonged recovery, a learned response that affords a host of secondary gains. They suggest it is valuable to use antidepressants and counseling therapy in treating patients exhibiting this behavior. Brink (Mundy et al., 1994) coined the term Workers' Compensation syndrome, describing it as a power struggle. The dynamic is between the worker who is injured and those who question the pain of the worker and attempt to bring the worker back to work. The worker fears continued suffering related to returning to work too soon and, therefore, tries to avoid returning to work too soon. At the same time, the nurse who is attempting to bring the worker back to work fears that an early return to work will prolong the worker's disability and produce a delayed recovery response that could disable the patient permanently. Significant secondary gains can develop as the injured worker is paid Workers' Compensation, typically at two-thirds full pay, tax free.

Brink suggests that nontraditional therapeutic strategies such as guided imagery and hypnosis are valuable in treating chronic pain syndrome, and he supports family involvement in the rehabilitation process. Mundy et al. (1994) provide a comprehensive review of this subject. They discuss the specifics of the phase of care when drugs and lack of activity contribute to the patient's poor adaptation to chronic pain. As a result of this poor adaptation, the patient remains in pain rather than moving through this stage. This, in turn, affords certain financial, social, and political secondary gains, thus preventing a successful recovery process. The suggested intervention is increased rehabilitation counseling with a trained professional in an effort to bring about effective disability resolution and return the patient to work. One of the most significant issues is when to begin rehabilitation. Mundy et al. (1994) suggest, "It may be more effective to begin the rehabilitation process concurrently with the medical assessment and treatment phase"(p. 382). This approach suggests a new time line for the tertiary phase of prevention, starting in parallel with the secondary phase with the intention of keeping the patient connected to the nurse and the treatment goals.

The demands and the diversity of skills required in primary, secondary, and tertiary clinical care are enormous. The clinician must have excellent communication skills, build a powerful therapeutic relationship, practice counseling skills, understand human motivators, and compliance and rehabilitation theory, and have excellent assessment and treatment skills. The demands are great. Often, a clinician will be more skilled in several of these areas than in others and, thus, turn to community resources for assistance when necessary.

Summary of the Clinical Nurse's Role. One way to determine a decision making process for any nursing situation is to examine the process using a four-quadrant decision tool. In such a tool, the client is on one axis, the clinician on the other. Each must decide whether the current state of treatment is effective and no further care is thus needed or the client is not well and needs further care. This decision process is easy when the clinician and client are in agreement. Problems arise when the two disagree about the client's status. Some clinicians take the position that the client knows best, and, thus, surrender to the client's decision making process. Other clinicians believe that the professional knows best, and, thus create even greater tension between themselves and their clients. The Occupational Health Clinician Decision Making Model in Table 12.2 illustrates strategies for reaching a successful resolution. The different quadrants in the table offer hints for how to build consensus between

Table 12.2 The Occupational Health Clinician Decision Making Model

	Clinician's Data and Judgments	
	OK or Well	Not OK or Not Well
OK or Well	Everyone believes the client is OK and should return to work.	Objective data, possibly including expert opinions, must be increased to rectify significant judgment conflict.
Not OK or Not Well	The client does not believe that he/she is OK. It will take significant objective testing and relationship building to establish consensus. If an expert opinion is to be used, try to pick the expert collaboratively.	For best results, pursue effective care that meets the needs of both the client and the clinician.

Client's Data and Judgments (row axis label)

Source: Used by permission of D. Ondrejka, 1982.

client and clinician regarding what, if anything, is needed. This model also helps to clarify the issues when conflict exists between the clinician and client.

CM IN THE WORKPLACE

The subspecialty of CM, already discussed as a function of OHN and EHN practices, is currently a growing specialty unto itself. As noted in Chapter 7, the demand for CM has been rising, and its uniqueness is beginning to be recognized within nursing.

The Need for the CM Specialty

Rogers (1994) discusses the *USDHHS report No. 91-50212* of 1991 on "Healthy People 2000." This report lists the average costs of many chronic and acute illnesses and injuries affecting Americans. Most of these persons are in the workforce and have insurance that is provided by companies in addition to Workers' Compensation. The report documents staggering costs, for example, the 7 million Americans with coronary artery disease resulting in 500,000 deaths and leading to 284,000 bypass procedures each year at an average cost of $30,000 each. The report lists only those costs related directly to health care and does not include the indirect costs related to loss of expertise and the training of replacement personnel.

Gropper (1983) writes about the corporate movement to confront the dramatic health care costs in industry, which approach 10% of the Gross National Product (GNP). Gropper states that health care costs have become a top priority for most major corporations. In its 1985 corporate report General Motors, for example, cited its 1984 health care bill as $239,000,000 with an additional $456,000,000 in life, disability, and Workers' Compensation costs. The total health care costs to General Motors exceeded the cost of the raw materials it used to make vehicles. Other major companies were facing similar challenges. CM was a natural outgrowth of this problem and an attempt by employers to control costs.

Nan Bertone, director of CM at Montgomery Hospital in Norristown, PA, cites nine axioms to live by while trying to run an effective CM program in the workplace (Stanchfield, 1995, p. 17).

- The CM's role is to ensure provision of quality medical care that is prudent and pertinent to the injury or illness involved.

- Although the "whole" patient must be treated, becoming involved in workplace politics is inappropriate and unwise.

- Workers' Compensation was designed to assist employees injured at work—not to give them unlimited paid vacation.

- The employee's primary responsibility while on Workers' Compensation is to make every effort to improve his or her condition and follow medical treatment recommendations.

- Return to work, however limited, speeds recovery and provides a sense of worth to the majority of patients.
- A small percentage of employees injured at work create a great percentage of the work and cost of Workers' Compensation.
- Creating a nonadversarial atmosphere fosters good will between all parties and is more valuable than dollars spent on promotion.
- Prevention programs are worth the effort in any loss-control situation.
- You can't win them all.

CMs perform time-consuming tasks including preventing the health care system from dropping the client and thereby either delaying recovery or decreasing the chances of an effective recovery. The CM nurse must have special skills in psycho-social-motivational theory so as to engage the client in participating actively in rehabilitation and successful recovery. Achieving these outcomes requires special skills in reducing secondary gains, thus preventing what has been termed *disability syndrome*, or delayed recovery.

The standard of the CMSA (the professional organization for CMs) is for the CM to serve as an advocate for the client. When practicing CM in the workplace, however, the nurse is challenged to advocate for *both* the client and the employer. An effective CM program comprises strategies and actions based on the level of patient advocacy and the level of control employed by the CM. For the workplace, the model assumes that a high level of patient advocacy is consistent with the nurse's responsibility to also advocate for the legitimate interests of the employer. Level of patient advocacy and level of control employed by the CM are inversely related, as illustrated in Table 12.3.

The advocacy scale is used as a framework to help the CM determine which approaches to take regarding particular cases. The scale also helps clarify the CM philosophy. At the -4 level, CMs will follow the lead of the client and will serve strictly as data collectors. At the other extreme, the 4 level, the CM will avoid face-to-face contact with the client and will instead perform the majority of interventions via mail, certified letters, use of private investigators, or confrontive phone calls,—and will usually end up working through

Table 12.3 Advocacy/Control Scale for Case Management Assessment

High Level of Patient Advocacy									Low Level of Patient Advocacy
Low Level of Control Employed by the CM	-4	-3	-2	-1	0	1	2	3	4	High Level of Control Employed by the CM

Developed by Dennis Ondrejka for this project, 1995.

the client's attorney. At the 0 level, the CM will try to maintain a balance between cost-control techniques and the client's needs, with the goal of obtaining desired health care outcomes efficiently and effectively.

It is possible to be at a different place on the advocacy/control continuum depending on the client, but this is a high-risk approach because of the informal network of any organization and how quickly word spreads regarding actions being taken to control claims. The actions taken at each level of the advocacy control scale might be as follows (as defined by this author):

Level Actions

-4 Never question the action desired by the patient, do not set up independent exams, follow only those recommendations of the attending physician's, and document visits and return the patient to work when the patient indicates readiness.

-3 Same as at level -4 with the addition of requesting more information and scheduling the patient for more regular CM visits.

-2 Same as at level -3 with the addition of suggesting more effective care and discussing return to work with restrictions and when the client is ready, and trying to increase objective data for the patient to use in making a decision.

-1 Same as at level -2 with the addition of asking the client's physician for specific information and clarification regarding various questions through the patient, but making no such formal requests.

0 Creating a balance between the treating physician and the company physician via information sharing, suggesting alternative treatment when results are not effective, documenting the case and discussing it at staffing meetings, and scheduling the client for regular visits and updates.

1 Same as at level 0 with the addition of asking for formal documents from the attending physician so as to resolve specific questions, holding staff meetings to offer additional suggestions regarding care, and encouraging the patient to think about returning to work with restrictions.

2 Same as at level 1 with the addition of obtaining independent examinations to determine work ability as measured against a functional standard and then have a return to work assessment with any limitations specified, following up on any missed appointments by calling the patient to discuss the patient's status and treatment plan and to immediately reschedule the missed appointments.

3 Same as at level 2 with the addition of performing highly controlled independent examinations, obtaining a release to examine the attending doctor's records in person and even meeting with the attending physician, and never letting the case go more than one week without a specific action being taken.

4 Same as at level 3 with the addition of hiring private investigators and using video surveillance when fraud is suspected, increasing by phone contact with the patient and possibly contacting the patient only through an attorney, always talking about objective data and facts, confronting the patient regarding any occurrences of fraud, and sending a video of the patient's job to the attending physician and any independent physician who will be examining the patient.

Obtaining a good panel or independent medical evaluation (IME) group is a challenging process, but is critical to a successful CM program. In many states, such a group may include chiropractors and other practitioners of non-traditional medicine. The CM program must comply with state regulations regarding who can perform such examinations and the roles of each of the participants in the process. The prevention aspect comes into play when CM or rehabilitation is started the first day of an injury. Prevention involves having excellent treatment facilities, developing a follow-up schedule, talking to the employee's supervisor within twenty-four hours regarding which return-to-work limitations will work for the department, displaying concern for the patient, being responsive in getting payments to the patient on time, listening more than talking, and visiting the patient in the hospital (if hospitalization occurs) and talking only about the patient's needs. When visiting a patient who has suffered a severe injury, leave your card and send a gift or book focusing on positive attitude. Such actions can produce great results while staying at the 0 level on the advocacy/control scale, but are extremely time consuming.

FUTURE OPPORTUNITIES IN OHN, EHN, AND CM

The descriptions of the subspecialties discussed in this chapter suggest a need for solid clinical skills along with specialized training. These nursing positions are best filled by experienced nurses, but nurses who have minimal experience may also find opportunities to enter these fields.

Nurses with minimal professional experience are less likely to find opportunities in small or single-nurse units in these subspecialties, because of the high level of independence and the skill depth necessary to deal with complex situations. The clinical practice and skill level are unique, broad, and demanding. The nurse must have excellent assessment and counseling skills, and must be self-assured regarding clinical skills. A multinurse unit is the best place for the beginning nurse to gain knowledge and experience in these subspecialties. The multinurse unit affords more support and opportunity to develop these unique and diverse skills over time. Although a group of nurses might work in the unit, each nurse is still required to have a highly independent level of skill and knowledge about diseases, injuries, medical procedures, and CM strategies. It is very unlikely that a nurse could survive in the CM role without having broad-based nursing and health care knowledge.

The general practices of OHNs and EHNs offer diverse nursing opportunities and independent practice. Certain past nursing experiences are better suited than others for performing within these roles. An excellent way to move into one of these subspecialties is to float or work part-time with other nurses in the field.

Some settings and employers provide for limited client contact on the part of the nurse, while others heavily emphasize the practitioner component. In some settings, nurses must have expertise in Workers' Compensation, while in other settings, only solid expertise in current medical-surgical nursing and current knowledge of clinical practice standards are necessary. Certain OHN and EHN settings find ER and triage skills valuable. However, ER nurses do not typically provide care to the same type of nonacute patients and/or practice with the diverse clinical independence found in OHN and EHN practice. Also, ER nurses usually use more specialized assessment skills in life-saving and crisis management.

EHNs will continue to operate mostly in single-nurse units and under very heavy caseloads and extensive surveillance programs. They must increase their use of technology in order to become more efficient. OHN continues to struggle, and has in fact seen a drop of membership in the professional association from 19,000 in 1972 to 12,000 in 1994. This drop in number could be the result of the other specialties splitting off or of nurses supporting priorities other than organizational involvement.

OHNs appear to be holding their own, demonstrating steady numbers over the past few years. This author believes that a greater impact can be made by OHNs providing more rehabilitation strategies and continuing to invest in internal CM programs as a way to provide cost benefit for the organization. This will keep the value of the OHN and EHN at the forefront and in step with the trend toward CM.

SUMMARY

OHN, EHN, and CM in the workplace represent important opportunities for nurses, as employers focus attention on health care costs. Insurance companies and health care providers will continue to increase their use of CM in an attempt to control costs and, thereby attract more business. Nurses are playing a vital role in the fast-changing health care marketplace because their unique skills offer immediate financial return to the employer. Nurses filling these subspecialty roles discussed in this chapter must be independent, and must possess broad-based assessment skills and thorough understanding of the work environments in which they provide their professional services.

REFERENCES

American Health Consultants. (1982). *Hospital employee health: Practical solutions to current and potential problems.* Atlanta, GA: Author.

Brown, M. L. (1981). *Occupational health nursing: Principles and practice.* New York: Springer Publishing Company.

Cahall, Jean. (1981). The history of occupational health nursing. *AAOHN Journal, 29*(10), 11–13.

CMSA. (1995). *CMSA's standards of practice.* Little Rock, AR: CMSA Publications.

Davidson, G., Widtfeldt, A., & Bey, J. (1992). On-site occupational health nursing services. *AAOHN Journal, 40*(4), 172–181.

EEOC. (1992). *A technical assistance manual on the employment provisions (Title I) of the Americans with disabilities act* (EEOC-M-1A). Washington D C: Federal Document Publications.

Gropper, D. (1983, July). Cutting the company medical bill. *Institutional Investors, 3,* 130–137

Hamory, B. (1991). Report 1: Employee health fundamentals. *Journal of Hospital Occupational Health, 11*(2), 5–7.

Hunter, D. (1978). *The diseases of occupations* (6th ed.). London: Hadder and Stroughton.

Leavell, H. H., & Clark, E. G. (1965). *Preventive medicine for the doctor and his community* (3rd ed.). New York: McGraw-Hill.

Manchester, J., Summers, V., Newell J., Gaughran B., & DeCourcey-Spitler, D. (1991). Development of an assessment guide for occupational health nurses. *AAOHN Journal, 39*(1), 13–19.

Massante, L. (1995). Employee health department model. *Journal of Hospital Occupational Health, 15*(1), 24–31.

Mundy, R., Moore, S., Corey, J., & Mundy, G. (1994). Disability syndrome: The effects of early vs. delayed rehabilitation intervention. *AAOHN Journal, 42*(8), 379–383.

Rogers, B. (1994). *Occupational health nursing: Concepts and practice.* Philadelphia: W. B. Saunders Company.

Rogers, B., & Hayes, C. (1991). A study of hospital employee health programs. *AAOHN Journal, 39*(4), 157–166.

Stanchfield, K. (1995). Case management and worker's compensation (presented by Nan Bertone). *Journal of Hospital Occupational Health, 15*(1), 17.

United States Department of Health and Human Services (USDHHS). (1991). *Healthy people 2000,* report no. 91-50212. Washington, DC: author.

Chapter Thirteen

Entrepreneurial Nursing

Kay Davis

INTRODUCTION

Nursing has changed. Being a nurse in the 1990s presents a greater variety of opportunity than ever before. Although many people still hold outdated stereotypes of nurses, more and more people are realizing the tremendous diversity and contribution of nursing professionals.

The percentage of nurses working in acute care settings has been decreasing steadily, a trend reflecting the continuing shift from inhospital care to community-based settings. Nurses are recognizing the many different career options available to them, many of which were never discussed in nursing school trends class. One very exciting and challenging option has been named *entrepreneurial nursing*. As you read further, you'll find this to be a very general label, one which seems to group together those nurses who are pursuing their professional practices in very nontraditional ways and one which branches into business in a manner not typical or customary for clinicians.

Entrepreneurial nursing is really not a distinct career, but, rather, a somewhat new manner whereby nurses perform selected roles. In other words, nurses stop working for someone else and choose, instead, to work for themselves. Historically, the overwhelming majority of nurses have been employees. Today, the small percentage of nurses who practice their professions differently, if only by nature of who writes their paychecks, are deemed entrepreneurs. Entrepreneurs practice as self-employed persons or persons in partnership with others. Entrepreneurial nurses work for themselves or with their partners on a fee-for-service or contract basis. Many of these entrepreneurial nurses assume business roles far beyond those presented by nursing schools as aspects of professional expectation.

It is typically after graduating from school and gaining some experience that a vision of entrepreneurial practice develops. Entrepreneurial practice builds on specialized practice and experience. RNs typically discover their skills and interests through their practices. When they then match their skills and interests with marketplace needs and develop independent businesses in response, they arrive as entrepreneurial nurses. Matching perfected skills with consumer needs leads nurses to develop niches—specialized services or products that address the needs and wants of potential customers. Thus, most entrepreneurial nurses primarily practice nursing; but they deliver health care in nontraditional manners. This difference brings them both praise and criticism, as they push the envelope of the paradigm surrounding the word *nurse*.

DEFINING ENTREPRENEURIAL NURSING

Entrepreneur is used as a label for self-employed nurses who are doing either the same thing they did as employees or something unique and revolutionary within the role and definition of nursing, specifically with regard to how they provide health care services or information to people. The term *entrepreneur* thus describes a new vision of professional practice. As more nurses choose the entrepreneurial path, some roles will merge, such as business owner and consultant/practitioner. Several other already common roles such as educator and advanced practice nurse are increasingly moving toward an entrepreneurial work structure.

Downsizing of education departments in many hospitals and the related downsizing of nursing faculty create episodic needs for outside assistance in designing and implementing educational programs. As advanced practice nurses take their places as primary care providers, many will move into the entrepreneurial arena. Not everyone will need or desire to be in entrepreneurial practice. But for many nurses, entrepreneurial practice offers the opportunity to pursue a committed and active practice in nursing as an alternative to leaving the profession because of fatigue, frustration, financial limitations, or boredom.

Identifying just how many nurses are pursuing entrepreneurial nursing practice is difficult for several reasons. One reason is that unlike some roles, the boundaries of entrepreneurial practice are not clear. For example, if a nurse were to implement an innovative program within an organization as an employee *and* assume responsibility for generating revenue to support the program at a break-even or profit-making level, the term *intrapreneur* would best describe the role. Whereas, the intrapreneur relies on the resources and security of the organization, entrepreneurs rely on their own resources and/or those of their partners. Because the overwhelming percentage of nurses are employees, however, intrapreneurial endeavors are not commonly recognized and, thus, often are not counted as such.

There are also numerous examples of overlapping roles. A nurse practitioner (NP) working in private practice, for instance, is certainly counted as an advanced practice nurse but less commonly as an entrepreneur—although managing the business aspects of a private practice in addition to delivering patient care is clearly entrepreneurial. There are also those nurses whose expertise and experience lead them to educational roles, often marketing educational products and services. Nurse educators have developed many businesses including CPR certification agencies, consulting practices in competency assessment and validation, and educational enterprises to prepare nurses at all points along the nursing education continuum—from preparing for the NCLEX examination to preparing for advanced certification. Some offer their services as consultants while remaining employed. Thus, while they are educators, they are also entrepreneurial nurses. Yet other nurses with clinical expertise are increasingly being called to the courtroom and paid as expert witnesses. Some, in fact, have established lucrative businesses for themselves as well as for other nursing experts.

Many successful and established entrepreneurial nurses do not consider themselves as such, partly because basic nursing education does not prepare a nurse for entrepreneurship. Rather, basic education prepares a nurse to enter a practice arena. It is in this arena that the nurse will perfect skills that can lead to entrepreneurial practice.

Some entrepreneurial nurses say they are no longer nurses but, rather, businesspersons. Although their businesses involve health care, and their clinical expertise was essential in forming these businesses, some have found few role models to suggest that linking their current practices to their nursing clinical experience is of any value. This scenario fortunately is changing. As nurses become more comfortable with nontraditional roles and the idea that there is much more to the nursing profession than employment in clinical roles, they will be more likely to establish their credibility as health care businesspersons partly based on their nursing expertise. For example, many nurse attorneys specialize in health care law or medical malpractice. The nursing education and practice of these nurses certainly contributes to their expertise in their current practices.

As any new role evolves, it creates some controversy. The nurse entrepreneur is no exception. Debates abound regarding whether nurses are able to function independently and whether they better serve patients as employees. Such debates are especially prevalent among physicians. As a nurse entrepreneur during nursing shortages, this author has heard administrators blame "nurses like me" for the nursing shortage. I was told that if I'd stop thinking so much about business and get back to the bedside, there wouldn't be a problem. In other words, if I'd just be a nurse, there would be no nursing shortage.

The problem with such an argument rests in the differing perspectives regarding what nurses are and what they do. Providing nursing care at the bedside is not the only way to be a nurse. As our profession struggles with defining roles and practices, misperceptions abound not only among the other disciplines involved in health care, but also within our own ranks. As a profession, nursing has been very reluctant to embrace new approaches toward nursing education, nursing practice, and nursing roles. *Nursing Outlook* editor Carole A. Anderson (1994) cites the nursing profession's enemy as being within when she speaks of nursing infighting as an old phenomenon within the profession. She questions, "But why do we do it? Why do we fight with one another for the dubious privilege of retaining the lowest educational entry requirement among all health professions? Why is it that after this fight, which has prevented the profession from moving in the way that others have moved, we wonder that other professions don't think of us as their colleagues?" (p. 149). The struggle to establish a unified voice for nursing continues, with the optimistic view being that progress is occurring. Nursing has room for many ways of practicing, each of which emphasizes different dimensions of practice. Nurse entrepreneurship offers opportunity to those who choose to develop self-employment business skills and leverage their nursing expertise.

Regardless of your place on the political continuum, there is no doubt that the Health Care Reform debate of 1994 impacted the health care system. The inability of politicians to reach consensus regarding the way whereby the system should or could be changed certainly invigorated the health care industry. Costs associated with the health care industry account for nearly 14% of the Gross National Product (GNP). In response to the Health Care Reform debate, the industry has modified practices in an attempt to reduce the cost of delivering health care. Though problems remain, one positive outcome of this process has been recognition of the unique and diverse contributions of the nursing profession. Old ideas of a singular nursing role are fading fast. The ability of the advanced practice nurse to provide high quality, cost-efficient, and effective care is being noted. The creativity of entrepreneurial nurses in delivering services to people is being recognized. The excellence of nursing educators and managers is being discussed. Health care reform, though not completely implemented, has thus opened many minds to the changing roles and contributions of the individual nursing professional. This open-mindedness is much like the opening of a box of opportunities. Like Pandora's box, it releases many unforseen possiblities—in this case, exciting new opportunities. Envisioning these new opportunities frees the nurse who has felt trapped and unfulfilled professionally. The opportunities abound, and nurses will not let the lid slam shut now.

Entrepreneurial practice, then, is a state of mind—a level of independence not commonly found as an employee, and one that is limitless in possibilities. Nursing entrepreneurialism does not necessarily imply a nurse in a distinct role, but, rather, implies an approach to practice. It is how the individual nurse, whether clinician, educator, or manager, "realizes" his or her own nursing practice.

Being an entrepreneur requires first envisioning a service or product and then establishing a mechanism to bring that service or product to the client. There are also increased responsibilities related to decision making, financial planning and follow-through. The nurse must be financially responsible and attentive to the need for cost-effectiveness in order to be successful.

The term *entrepreneur* comes from the French verb *entreprendre* essentially meaning "to do something." Writings about entrepreneurialism have been traced back to as early as the twelfth century. Although modern entrepreneurial theory is characterized by variation and lack of consensus regarding how one becomes and what one does as an entrepreneur, there is one point on which all modern theorists seem to agree: the essence of entrepreneurship appears to be innovation and an alertness to opportunities (Herron & Herron, 1991).

BEING AN ENTREPRENEUR

Most of the literature regarding entrepreneurship focuses on personal characteristics of the individual. There have been numerous attempts to differentiate the entrepreneurial personality from the nonentrepreneurial personality. Such studies are found throughout the economic and management literature. In 1988, Gartner reviewed thirty-two studies and found much variation in the definition of entrepreneurship as well as lack of consensus regarding the characteristics and traits typical of the entrepreneur (Gartner, 1988).

Common, well-documented beliefs regarding characteristics of the entrepreneur include (1) a risk-taking propensity, (2) a need for achievement, (3) a tendency to have higher internal loci of control than do others, and (4) a tolerance for ambiguity (Herron & Herron, 1991). Other work has focused on skills more than characteristics. Herron (1990), for example, identified the following as essential skills: (1) leadership, (2) knowledge, (3) networking, (4) planning, (5) design development, (6) business capability, and (7) opportunity recognition with subsequent action.

The literature also includes numerous discussions of the intrapreneur. Within nursing, the primary difference between entrepreneurship and intrapreneurship is whether the nurse remains with an organization (the intrepreneur) or steps outside an organization to independently form a new endeavor (the entrepreneur). Intrapreneurship combines the resources and security of an organization with the freedom and creativity of the entrepreneur. Some people need an organizational environment and will not flourish in a home office or other unfamiliar work setting.

Whether entrepreneur or intrapreneur, certain personality traits have been explored in attempt to predict which individuals will succeed. Although personal characteristics do influence success, this author believes that because the necessary skills and characteristics vary tremendously among entrepreneurial endeavors, individuals can acquire what they need. It is not the personality that predicts success as an entrepreneur, but, rather, initial desire and commitment combined with subsequent skill and knowledge acquisition. Decisions based on careful consideration of the ramifications of various alternatives combined with periodic review is thus perhaps a stronger predictor of satisfaction, effectiveness, and success.

Nurses who choose to become entrepreneurs change the paradigms of their nursing practices. The Greek word *paradigm*, originally a scientific term, commonly is understood today to mean a perception, frame of reference, model, theory, or assumption. Entrepreneurial nurses have different frames of reference regarding nursing practice than the traditional ideas regarding what nurses do. They perceive their roles as nurses from a different vantage point. They choose alternate ways of practicing their skills and knowledge, and thus impact health care delivery from a very different model than do most health care professionals. The term *paradigm shift* was introduced by Thomas Kuhn, who demonstrated ". . . how almost every significant break through in the field of scientific endeavor is first a break with tradition, with old ways of thinking, with old paradigms" (Covey, 1989, p. 29). Paradigm shifts are occurring not only in the profession of nursing, but in health care delivery itself. There are new approaches to care, new methods for managing resources, and new alternatives for intervention. All represent new paradigms for the health care system in the United States.

Stephen Covey (1989) uses the framework of paradigm shifts to introduce his now famous *The Seven Habits of Highly Effective People*. He defines a habit as the intersection of knowledge, skill, and desire. "Knowledge is the theoretical paradigm, the what to do and the why. Skill is the how to do. And desire is the motivation, the want to do" (p. 47). The seven habits enable the individual to move from dependence to independence to interdependence. Dependence is the paradigm of someone else taking care of "me" of someone else either coming through for me or not, of someone else being responsible for me. The paradigm of independence involves "I"; I can do this, I am responsible, I am self-reliant. Interdependence involves "we": we can combine our abilities and talents, we can do it together and create something great.

Entrepreneurial nursing requires the individual to shift from a dependent paradigm to an interdependent paradigm. As the profession of nursing struggles with this shift, some entrepreneurs are getting stuck in the independent paradigm and are not moving toward interdependence. This may permit success in the short run, but ultimately contributes to isolation, anger, and poor colleagueship. This author believes that the independent nurse entrepreneur needs collegial ties now more than ever. Through interdependence, nurses can continue to emerge with valued and powerful voices in the ongoing health-policy debate.

Another influential business writer, Denis Waitley (1995), discusses new leaders as individuals who ". . . will welcome change rather than try to resist it. They will have learned to make change work for them rather than against them. And they will have developed unique strategies and skills that enable them to create opportunities from challenges" (p. 7).

Nurse entrepreneurs are becoming the new leaders in nursing. They have taken frustration and lack of power and transformed these things into opportunities to change their practices and futures. They have learned to work with the new realities of the health care system rather than allowing those realties to further dampen their efforts and ideals.

Waitley (1995) also speaks in favor of interdependence. He advocates that leaders of the present be "champions of cooperation more often than of competition" (p. 8). Furthermore, he maintains that while access to resources will remain important, the old adage of survival of the fittest will change to "survival of the wisest" (p. 8). He believes real leaders will succeed by helping others succeed as well.

Nurse entrepreneurs, thus, must reinvent themselves. They must change their paradigms of role relationships within the existing system, and they must take advantage of the numerous opportunities to reinvent health care delivery. Collaboration with nursing colleagues as well as with members of all other health care disciplines will facilitate an improved level of care for consumers.

Nursing Qualities Favoring Entrepreneurship

In many way, nurses already qualify to succeed as entrepreneurs. The foundations of nursing education provide critical elements for approaching and managing situations. The critical analysis needed for independent decision making is really the heart of the nursing process. The assessment, planning, intervention, and evaluation cycle that directs nursing practice can be readily transferred to the business environment. By applying this decision making model to any set of circumstances, a nurse is well on the way to success as an entrepreneur. Other qualities and skills essential for success as an entrepreneur are also inherent in nursing education and transferable to other realms. Some of these are discussed following.

Judgment. Nurses all know that there are times when they must make critical decisions. Sometimes a nurse cannot let time pass without proactively seeking medical decisions and interventions. There are also circumstances that permit less aggressive action. Many instances warrant the use of nursing judgment. Through consideration of various pieces of information, including clinical signs and symptoms, nurses use their judgment to determine subsequent actions.

Entrepreneurs also rely on judgment. Numerous decisions must be made at all steps of the process of selling a service and/or product. The entrepreneur judges when to move forward, when to seek consultation, when to wait patiently, and when to revise plans. All these decisions demand judgment.

When nurses incorporate their information gathering, planning, and evaluation skills and knowledge into entrepreneurial thinking, they prepare for roles in business. Nurses must incorporate these skills and ideas, and then expand their application. Successful business endeavors are most commonly predicated after careful information gathering, careful planning, and periodic evaluation. In business jargon, a thoughtful business plan is created. Nurses have these skills and are experienced in using judgment as part of the decision making process.

Communication. If there were only one characteristic that could make or break the entrepreneurial endeavor, it would likely be communication skills. Nurses are taught to pay attention to both verbal and nonverbal communications. They watch closely for indications of incongruence between these communications so as to ascertain the real meaning. Nurses are taught to probe for information when it is not forthcoming, to clarify when information is ambiguous, and to follow up an order to ensure mutual understanding. These aspects of communication are all crucial in successful businesses.

Nurses communicate with their clients under both comfortable and trying circumstances. Sometimes, nurses must help patients overcome limitations to communication, whether those limitations be deafness, aphasia, confusion, blindness, or emotional distress. Other health professionals as well as family members also depend on the skills and creativity of nurses to enable effective communication. Nurses often must modify their styles according to the intended receivers, and it is rare that only one attempt at explanation is required.

Perhaps one of the biggest challenges for the entrepreneur is finding effective and efficient ways of communicating with colleagues. Attempting to keep each other informed about clinical issues and operational procedures can present daily challenges. Whereas the nurse as employee learns new clinical and operational information every day, entrepreneurs operate on their own, and therefore must develop means of keeping their clinical and operational knowledge and skills current. After leaving employment in a health care organization, the entrepreneurial nurse must accept the responsibility for devising ways to remain current.

Proficient communication is essential in pursuing entrepreneurial endeavors. The ability to seek answers to known questions as well as to probe for questions not anticipated is critical. The ability to interpret nonverbal signals can also be crucial in knowing when and how to make decisions. Numerous individuals will provide information and will represent varied professions. Nurses' communication skills can enhance their abilities to find out those things that they need to know.

Most entrepreneurial endeavors involve selling a product, service, or process; all require communicating effectively with clients and customers. Many times the thing that makes a new idea work is having its value communicated. Nurses can tap their years of communication experience and easily transfer their communication skills to the business environment.

Homeostasis and Change. Basic nursing education programs include course work exploring the ideas of homeostasis and change. Nurses are taught to assist the patient in maintaining a homeostatic environment, both internally and externally. They are also taught about the reality of change and how it impacts the homeostatic condition. Changes occurring too rapidly or too severely trigger some type of intervention. Nurses are taught to pay attention to the subtle changes as well and to always consider how each change impacts the overall person.

Businesses also need homeostatic balance. Things that are secure and stable one day can become fragile and brittle the next. The need to watch closely for subtle indicators cannot be overemphasized. Just as the human body can build resistance and resilience to illness, so too can a business develop a firm foundation that, with care and attention, can weather difficult, changing conditions.

Again, the nurse has honed the eyes, ears, and tactile sense to anticipate changes and their effect on homeostasis. This ability can also be applied in a different context. Caring for an entrepreneurial endeavor is very much within the nurse's abilities.

Ethos. In Greek, *ethos* refers to the rightness or wrongness of an act. Nurses often are exposed to difficult ethical dilemmas that can strain the often delicate balance between personal ethics and professional ethics and responsibilities. It is not unusual for health care providers to choose the environments in which they work based on personal ethics. Problems can still arise, however, when patients in crisis desire different alternatives than those with which the nurse is comfortable. The nurse must sometimes find a method of maintaining personal ethical integrity while respecting the ethical decisions made by patients and colleagues.

In business, countless circumstances emerge that require ethical decisions. Entrepreneurial nurses must therefore have a strong sense of what they consider to be right, and will be disappointed if they expect to escape difficult ethical situations by moving into the entrepreneurial realm. The stakes may be different, but the demanding need to consider often conflicting alternatives is essential in managing an entrepreneurial practice.

Collaboration and Colleagueship. Effective delivery of health care requires collaboration and colleagueship, both of which have often been absent among nurses as well as among members of other disciplines. In order to succeed in entrepreneurial endeavors, however, nurses must master skills related to collaboration and colleagueship.

Although businesses are often managed by individuals, success requires the help of many. Business, financial, and legal consultation are but a few of the areas often requiring outside assistance. Furthermore, establishing a client base occurs only through marketing and networking. A good idea without someone to buy it will quickly fail. Support from colleagues can go far in establishing and maintaining an entrepreneurial practice.

GETTING STARTED AS AN ENTREPRENEUR

A commonly asked question regarding entrepreneurial nursing is, "How or where do I start?" Several critical elements must first be in place. A level of discontent with existing conditions and options many times prompts nurses to look for something different. Perhaps there is a general, underlying sense of low satisfaction combined with a desire to make a change. Perhaps the nurse identifies a need for change. Perhaps the nurse identifies a personal or professional unfulfilled need.

Another critical element is the acquisition of necessary knowledge, skills, and, possibly, credentials. Rarely can a person become successful in a new role without some preparation. The amount, extent, and type of preparation required, however, can vary tremendously. Many nurse entrepreneurs are self taught and explain their evolutions as including reading, reading, and more reading.

Through the course of nursing practice, a nurse may discover a societal need that is not being met. This need may directly involve a patient or may be related to the health care system itself. When faced with an obvious deficiency, an entrepreneurial thinker starts imagining ways to solve the problem, focusing on resolution strategies rather than on the problem itself. One way for a nurse to stop playing the "ain't it awful" game and, instead, start making changes is to pursue an entrepreneurial path.

A key element in getting started in entrepreneurial practice is having the courage to be different. The entrepreneurial nurse is unfortunately still considered "nontraditional." If this label bothers you, you may either want to rethink your future in this type of practice or consider why you are hesitant to try something considered by many to be nontraditional. Fear often is the reason for such a hesitancy. Fear of the unknown or insecurity stalls many potential entrepreneurs. You can, however, find ways to resolve such fears. Many successful nurse entrepreneurs developed their businesses slowly, maintaining some security in a known, part-time role while pursuing their entrepreneurial efforts on the side. After success is experienced, fear tends to dissipate. Whether it comes sooner or later, however, courage to try something new and different is essential.

Beyond the initial decision to strike out as an entrepreneur, the second single most important decision you must make relates to what you will sell. What will you make or do for people? In other words, what will be your niche? You must consider what you have that other people will be willing to pay for in order to get.

In deciding what you will sell, you must also consider the type of role you seek. Are you seeking to be an advanced practice clinician (e.g., an NP), an educator, a business owner, a product developer, a media or communications professional, an author of or contributor to written or multimedia products, or, perhaps, a consultant and speaker to organizations? To help you decide, talk to people who are doing these things. Nurses have been active in all these roles for at least a decade, and most are very happy to talk to aspiring entrepreneurs.

After you get a sense of what you will sell and in which role you plan to market this product or service, you must next consider the financial and legal decisions regarding business and tax structure. Numerous options exist, ranging from sole proprietorship to corporate structures. No single option is correct, and advantages and disadvantages to each abound and are influenced by many variables. To make the best choice, some study of tax and business structures is essential. Readily available resources include inexpensive monthly periodicals, hundreds of new books published annually, and eager accountants, attorneys, and business consultants. You may also find help from your current bank and your tax accountant. Learning about the parts of a business and the way they function is much like learning anatomy and physiology of the human body. Although doing so takes some effort, learning about business is actually less complicated than much of the learning that has already been required of you as a nurse.

A good way to get started as an entrepreneurial thinker is to listen to nurses who have already successfully launched entrepreneurial practices. Storytelling is a very effective way to illustrate the application of theory. Hearing the real stories of real nurses can be more beneficial than hypothetical scenarios or long lists of "should" and "should nots." The stories that follow are told in the words of the nurses themselves and were originally published in *How I Became a Nurse Entrepreneur* (1991) by the National Nurses in Business Association.

The Courage to Take the First Step
by Beverly J. Zeiss, RN, BS, CCRN

Have you ever had an overwhelming urge to change careers or to create a niche within your career that might be more exciting and challenging? I did, and in responding to this urge, I created an opportunity for myself that has been both exciting and challenging. All it took to get started was the courage to take the first step.

After spending fifteen years in critical care and two years in nursing administration, I finally realized that I was no longer able to deal with the constraints and political climate of hospital nursing. But just what does a critical care nurse turned nursing administrator do outside of the hospital setting? This was a tough question, but one evening, over a bottle of wine, my husband, John, and I searched for an answer.

We took a personal inventory of our skills, and decided that with my background in nursing and management, and his business and computer expertise, a health care business would be ideal. We soon focused in on a private employment agency specializing in the referral of critical care nurses into the critical care units of area hospitals, one that gives excellent service to both hospital and nurse clients. Meeting these criteria became the mission of Critical Care Associates.

Tip 1: Quality is your competitive edge. Always strive to be the very best.

We were now ready to make a commitment and to take that first step.

To test our business hypothesis, I conducted an extensive market survey of all the hospitals in my area. This was my introduction to what is referred to in marketing as the "cold call." It is the process of calling someone you have never met before for the purpose of gaining information, making an appointment, or making a sale. Although I was apprehensive, I found the hospitals to be very responsive, confirming our perceived need.

We also surveyed our competition and found that there was only one other specialty agency out there, and that they were experiencing quality problems. There were, however, many agencies that placed nurses in all areas of hospitals as well as in home care and private duty. We had apparently found an optimal market niche.

Tip 2: Get to know your competition, and never, never underestimate them.

It was important for us to determine the external governmental controls on this type of a business. I have always had a very strong belief in the professionalism and autonomy of nurses; therefore, I opted to treat the nurses as independent contractors (ICs) rather than employees. We had our attorney survey the industry, and he confirmed my belief that the use of ICs has been, and continues to be, a long-standing practice within the industry.

We discovered that the state of New Jersey Department of Labor (DOL) was beginning to question the right of nurses to function independently as licensed by the state of New Jersey under the Nurse Practice Act. We also learned that the DOL had been auditing nursing registries, agencies, and staffing services. After researching the state of New Jersey "ABC Test" and federal "Common Law Factors" for determining ICs, I felt confident that we met all of the requirements; thus, we proceeded in scheduling only self-employed ICs.

Of course, I didn't know at the time that I would be spending at least three years in legal battle with the DOL, fighting for the right of nurses to practice autonomously. We went through an audit and several appeals, and, finally, instituted a lawsuit against them. I realized the magnitude of the situation when we received our docket number with the words "Critical Care Associates vs. the New Jersey Department of Labor."

By May of 1990, we were one of three firms awaiting trial to appeal the DOL decision. The first firm to go to trial won the decision in Appellate Court, thereby setting a precedent for all of us.

Tip 3: Sometimes you can fight City Hall!

We were fortunate to retain a friend as our attorney. Not only is he comfortable to work with, we knew from the beginning that he would always do an excellent job; and he has never disappointed us. We initially thought that we would require his services only for incorporation and corporate advice—we never realized that we would all wind up becoming experts in tax and labor laws!

Our accountant was recommended to us by our attorney, and once again, we were fortunate. He is competent, easy to work with, and, through the years, has become a good friend.

Tip 4: Make friends with your attorney and accountant and heed them well, for they are the ones that keep you out of trouble.

We began our business in a one-room office of a newly renovated building, just five minutes from our home. The building also provided us with a shared receptionist to answer the telephone. This was an ideal situation for me when I was on marketing calls or covering a shift in a hospital.

Our entire floor consisted of start-up companies of varied types and purposes. This group of new entrepreneurs became a very supportive and positive environment. Although we often joked about wondering which companies would be remaining by the next year, we supported one another and helped each other in any way we could.

Tip 5: Surround yourself with positive people. Don't let the pessimists get you down!

When we began to design our stationery and business cards, we identified the need for a distinctive logo. Instead of approaching an exclusive advertising firm, I commissioned my teenaged son to work up some designs. He developed exactly the look that we wanted and charged us much less than an advertising firm would have charged. We have used his logo ever since, even after we redesigned and updated our stationery with a professional advertising firm.

Tip 6: Be creative. Recognize and utilize all the resources at your disposal.

Our initial marketing strategy consisted of a series of newspaper advertisements that became more and more sophisticated as we grew. As it was important for us to introduce our services to both nurses and hospitals, we found this form of the media an effective way to accomplish both. Initially, we wrote and designed our own ads, but later, when we could better afford to do so, we collaborated with an advertising agency for appropriate positioning within our industry.

Another major marketing component consisted of direct mailings to prospective nurse and hospital clients. Fortunately, John had a very strong computer background and set me up with the capacity to construct personalized introductory letters to both client bases. We then purchased databases from several sources of medical publishers. Hospital contacts and addresses were provided in a manual we purchased listing hospitals and hospital personnel.

Tip 7: Position yourself as number 1 in your field, and you may soon find that you are number 1.

Our first hospital client was a small community hospital that was a very desirable working environment due to its friendly, pleasant atmosphere. I was contacted by one of the supervisors, who was a friend of mine from a previous hospital. During an earlier conversation with her, I had mentioned that I was developing a specialty staffing service, and she remembered this when she was experiencing a severe staffing shortage in her critical care unit. As a result of this referral, this hospital has been a valued client for the past five years.

Tip 8: Network! Network! Network! You will find that important referrals will often come from friends and acquaintances that you've met and kept in touch with through the years.

In order to build the reputation of our agency, I found myself covering many shifts by myself, often working a night shift and covering the office during the day as well. Although I was beginning to believe I had jumped "from the frying pan into the fire," the excitement of building a business provided me with a great source of energy at those times when I needed it most. I can truly say that I've never worked harder in my life, but I must also say that I have never enjoyed it more.

Tip 9: Be prepared to work longer and harder than ever before, for the harder you work, the more opportunity you will create for yourself.

Inquiries soon started coming in from other hospitals that I had marketed, and over the next six months, we gradually began adding to our client base. At the same time, our roster of nurses also began to grow. Maintaining a balance of hospital clients and available nurses is perhaps one of the most frustrating aspects of this business. Another source of frustration was the development of the correct formula for client charges and nurse compensation, enabling us to make a modest profit as well. Initially, we accomplished this through trial and error, with market supply and demand strongly dictating all three factors, while pricing and compensation of our competition also had to be considered.

Tip 10: The old economic principles of supply and demand within the marketplace hold true in all areas of business.

We soon realized that operating a staffing service was a very capital-intensive business, and became even more so as we grew. Banks are wary about lending large amounts of money to start-up companies. Our solution was to personally finance our start-up and growth. With a second mortgage on our home and about twenty-six credit cards, we were able to meet our financial requirements. Although this was a great risk for us, we had a strong belief in our business and our ability to make it work.

Tip 11: At the essence of entrepreneurship is the willingness to take risks.

When we were able to demonstrate to a bank that we were willing and able to assume personal responsibility for financing our company, they were impressed. It wasn't until then that they seriously considered assisting with our financial growth needs. We now have an excellent relationship with a bank and an ongoing line of credit.

As our business grew, it was necessary to hire sufficient office staff to give quality service to both of our client bases. In order to maintain the quality that we desired, we decided to hire professional nurses to do the staffing and enhance our relationships with our clients. We selectively chose to offer positions to people who we knew were at the top of their fields and who possessed all the qualities required to be successful in their respective positions.

Tip 12: Your business is only as good as the people who are running it. Use care when selecting your staff.

By the end of our second year, we were growing so rapidly that administrative tasks were becoming out of control. With little persuasion, John decided to resign from his position at a large pharmaceutical company, after seventeen years with them. Although the decision was not an easy one, it worked out beautifully. John took over all the financial and computer aspects of the business, and I was able to concentrate on the nursing, staffing, and customer service aspects.

Tip 13: Yes, a husband and wife can work together twenty-four hours per day, and enjoy it!

Today, Critical Care Associates, Inc. serves more than forty client facilities throughout New Jersey through the referral of qualified, caring, critical care nurses. Our facilities include a home office and two satellite offices. We have many preferred provider contracts and are the sole provider for the largest and most specialized critical care facility in the state.

We project sales in excess of $6 million for this year; we anticipate that our growth pattern since start-up will qualify us for the inclusion in the Inc. 500 listing of top companies. This was one of our goals at start-up, and has served as a major motivation factor throughout the past five years.

We will begin our sixth year of operation with the same commitment to quality service, the same ideals for independent nursing practice, and eager anticipation for further growth through diversification.

Through the establishment and operation of CCA, Inc., I have learned that we have within ourselves a tremendous capacity for personal growth and accomplishment, far beyond what we ever imagine. I have been amazed at times by the large reserves of energy, knowledge, enthusiasm, and management skills that have surfaced when I needed them most. I have learned to stretch myself as far as I could—and then yet farther when necessary.

One question that I am most frequently asked is, "Do you still consider yourself a nurse?" My answer is always unequivocally, "Yes!" Although I no longer choose to practice in a full-time clinical setting, I use many nursing principles on a daily basis. The problem-solving and decision making skills that I have acquired in the critical care setting, along with the practice of the nursing process have enabled me to "think on my feet" and make complex business decisions that have led to the success of my business.

Nurses, by nature of our training and experience, are naturals in the business world.

A Roller Coaster Ride into Business

by Pamela M. Buckman, RN, MS

I would love to be able to say that I started my own business based on a well thought out plan for success, but it simply isn't true!

A Harvard MBA always sounded to me like a lab test for an exotic disease. During my twelve years of clinical nursing, I have never attended a business class, never raised capital, never written a business plan for my own company, and never been able to fully grasp the nuances of an intricate financial statement without significant hand holding from my accountant. Even so, I have been in business for ten years and never known a month "in the red." In retrospect, I recognize that I have what it takes to start a business and make it successful.

The word that leaps to mind most readily to describe my entrance into business is *survival*. My nursing career was a predictable eighteen-month roller coaster ride through changes in specialties, areas of employment, positions, and responsibilities. I spent six months learning a new job, six months doing the job, and six months looking for the next challenge. I always loved what I was doing because it was constantly new. I made sure I didn't get bored. Whenever the challenge and/or fun began to wane, I made a change, although starting a business did not occur to me during those years. I was merrily working away, just like everyone else I knew. I married, had two children, and became the stereotypical, second-income wage earner.

And then two things happened. I chose to place myself smack dab in the middle of one of the most prevalent of women's problems in America today. I became a single mother with two preschool children, and the primary (sole, more often than not) breadwinner. I could no longer live with rotating shifts and weekend and holiday work with financial disaster as my reward. Even more importantly, I couldn't see it would ever be any different if I didn't make a significant career change, and so I did.

I am forever grateful to my mom, who saw an ad from a local medical device firm in the classified section of the Sunday paper. They were looking for a master-level nurse who was familiar with research and cardiovascular and orthopedic nursing. (Thank goodness for that extra two years in school and all those specialty changes during my roller coaster days.) I threw together a résumé (never having done one before) and submitted it to the company. They sent me an application for employment, which I completed and hand delivered to a receptionist one morning. I was wearing jeans and tennis shoes, because I had little confidence this would actually lead to anything. Much to my surprise, two weeks later I hung up my white uniform for the last time and joined the business world.

My position involved the management of clinical trial programs to evaluate company products in satisfaction of Food and Drug Administration regulations. I was inundated with information—all of which was brand new to me. I not only had to learn my job, I had to learn to do my job in a foreign country, i.e., an office. As if traveling to a foreign country, I read, watched, and listened with a renewed interest in work that I had not realized was being done. I felt challenged and motivated to learn, produce, and do whatever was required to excel—whether or not the work could be done in forty hours a week.

I also learned to travel and juggle a home life at the same time. This is not an easy task for anyone, and indisputably impossible without a supportive family, which, luckily I had.

The occupational hazards of working for someone else in the business world soon came my way. Within two years, the company was sold and relocated. I went to work for another medical device firm doing essentially the same thing. That medical division was below the acceptable profit margin level for the board of directors of the parent company, and the division was dissolved.

At this point, I decided it was time to stop putting myself in dependent situations. This time, I entered into a partnership with a colleague with whom I had worked very well in both previous firms.

Our business focus was to provide clinical trial management services to many medical device manufacturers on a consulting basis. The concept was that my colleague had the industry contacts, and I knew how to do the work once he sold the account. Sounded good but...! I soon came to resent doing all the work (shades of my nursing days kept leaping into my mind) while someone else got all the credit. And so the business went well, but the partnership did not. We went our separate ways, and I was once again "between opportunities."

In the meantime, I had remarried. My husband (whose background was medically related) and I opened a retail business in art framing and supplies. It was alot of fun but a distinct diversion from what we both knew well, and the timing was poor because the country was in an economic recession. As a result, we had no family economic security and no strong prospects of any. It was a lousy time for me to start a business of my own, but I did it anyway.

I talked with one of the clients with whom I had worked closely during the days of the ill-fated partnership. The client encouraged me to take on his project as a sole proprietor, and I agreed. I converted a part of the garage to my office. The conversion consisted of a carpet remnant, someone else's discarded furniture, a used typewriter, and a telephone.

Within a few weeks, there were three clients; and within a few months, I was swamped with work. My husband was still operating the retail business all day and coming home to help me in the garage every evening. We operated this way for eighteen months or so, at which time he sold the retail business and joined me full-time. We bought our first computer system, squeezed it and another secondhand desk into the garage, and installed another phone line.

After three years, we incorporated and hired a part-time secretary. Our first office out of the garage was one room in the back of a bank—rent: $100 a month. Clients kept coming, and we kept working more hours to see that they were satisfied. All of our work came to us via referral. We never ran an ad or conducted a direct-mail program. In a sense, we never directly marketed our services.

And so, there I was, still working weekends and holidays. The difference was I now worked fourteen- to sixteen-hour days and six to seven days a week. But that was not the only difference. More importantly, I was no longer bored. I thoroughly enjoyed entering into a contract to do a job; completing that job with integrity, on time, and within budget; and being handsomely rewarded for my efforts.

It is now ten years later. We have a staff of seven; a very nice, but not extravagant, fully equipped suite of offices; an extensively networked computer system; and multiple opportunities for further expansion.

Have we made mistakes along the way? You bet, and plenty of them! We sold a piece of the company to an accountant because we were naive to the telltale signs of manipulation. It cost us dearly to buy back that piece of the company. We hired the wife of a friend. The wife turned out to be incompetent. Firing the wife cost us the friendship. We loaned money to friends, never dreaming we would have to threaten legal action to be repaid.

But we obviously did more things right than wrong. We controlled our overhead with a vengeance and continue to do so. We put money into people—not furniture. We were patient. Our slow, constant growth was controllable and therefore predictable. We never hired an employee until we exhausted every possibility of doing the work ourselves. We watched and listened to other successful small business owners—and learned from them.

In the early days, I personally had many opportunities to meet with small groups of nurses who talked about wanting to start their own businesses. Some of them had taken the first steps to establish themselves. I remember being amazed at comments such as, "I won't travel over a weekend," or "I won't travel at all," or "My hours are 8:00 to 5:00," or "I won't work with someone I don't like."

These comments do not embody the entrepreneur spirit. In contrast to the preceding, my philosophy has always been; "Work wherever the work is and whenever the work needs to be done." To borrow a saying from a successful friend of mine, "Where is it written that associates must always be friends? It is only necessary to do good business." This doesn't mean you should agree to work with unethical or otherwise undesirable individuals. It does mean that you must develop the proper perspectives. Business associates do not have to stand up to the same scrutiny as candidates to date your daughter. By the way, among those nurses I met who made the remarks I found so amazing, none have been successful in their own businesses. Owning your own business involves long, hard, endless hours of work and responsibility. Being willing to work that hard is not enough. You have to thrive on it. It has to be fun!

Would I do it again? You bet. Could I work for someone else again? Of course—I am a survivor—but I don 't plan to have to make that choice.

If I were to use one word to capture the feeling that embodies being an entrepreneur, it is *caring*. The successful owner conceives, delivers, nurtures, and develops the business like a lioness does her pride. She is protective and defensive. Success depends on delegation of authority and responsibility to others. But, in the end, no one benefits and no one fails any more or any less than the extent to which the entrepreneur cares.

The Evolution of a Nurse Entrepreneur

by Gail Wick, RN, BSN, CNN

How does a nurse start and develop a business? How does one become a consultant? Neither question has a short, clear-cut answer, so let me share the evolution of my business and career with you as a stimulant for creative brainstorming.

In 1970, straight from nursing school, I jumped into what was emerging as an exciting specialty: nephrology nursing. I became a staff nurse in the renal ICU and transplant unit at Grady Hospital in Atlanta. After six months, I left the specialty for approximately three years, returning finally to become a staff nurse in the subspecialty of dialysis. Quickly, I subspecialized again, as a teacher. I was first a home-training instructor and later the education director for three large, non-profit dialysis facilities in Atlanta. My specialty niches of nephrology nursing and teaching were created.

When I chose a specialty in nursing which I truly loved and found exciting, and which met the needs of a large health care consumer population, I began the development of what I now call the "strategic plan" for my career. Nephrology nursing with a focus on teaching became my first career path. All else would come from this focus. As part of the plan, I became very knowledgeable about my specialty and consistently worked to develop my teaching and lecturing skills. I read books, attended hundreds of seminars and meetings, and practiced what I learned on a regular basis.

I began to network at every opportunity. Through my attendance at meetings and networking opportunities, I chose role models to learn from, and developed a mentor relationship with a highly respected nephrology nurse, author, and teacher. Later, as I developed a serious interest in the business issues of health care, I found nurse/businessperson role models as well as nonnursing role models in the business world.

I joined professional organizations and actively worked on committees. Eventually, I became an officer in many of them, thus increasing my visibility. Although I gave a lot of volunteer time and effort, I gained as much or more than I gave. Through my involvement, I met my colleagues and the businesspeople in my specialty, gained credibility as a specialist, and, importantly, kept a pulse on the state of the art and the needs of the specialty community.

I began speaking at meetings, first presenting abstracts, later as an invited speaker and seminar leader. For a long time, I wasn't paid; but as time passed, my skills and uniqueness as a speaker enabled me to ask for compensation. This was in actuality the beginning of my consulting/education business, which I began officially in 1983. My business and marketing plans still call for speaking engagements because they provide income, exposure, and free marketing opportunities.

In the early 1980s, I began to realize that I had a serious interest in not just the health care business, but business in general. This insight came from a number of sources. I began to work as a part-time consultant for a catheter company, and realized that I had a knack not just for teaching about the product, but also for selling the product. I didn't officially pursue sales as a career, but did begin to learn as much as possible about selling. I began to attend sales and business-related seminars to develop the knowledge base I lacked. I observed salespeople and businesspeople in as many settings as possible. I also focused on customer service and satisfaction, fee structuring, and basic marketing principles. This knowledge base later helped me sell my company's services for a reasonable profit and keep my customers satisfied.

While I was testing the waters of the corporate health care setting, I put another of my talents—designing—to work, and bought a small, wholesale, home-decorative-accessory business. I didn't make a lot of money, and I worked far too hard; but I gained valuable experience in marketing, sales, budgeting, management, and business partner relationships. Because I only focus on the positive aspects of the experience when I discuss that business, it has helped me gain credibility as a businessperson with my corporate clients today.

Today, my company is officially identified as Gail Wick & Associates, offering health care consulting, placement, and education services. Although many of my presentations and seminars have universal appeal, the consulting and placement services are specific to nephrology. We service both manufacturers and health care providers. Seminars and meeting management round out the education services.

The name of my company serves three main purposes—use of name recognition from years of visibility within my target market, identification of the company's primary focus, and flexibility to expand services and focus as opportunities arise. I believe that an entrepreneur must always be alert to exciting opportunities and needs which identify themselves in amazing ways. For the present, though, by concentrating on an area in which I am knowledgeable, known, and have an extensive network, I have been able to find a profitable niche quickly.

As I look to the future, I recognize a need to increase and refine my knowledge of the business of health care. Improved negotiation skills, more sophisticated marketing techniques, and development of a long-range business plan are immediate needs. Networking activities and involvement in organizations will become increasingly important. And perhaps most importantly, my commitment to nurse-owned organizations will continue to fuel my drive and commitment to nurse entrepreneurship!

From reading the preceding, it sounds like the development of my career path was very well thought out, smooth, and calculated, doesn't it? Hardly! What you have read above is sixteen years of hindsight talking. The actual development of my career and current business was actually part luck, part accident, and part design.

Probably the best things that I have had going for me over the years are my true belief in what I'm doing, my love and respect for nursing and nurses, the insight to identify what I wanted from my career early, the ability to "fake it while I'm making it," and the guts to go for what I want.

ENTREPRENEURIAL INTERACTION AND COLLABORATION

All entrepreneurial nursing roles entail differing needs and modes of collaboration. Pursuing entrepreneurial practice can either greatly increase or greatly decrease the amount of interaction with colleagues. When interaction decreases, some entrepreneurs feel isolated and disconnected from the profession. Individual nurses in entrepreneurial practice are free to create their own environments, however, and must work to find the correct balance for their personalities and professional goals. To explore this issue further, four common entrepreneurial roles are discussed following: advanced practice nurses in private or collaborative practices, educators, business owners, and consultants.

Advanced Practice Nurses in Private or Collaborative Practices

Experienced NPs, clinical nurse specialists (CNSs), nurse anesthetists (CRNAs), and nurse midwives (CNMs) who establish private practices generally do the same things as they would as employees. If their shifts to entrepreneurial practice are intended primarily as a way to accomplish improved financial prospects and higher degrees of autonomy, chances are that these nurses will continue to practice nursing as advanced practice nurses. With increased financial independence, however, also come the responsibilities of marketing services, understanding fiscal and legal matters, and developing long-term plans. Two common benefits of entrepreneurial practice are enhanced self-esteem and a strong sense of and accomplishment, resulting from increased autonomy and responsibility.

Collaboration is increasingly important in order to secure a client base and be able to provide safe, high-quality care. Physicians become key colleagues in efforts to establish the collaborative protocols necessary to address legal and ethical realities of the system. In addition, referrals to other providers may be the responsibility of the advanced practice nurse, necessitating crucial relationships with members of other disciplines, such as physical and occupational therapists, dietitians, pharmacists, and social workers.

With the increasing shift to managed care networks, the case manager (CM) role will be an essential link for the advanced practice nurse in independent practice. The advanced practice nurse must understand the CM role and work diligently to establish contractual relationships to ensure a client base.

Other interactions involve representatives from insurance companies and government agencies. Most Americans pay for services through their insurance carriers, whether those carriers be private companies or state or federal government programs. Advanced practice nurses must either build this function into their roles or contract with others to provide this service. Even when the highest quality of care is being delivered, billing and receiving money are essential for a private practice to succeed and remain in business.

As most nurses know, the health care system is heavily regulated. Responding to state and federal regulations and voluntary accrediting bodies requires an ability to interact effectively with surveyors. Because nurses in private, independent practice are still considered to be outside the norm, they must be prepared to encounter increased scrutiny and evaluation.

Lastly but no less important are interactions with a knowledgeable attorney and accountant. The entrepreneurial advanced practice nurse should not rely on a brother-in-law's or a next-door neighbor's favors. Health care law and finance are unique and complex. Thus, services must be obtained from individuals who know how to establish, maintain, and assist a health care provider in independent practice. People with these skills are available; they have been well serving physicians for years.

Educators

Many beginning entrepreneurs start in some sort of educational role. Because of their expertise, they may be asked to serve as guest speakers, for example, and receive honoraria for this service. As a result, these nurses may realize that they can get paid for sharing what they know, they begin to understand both the value of their expertise and the willingness of others to pay for that expertise.

The ways whereby an educational product is packaged and marketed are key variables in success. Some entrepreneurial nurse educators serve as guest speakers in a variety of forums and settings. Some present longer, more elaborate educational programs, often directed toward colleagues seeking new role alternatives. Still others focus their efforts on written materials, contributing new resources and texts as well as self-directed learning materials and multimedia products.

A small but growing number of nurses are embracing opportunities in the media by hosting or producing radio and cable programming geared to health care issues and strategies to assist consumers in navigating the health care system. Through these efforts, nurses strengthen their position as strong patient advocates; they are educating the public.

Nurses who develop entrepreneurial practices as educators make numerous choices that impact collegial interaction. The diverse settings in which educators can function allow for a wide variety in amount and type of communications with other health care providers. The entrepreneurial educator typically focuses educational efforts toward one of three specific learner groups: consumers (commonly referred to as *patient education*), entering nurses (student nurse and new graduate education), or colleagues (continuing education and staff-development).

Consumer-Focused Educators. In consumer-focused education, content is directed toward the public. Increasing client understanding of pathophysiology in order to change health care behaviors is typically the goal. To be successful in this type of entrepreneurial practice, the nurse must rely heavily on the foundations of nursing practice, including physiology, pathology, and communication. Mastering instructional strategies such as program development, teaching techniques, and evaluation is also essential.

Relationships with colleagues from varying disciplines often serve as the means of establishing a client base. Client education often happens in direct connection with medical care. Although more nurses are venturing into community education without establishing some tie to the medical community, much of the public remains skeptical about health care education not associated at least indirectly with a member of the medical profession. Therefore, referrals from physicians and/or joint efforts often are preferable.

Student Nurse and New Graduate Educators. When the entrepreneurial nurse educator focuses efforts toward the new nurse or toward nurses having novice-level skills, collaboration with academicians is common. It is important to understand the current curriculum content of basic, entry-level nursing programs in order to effectively educate nurses as they transform from what Patricia Benner (1984) describes as novice to expert. It takes special skills to mold effective and safe nurses from graduates who emerge from nursing schools with varying levels of knowledge, clinical experience, life experience, and motivation. The long-discussed "reality shock" of professional nursing practice is alive and well. Because of technology, shorter hospital stays, chronic and complex interactive medical conditions, and drastic changes in the settings where nurses have traditionally begun their careers (i.e., hospitals), the enormity of that shock is greater than ever before. The entrepreneurial nurse who enjoys developing skills and confidence in others is a much-needed resource in nursing. Businesses focusing on mentoring new nurses are thus welcomed by both the profession and employers.

Continuing Education and Staff Development Educators. Education of colleagues can be quite varied. Sometimes the educator provides staff development for nurses only. Other efforts may be directed at all health care professionals and disciplines. Regardless of the target audience, the entrepreneur typically must interact with colleagues responsible for organizing and coordinating continuing education and staff development programs. Traditionally, this role has been filled by a nurse with the title of inservice director or staff development coordinator. Today, in addition to these positions, some organizations have entrusted staff development to human resource departments, which may or may not be headed by nurses. Likewise, conferences are often coordinated by marketing professionals, who may see the selection of speakers and presenters from a "drawing card" approach. The ways whereby entrepreneurial nurse educators present themselves in person and through oral and written communications can often be deciding factors; appearing organized, knowledgeable, and informed to the person responsible for coordination is tantamount to success in this arena.

Business Owners

Being a business owner perhaps entails the most uncommon application of nursing skills as compared to the previously discussed roles. It also illustrates what sets nurse entrepreneurs apart from their colleagues in other nursing realms. Leadership abilities and resource management skills are especially critical to success. The entrepreneurial nurse business owner must take full responsibility not only for daily operational issues, but also for growth and maintenance planning. The more employees involved, the more complex the issues. The fewer the management resources, the greater the need for the owner to have a broad understanding of fiscal and legal issues.

The thought of having complete authority over and responsibility for a company that may have as few as 5 or as many as 500 employees may sound overwhelming to some nurses. Yet, others welcome the associated legitimized decision making power. The past twenty years have required many nurses to develop their practical and theoretical understandings of resource management. Many nurses who tired of clinical practice or felt compelled by a sense of wanting to change the rules and standards have excelled as nurse managers and executives. Managing a self-owned service can, in fact, be as easy or even easier than managing a service owned by someone else. This is not to say that owning and growing a business is easy by definition. But doing so is possible and offers a more natural transition than might generally be believed. Collaboration skills are essential to success. Unless there are unlimited financial resources to hire and delegate authority, the business owner must be able to negotiate, plan, manage, and lead. Knowing not only with whom to connect, but also how and when to do so, is crucial to stabilizing productivity and effectiveness.

If the business owner sits alone in an office and has little telephone or electronic contact, the owner's great idea most surely will die. The entrepreneurial nurse must believe wholeheartedly in the business and commit to communicating this vision to the potential customers of the business. Rarely does business come to you. You must establish a plan and method of marketing your service or product, or at the very least, have access to individuals who will provide you with referrals.

When a business becomes successful, the nurse entrepreneur often must hire other people. Interviewing skills and professional contacts thus also are critical to success. Losing contact with colleagues makes finding needed people more difficult.

Consultants

The term *consultant* elicits very diverse reactions. Some think a consultant is a person who cannot find a job or who is seeking a method to minimize tax liabilities. Although each of the aforementioned drive some individuals toward consulting, the reality is that consultants provide extremely valuable services for organizations and industries. There is variety not only in the expertise of consultants, but also in the manners and types of consultation provided. There are also numerous methods of reimbursement.

Natural consultation avenues for nurses are those that involve applying nursing knowledge and skills. Because of already established credibility, others are willing to buy such expertise from a nurse consultant. These nurses can provide education, legal testimony, opinion, and experience. Further, the value of replicating successful services or processes in multiple organizations is becoming more wildly recognized. When management knows something has worked somewhere else, they are more willing to commit time, effort, and resources to the changes required to initiate that thing in their organization. The individual who can not only talk about change, but who can implement it is a very valuable commodity in today's workplace. Organizations are interested in producing efficient and effective operations, and consultants can facilitate new ideas and changes in organizations where managers are overcommitted and overtired.

Consultation efforts primarily focus on either process or outcome. Some nurse consultants build their practices through providing services that result in specified outcomes (e.g., the opening of a new pediatric service). The consultant provides content expertise as well as experience relating to all the elements necessary for implementation. Such elements may include needs assessment, staff education, needed supply purchases, contractual arrangements, and other numerous considerations.

Process consultants, although also interested in outcomes, often are hired to facilitate the interactions of various employees toward a predetermined outcome. For example, if an organization recognizes that there is a need to improve collaboration between nurses and physicians in order to institute critical pathways, and that a neutral, objective individual is needed to facilitate the process, a process consultant is appropriate. A lack of expertise in the organization is not necessarily the problem that must to be remedied; instead, the collaborative efforts of the existing experts must be facilitated.

Consultants must to be strong oral and written communicators. Consultants make numerous presentations to clinician colleagues and management staff. Nurse consultants may find themselves surrounded by colleagues with like experiences; or, they may find themselves working with nurses and others who have dissimilar experiences. The nurse consultant also faces the challenge of responding to clients whose goals differ greatly depending on the types of facility and the regions they represent. Some nurses serve as consultants to nonhealth care organizations struggling with employee health issues, health insurance choices, regulatory bodies, or the general trend toward consumer awareness of healthful living practices.

Consultants interact with diverse groups of individuals with varying interests and needs. Again, maintaining connections to professional colleagues enhances business opportunities. An understanding of marketing strategies, associated regulations and standards, and means of remuneration also is crucial to success.

SPECIAL CONCERNS IN ENTREPRENEURIAL PRACTICE

As in most businesses, regional differences are important to understand. Knowing whether your service or product is needed in your immediate market is essential. Having a sense of appropriate fees to charge is also important in growing and maintaining a business. Certainly, there must be people *somewhere* who are willing to purchase your service. And today's technology makes possible managing a service from a distance. Whether or not a long-distance approach can work for your idea, however, will take careful consideration.

What is the potential for financial reward? Of course, it varies tremendously depending on the type of entrepreneurial practice and the amount of risk and leverage assumed by the individual. Some entrepreneurs operate on a fee-for-service basis; others are compensated by the hour; and still others work for monthly retainers. If a product is being developed and sold, profits and royalties can be significant. The key to success is for the entrepreneur to calculate how much money is needed to compensate for the time and expertise required to provide the service—and then find the buyer who is willing to pay that amount. Negotiation and flexibility are important. Trial and error also contribute to setting fees that will allow you to feel fairly compensated while allowing your clients to feel that they have gotten their money's worth.

The profit motive undoubtedly steers many nurses toward entrepreneurial practice. But you must carefully consider the nature of any profit. When you are self employed, many of the "givens" you enjoyed as an employee vanish. No one issues you a fixed-amount pay check on a regular pay schedule. No one withholds your taxes, enrolls you in a retirement plan, or structures your health insurance benefits. Instead, you control and must manage all these benefits. At the same time, you will likely enjoy more control over your time and, perhaps, your attire. These, then, are the realities. If you have the courage and enthusiasm to accept such challenges, nurse entrepreneurship may be a good choice for you. Other nurse entrepreneurs will likely be glad to help you establish yourself in these areas.

Another concern related to entrepreneurial practice is the business structure adopted. This often is a financial and legal decision based on the objective of the desired business, but may also be a function of the community or state in which the entrepreneur resides (i.e., because of local or state ordinances). Examine these issues carefully with a trusted accountant and attorney.

Yet another concern related to entrepreneurial practice is whether to operate as a specialist or generalist. It has been said that fame accompanies the specialist but fortune accompanies the generalist. This certainly does not mean that a specialist cannot make a good deal of money. However, the entrepreneur focusing on a very specific product or service had better be in the right place at the right time. Furthermore, the ability to diversify and adapt is important to long-term success.

As discussed earlier, nurse entrepreneurs are still rather uncommon. It is thus important to consider how different you want to be. Do your current environment and living conditions allow you to accept the risks and ambiguities of entrepreneurial practice? How nontraditional are you willing to be?

RESOURCES FOR FURTHER INFORMATION

Any bookstore offers dozens of books about business. You can also find valuable information in the business sections of local newspapers. Several monthly periodicals are devoted specifically to individuals interested in entrepreneurship. Browsing your newsstand will introduce you to many of these. Several that nurse entrepreneurs commonly read include *Inc., The Executive Female, Money*, and *Forbes*.

The National Nurses in Business Association (NNBA), founded in 1988, is dedicated to promoting nurse entrepreneurs in developing, growing, owning or managing businesses in the health care industry. NNBA's mission is to integrate the art of nursing and the world of business in order to help nurses reach their personal career goals and, concurrently, elevate awareness of the unique contribution of nurses in the business of health care. As NNBA works with its approximately seven hundred members nationwide, assisting them with networking and educational needs, local health care consumers also benefit. Approximately one-half of its members already own and operate health care-related business; and the other one-half are exploring entrepreneurial options and seeking nurses with like ambitions and ideas. You can reach the NNBA in Staten Island, New York, by calling (800)-331-6534.

SUMMARY

Becoming a nurse entrepreneur can be exciting and satisfying. Although you will face many challenging decisions, the opportunities and role options are tremendous. Any nurse who wishes to explore this professional alternative must remember the following critical elements: the courage to be different, a feeling of discontent with existing options, an identified niche, a desire to fulfil an obvious need, and the necessary knowledge, skills, and credentials. If you currently possess or—in the case of knowledge, skills, and credentials—are willing to obtain these elements, entrepreneurial practice can greatly reward you.

REFERENCES

Anderson, C. (1994). The enemy within. *Nursing Outlook, 42*(4), 149–50.

Benner, P. (1984). *From novice to expert: Excellence and power in clinical nursing practice.* Menlo Park, CA: Addison-Wesley Publishing Co.

Covey, S. (1989). *The seven habits of highly effective people: Powerful lessons in personal change.* New York: Simon & Schuster.

Gartner, W. B. (1988). "Who is an entrepreneur?" is the wrong question. *American Journal of Small Business, 12*(4), 11–32.

Herron, D., & Herron, L. (1991). Entrepreneurial nursing as a conceptual basis for in-hospital nursing practice models. *Nursing Economic$, 9*(5), 310–316.

Herron, L. (1990). *The effects of characteristics of the entrepreneur on new venture performance.* Unpublished doctoral dissertation, University of South Carolina, Columbia

Norris, D. (editor) (1991). *How I became a nurse entrepeneur.* Petaluma, CA: National Nurses in Business

Waitley, D. (1995). *Empires of the mind: Lessons to lead and succeed in a knowledge-based world.* New York: William Morrow and Co., Inc.

representing a plaintiff in a Workers' Compensation case may need clarification about a particular procedure that the client underwent. Or an attorney may need an explanation of the type of nursing care necessary after a particular injury. The nurse legal consultant's input and evaluation can aid the attorney in obtaining an award of necessary compensation and benefits for the client.

Familiarizing an Attorney with Medical/Nursing Terminology

Although attorneys who represent individuals with personal injuries of any kind are, as a rule, familiar with medical and nursing terms, new procedures, new theories of treatment, and innovative health care delivery systems regularly emerge. The nurse legal consultant's ability to keep the attorney up to date on such developments, as well as to reinforce traditional health care knowledge, constitutes an invaluable service.

Testifying as an Expert Witness

When a nurse legal consultant acts as an expert witness in a professional negligence case, the consultant is educating the jury regarding the applicable standard of nursing care and whether the nurse whose conduct is in question in the case met that standard (Bernzweig, 1990). Specific requirements for expert witnesses vary among states. Generally, however, an expert witness must be someone who can demonstrate that through training, education, and experience, he or she has expert knowledge concerning the specific area forming the basis of the lawsuit (Bernzweig, 1990; Iyer, 1994).

Qualifications

To begin with, the nurse legal consultant must be someone who has extensive experience in the practice of nursing (Faherty, 1994). In addition, prior experience as a legal consultant or at least some type of experience in the legal system is helpful. For example, many legal consultants begin their careers by first reviewing medical records. As they gain more experience with that aspect of consulting, they then decide to expand their services to also include testifying.

It is helpful for the nurse legal consultant to have advanced educational preparation. This might include a graduate degree, certification in the nurse legal consultant clinical specialty, or both (Faherty, 1994).

The nurse consultant must also be able to communicate effectively, both orally and in writing. In addition, the ability to handle stress and meet deadlines is essential.

An additional qualification for the nurse expert witness is the ability to be comfortable giving an opinion that will be carefully scrutinized by attorneys representing the other parties in a particular case. Because the purpose of any trial or hearing is to obtain a verdict in favor of the client being represented, cross-examination during the trial can be a grueling and uncomfortable experience. In a professional negligence case, this is particularly true, because the expert's opinion must be discredited by the other side, if possible. Thus, the ability to tolerate such discomfort without taking it personally is absolutely vital.

Some nurse legal consultants work part-time for particular attorneys or firms. Others, however, start their own businesses, either on full-time or part-time bases. For nurse legal consultants wanting to start their own businesses in legal consulting, additional desirable qualities include the ability to take risks, self-confidence, and physical and mental stamina (Vogel & Doleysh, 1994).

The Need for Nurse Legal Consultants

The evolution of nursing and the nursing profession clearly indicates that from legal, educational, societal, and legislative perspectives, nursing has and will continue to change to meet the ever-changing demands placed on it (Weiss, 1994). Because more and more cases being filed involve alleged injury due to professional negligence, disability, or other actions involving personal injury, there is no doubt that some of those cases will involve nurses and nursing in some way.

Nurse legal consultants will be increasingly needed to meet the demands that new and current cases will place on the attorneys handling those cases. The nurse interested in becoming a nurse legal consultant can prepare to do so in the following ways:

- take seminars or continuing education courses on legal consulting
- join professional nursing organizations established specifically to help nurses in this role (e.g., the American Association of Nurse Legal Consultants)
- network with nurse colleagues already in the role of the nurse legal consultant
- keep clinical skills current
- obtain advice from necessary experts before starting a business in nurse legal consulting
- consult with nurse legal consultants to better patient care and the nursing profession as a whole by practicing with greater awareness of legal implications

THE NURSE RISK MANAGER

Risk management has been defined as a "systematic program designed to reduce preventable injuries and accidents and minimize the financial severity of claims" (Pozgar, 1993, p. 519). The process of risk management includes four components: risk identification, risk analysis, risk treatment, and risk evaluation (Brent, 1989).

An effective risk management program is proactive and based on loss prevention. After risks have been identified (most commonly through the use of occurrence reports) and analyzed, they are managed by initiating necessary actions to prevent them from occurring and then evaluating the actions implemented (University Hospital Consortium, 1992).

Managing risks in any health care facility is no simple task. Risks that risk management programs focus on include client-related risks (e.g., direct client care privacy and confidentiality of patient information), medical/nursing staff-related risks (e.g., licensure, staff privileges), employee-related risks (e.g., termination, on-the-job injuries), and visitor and family-related risks (e.g., falls) (Hagg, 1990).

Risk management may also include aspects of risk financing (e.g., purchase of professional liability and other insurance needed by the facility) and handling liability claims (University Hospital Consortium, 1992).

If a health care facility is large, the risk management department is given the task of carrying out the system's risk management requirements. If a facility is small, a risk manager, perhaps in conjunction with a risk management committee, may be responsible for administering the risk management program.

Qualifications

The qualifications for a risk manager, identified and compiled by the American Society for Healthcare Risk Management (ASHRM) in 1983 (Goldman, 1990), include the following:

- strong management skills
- knowledge of how a health care facility functions
- familiarity with laws, especially those pertaining to professional negligence and employment
- ability to guide and direct risk financing and risk control
- excellent writing and communication skills.

Experience in a health care profession is also strongly recommended. In fact, in the ASHRM study of 3,037 respondents, 385 possessed academic degrees in nursing or nursing administration, and 577 had previous experience of some form in the health care setting (Goldman, 1990).

Although an academic background concentrating in risk management is not required for a position as a risk manager, some colleges and universities do offer a bachelor's or master's degree in risk management. In fact, the ASHRM study revealed that 13 of the 3,037 respondents possessed academic degrees in this area (Goldman, 1990).

In addition to academic credentials, some form of certification in risk management is usually required. Many certification programs are available, including a professional recognition program offered by the ASHRM, an Associate in Risk Management certification offered by the Insurance Institute of America, and various programs focusing on the insurance business and its impact on health care delivery (Goldman, 1990).

Many law schools have recently established health law programs or institutes offering a master's degree in health law to nonlawyers. Although the offered courses do not focus solely on risk management, graduates of such programs will have been exposed to a solid background in many areas of the law, including professional negligence and other torts (e.g., defamation and false imprisonment), regulatory laws (e.g., Medicare and Medicaid) and medical and nursing staff issues. Academic preparation of this type provides a solid basis for beginning a career in risk management.

The Nurse as Risk Manager

Experienced nurses can make excellent risk managers. Because of their knowledge of health care delivery and patient care, nurses have much to offer their employers in the area of risk management. Knowledge of health care delivery and client care is not enough, however. Nurses must enhance these qualifications by obtaining additional academic preparation.

Because risk managers must also be "facilitators, educators, and enforcers" (Youngberg, 1994, p. xvii), the abilities to tolerate stress, productively handle confrontation and the fallout associated with unpopular decisions, and work long hours are essential to this role.

Experience in some aspect of risk management prior to seeking a position as a risk manager is also important. Such experience might comprise being an active member of a risk management committee while practicing nursing or being a risk management associate in a risk management department.

The Need for Nurse Risk Managers

Risk management is an essential component of health care delivery. Whether in the form of one person acting as the risk management "department" or a large department composed of many associates, risk management is "here to stay." The nurse interested in this role can act on this interest and pursue work in risk management in the following ways:

- explore available academic and certification programs in risk management
- seek experience in risk management while practicing nursing
- seek an entry level position in risk management before applying for a position as risk manager
- contact professional risk management organizations for further information about the role of risk manager
- obtain diversified experience in nursing to enhance personal and professional qualifications in preparation for the role of risk manager

THE NURSE ATTORNEY

An attorney is generally defined as an agent who is authorized to act in the place or stead of another (Black, 1991). In its common usage, however, the term means "attorney at law," "lawyer," or "counselor at law" (Black, 1991, p. 86). Thus, an attorney can be defined as one who is admitted to practice law in a particular state or states and is authorized to perform both civil and legal functions for a client (Black, 1991).

Attorneys practice law in various capacities, including for law firms (large or small), as in-house legal counsel for organizations (e.g., hospitals and long-term care facilities), as staff attorneys for public employers (e.g., as an Assistant States' Attorney or for the child welfare department), or as sole practitioners.

Many attorneys specialize or concentrate in particular areas while others describe their practices as "general" practices. General practitioners or firms provide a wide variety of legal services to their clients, including real estate closings, representation in criminal matters, and drafting and review of legal documents. In contrast, an attorney who specializes in a particular area of the law will handle only those legal problems related to that particular area. Examples of such areas are health law, criminal law, and family law.

The role most commonly associated with an attorney is that of litigator— that is, representative of a client in a trial or other type of judicial or quasi-judicial proceeding (e.g., an administrative hearing). Not all attorneys serve exclusively as litigators, however. Attorneys can also serve as risk managers, law school faculty members, negotiators for their clients (e.g., in relation to employment agreements or business purchases), and administrators in health care facilities.

In order to be licensed to practice law in any state, a person must be a graduate of an approved law school. Specific admission requirements are set by each school, but one requirement is universal: a bachelor's degree. At one time, it was helpful for the applicant to have an undergraduate major in prelaw or political science. Today, however, that is no longer the case. Thus, a nurse with a baccalaureate degree in nursing (or another field) has an equal chance of being accepted to law school as does any other baccalaureate-prepared applicant.

Although many law school applicants have graduate degrees (e.g., MS, PhD), a graduate degree is not required for admittance. Even so, the skills learned in obtaining a postbaccalaureate degree may help the applicant complete law school.

Another prerequisite for admission to law school is the Law School Admission Test (LSAT). The LSAT is given at various times throughout the year; information regarding test dates and locations can be obtained by calling any law school. The better an applicant does on the LSAT, the better the applicant's chances of being considered for admission. to law school. The test measures skills necessary for success in law school (e.g., reading comprehension and critical thinking). The multiple-choice format of the test should pose little problem for nurses because they are accustomed to this testing format.

In addition to the ability to think critically, law students must possess excellent communication skills, write clearly and concisely, be persuasive, and be able to withstand stress. Good organizational skills are also essential in order to complete assignments on time.

Nurses often begin law school with the skills necessary to complete the program. Because the practice of nursing requires the same skills needed to succeed in law school, the nurse who is a law student can adapt and begin to use those skills rather than having to learn them for the first time.

After graduating from law school, the graduate must apply for admission to the bar. This is a long and tedious process requiring, among other things, passing a character and fitness review and taking the bar examination. The character and fitness review is something familiar to a nurse. Although very different in scope and purpose, the graduate nurse undergoes a review in order to be certified to take the nursing licensure examination.

The bar examination is offered only two times each year: in February and July. Most law students prepare for the exam by taking a bar examination preparatory course.

Qualifications

As is true in law school, the skills and expertise acquired as a nurse can be helpful when beginning the practice of law. Independence, critical thinking, the ability to meet deadlines, active listening, and the ability to handle multiple situations (cases) at the same time are all essential. Continued education, whether through continuing education programs or an advanced law degree (e.g., an LLM [master of letters in law] in Health Law), is also essential.

Nurse lawyers must be able to accept the fact that they may often represent unpopular causes or clients. Personal desire to champion good causes or be accepted by others must yield to the professional obligation to represent one's client or cause to the fullest extent allowable by law.

The nurse lawyer must also keep in mind that legal ethics are very different from nursing ethics. Although both are grounded squarely on clear principles of right and wrong, the legal representation of a client is very different from the provision of nursing care, including patient advocacy as it exists within the practice of nursing.

The Need for Nurse Attorneys

The first nurse attorney, Eleanor McGarvah, was admitted to the Michigan bar after graduating from the University of Detroit in 1929 (Northrop & Kelly, 1987). From 1946 to when she retired in 1955, Ms.

McGarvah served as the Detroit Department of Health's Director of the Division of Special Investigations (Northrop & Kelly, 1987). Prior to graduating from law school, she held various nursing positions at the health department.

Many nurse attorneys have followed in Ms. McGaravah's footsteps. Perhaps the best known in recent years is Helen Creighton, whose text *Law Every Nurse Should Know* has been adopted for law courses in many nursing curricula. Other nurse attorneys began practicing law as well, albeit in quieter, less visible positions.

Although the exact number is not easily ascertained, there is little doubt that many nurse attorneys are practicing law today. They practice in large cities as well as smaller towns. Nurse attorneys often specialize in health law, malpractice defense, family law, criminal law, or elder law, to name a few.

In 1977, a nurse attorney named Cynthia Northrop saw the need to establish a professional association for nurse attorneys. Her efforts resulted in the establishment and incorporation of The American Association of Nurse Attorneys, Inc. (TAANA) in 1982 (The American Association of Nurse Attorneys, Inc., no date supplied). This not-for-profit association currently has a membership of over seven hundred fifty nurse attorneys, nurses in law school, and lawyers in nursing school. Its objectives include promoting the dual professions of nurse attorneys, educating its members, establishing a leadership role in health care and policy making, and educating the public about health law issues (The American Association of Nurse Attorneys, Inc., 1994).

Nurse attorneys' unique perspective on the practice of law will continue to be needed in the legal arena. Although the current overabundance of attorneys in some areas of the country (e.g., in large cities) often means too few positions available in those areas, the nurse attorney's dual preparation makes him or her a desirable candidate for any available position.

The nurse who is contemplating a career as a nurse attorney should obtain as much information as possible regarding law and the practice of law. Before making the change to nurse attorney, the nurse should do the following:

- attend an open house sponsored by the local law school
- talk to nurse attorneys about their practices and the practice of law in general
- evaluate the need for additional nurse attorneys in the community
- obtain information on classes offered through the health law institute of a law school
- contact TAANA to obtain information on nurse attorney practice and TAANA members
- take the LSAT as an initial indicator of abilities/capabilities for law school.

SUMMARY

It is clear that nursing as a profession can provide for additional careers in the area of the law, should nurses decide to explore new roles in this area. The nursing background allows nurses to make unique contributions to the legal arena in the roles of nurse legal consultant, nurse risk manager, and nurse attorney.

REFERENCES

Bernzweig, E. (1990). *The nurse's liability for malpractice: A programmed course (5th Ed.).* St. Louis, MO: C. V. Mosby.

Black, H. C. (1991). *Black's law dictionary (6th Ed.).* St. Paul, MN: West Publishing Co.

Brent, N. J. (1989). Risk management in home health care: Focus on patient care liabilities. *Loyola University of Chicago Law Journal, 20*(3), 775–795.

Faherty, B. (1994). Legal nurse consultants: Who are they? *Journal of Nursing Law, 2*(1), 37–49.

Goldman, T. (1990). The risk manager. In L. Harpster & M. Veatch (Eds.), *Risk management handbook for health care facilities* (pp. 37–53). Chicago: American Hospital Publishing, Inc.

Hagg, S. (1990). Elements of a risk management program. In L. Harpster & M. Veach (Eds.), *Risk management handbook for health care facilities* (pp. 23–33). Chicago: American Hospital Publishing, Inc.

Iyer, P. (1994). Mastering the expert witness role. *Journal Of Nursing Law, 1*(2), 35–45.

Noel, N. (1993). Historical overview: Policy, politics and nursing. In D. Mason, S. Talbott, and J. Leavitt (Eds.), *Policy and politics for nurses: Action and change in the workplace, government organizations and community.* (2nd Ed., pp. 36–46). Philadelphia: W. B. Saunders Company.

Northrop, C., & Kelly, M. (1987). *Legal issues in nursing.* St. Louis, MO: C. V. Mosby Company.

Pozgar, G. (1993). *Legal aspects of health care administration (5th Ed.).* Gaithersburg, MD: Aspen Publishers, Inc.

The American Association of Nurse Attorneys, Inc. (1994-1996). Endorsement Statement of The American Association of Nurse Attorneys. *Journal of Nursing Law.* _____. Informational brochure. Baltimore, MD: author.

University Hospital Consortium. (1992). *Nursing-legal survival: A risk management guide for nurses.* OakBrook, IL: Author.

Vogel, G., & Doleysh, N. (1994). Characteristics of successful entrepreneurs. *Entrepreneuring: A nurse's guide to starting a business* (2nd Edition). New York: NLN Press (Pub. No. 14-2635), 25–57.

Weiss, J. P. (1994). Nursing practice: A legal and historical perspective. *Journal of Nursing Law 2*(1), 17–36.

Youngberg, B. J. (Ed.) (1994). *The risk manager's desk reference* Gaithersburg, MD: Aspen Publishers, Inc.

Chapter Fifteen

Nursing Opportunities in the Public Sector: Military and Public Service

Sandra A. Holmes

INTRODUCTION

Some of the oldest, most time-honored career opportunities available to nurses exist in the public sector. The federal government began a health service for merchant sailors in 1798. Even though some might label it conventional or antiquated, the health care arena in the military, the U.S. Public Health Service (USPHS, or PHS) and the Federal Civil Service System evolve and change just as dramatically and rapidly as any other health care arena. These venues may not appeal to nurses who are perfectly content to settle and work in the hometowns where they were born and raised. However, the public sector is most definitely a viable option for the flexible individual with a sense of adventure.

The uniformed services consist of the U.S. Air Force, the U.S. Army, and the U.S. Navy, under the aegis of the Department of Defense (DoD), and the less publicized Commissioned Corps of the PHS, a component of the U.S.

Department of Health and Human Services (DHHS). A nurse in any one of the four serves in a dual capacity, as both a professional RN and a commissioned officer. Certain leadership and management responsibilities are inherent in being an officer, but along with these come increased autonomy in decision making as well as an emphasis on nurturing, developing, and educating junior personnel. Many may assume that the services are strict, rigid, and regimented. Yet, this is not the case! The central focus in the medical departments is on providing the highest quality patient care. Likewise, the standards and expectations of nursing and quality are the very highest. For example, the army has established standards of nursing practice, a comprehensive set of guidelines that is regularly updated to include the very latest developments in patient care.

MILITARY NURSING

With the exception of wearing a dictated uniform and meeting the eligibility requirements (as outlined in Table 15.1), the nurse's role in the armed forces is parallel to that of a civilian nurse. Military nurses, under most circumstances work forty hours per week and rotate shifts. Permanent shifts are sometimes available. Some military treatment facilities (MTFs) operate on eight-hour shifts, but units such as the ICU and ER may operate on twelve-hour shifts, with staff working thirty-six hours one week and forty-eight hours the next. There is no compensation for overtime or shift differential. By and large, the military utilizes team nursing in the nonspecialty areas.

Opportunities exist in ambulatory care, community health, managed care, computer technology, critical care, staff development, education, emergency/trauma, maternal/child health, medical/surgical nursing, neuropsychiatry, nursing administration, nursing research, orthopedics, perioperative nursing, and quality assurance. Expanded roles available include but are not limited to family nurse practitioner, midwifery, nurse anesthetist, OB/GYN nurse practitioner, and pediatric nurse practitioner.

Recent Changes

Similar to the civilian sector, the uniformed services are experiencing transformational times. Nurses are functioning in expanded roles, both clinically and administratively. Commanding officer assignments (comparable to private-sector CEOs) are now filled by nurses rather than just by physicians or health care administrators, as was the case in the past. There is also a shift from acute care to ambulatory care. Patients are being discharged earlier, and more surgery is being done on an outpatient basis. In all branches of the military, there is a continual need for critical care nurses.

So-called "mergers" in the military setting are taking the form of Tricare Health Service Regions. For instance, in northern California, Letterman Army Hospital has closed, and the Oakland Naval Hospital is slated for closure. David Grant USAF Medical Center will become the lead agent MTF for the entire region. In some locations, the MTF may be a bi- or tri-service facility staffed by personnel from the army, navy, and the air force, or by a combination of staff from any two of these. For example, the military hospital in Landstuhl, Germany, originally an army facility, is now a bi-service facility staffed by personnel from the army and the air force.

The end of the Cold War has had a significant impact on the DoD. Recommendations from the Base Realignment and Closure Commission have focused on several hospitals such as Fitzsimmons Army Medical Center, Long Beach Naval Hospital, and the base hospital at Castle Air Force Base, to mention a few. In addition, smaller, outpatient medical clinics located on military bases, are closed whenever nearby military bases are closed, such as the clinic at Mare Island Shipyard. Furthermore, the downsizing of the military has significantly reduced the health care staffing requirements. Fortunately, the demand for qualified nurses and nurse specialists such as nurse anesthetists remains high.

A cornerstone of military medicine has historically been—and continues to be—education. Balanced-budget, overall force-downsizing, and deficit-reduction efforts have all led to an increase in tri-service training initiatives, such as the Uniformed Services University of the Health Sciences. In some cases these initiatives take the form of service-wide programs, with a specific number of seats allotted to each DoD branch. In other cases, advanced cardiac life support (ACLS), advanced trauma life support (ATLS), or emergency medical technician (EMT) training may be coordinated on a regional basis. In some smaller less densely populated regions, training endeavors are also encompassing personnel at Veterans' Administration hospitals and other federal installations. Furthermore, other aspects of health care, such as a composite health care computer system for medical records, are being developed on a tri-service basis. Some free-thinking, nontraditional individuals have even gone so far as to predict that the future will bring a "purple suit concept" within the DoD, where all aspects of military medicine will be integrated and merged together as one.

Deployment

A significant aspect of military nursing that sets it apart from almost every other nursing career is operational readiness/contingency preparedness. For example, nurses were recently sent to the naval base on Guantanamo Bay, Cuba, to provide health care for Haitian refugees. Every member of the armed forces must also be available and willing to deploy (i.e., be sent on temporary assignment) in cases of conflict, such as those of Desert Storm, Somalia, or Bosnia.

The sixty-bed U.S. Field Hospital under the auspices of the United Nations (U.N.) in Croatia-Zagreb, for example, provides care for 32,000 U.N. troops from thirty-two countries. Located 200 miles from Sarajevo and the most hostile fighting, the hospital is staffed by 150 medical personnel including 21 nurses and 2 nurse anesthetists. Every six months, the staff is rotated, and another branch of the U.S. Armed Forces takes over. Aside from providing optimum care in a field setting, the other obvious challenge is the language barrier. The hospital serves military personnel from thirty-two different countries. It is common to have patients from Russia, the Netherlands, Egypt, Slovakia, Canada, the Czech Republic, and the Scandinavian countries. Sign language, interpreters, and dictionaries—not to mention other creative means of communication—are constantly in use. This represents the epitome of transcultural nursing! Ordinarily, patients are provided initial acute care and then are medevaced to their home countries for further treatment. One nineteen-year-old Russian who spoke no English was an exception to this rule, however. He had sustained a left below-the-knee amputation and remained at the hospital for 2 1/2 months to undergo physical therapy and prosthetic fitting. He finally returned to his battalion and to his job as a clerk. By the time he left, both he and the staff had learned enough words in each others' languages so as to communicate fairly easily. Getting to know him while providing him care was one of the most memorable experiences for the nursing staff during their entire deployment.

PHS

For nearly two centuries, the PHS has worked toward a single goal: improving and advancing the health of the nation's people. The PHS is the principal health agency of the federal government, and manages the largest public health program in the world. The 8,000 officers within the PHS help provide health care and related services to medically underserved populations (such as Native Americans and Alaskan Natives), and to other population groups having special needs. From inner-city clinics to remote, rural health centers, PHS nurses treat many disadvantaged patients who literally have nowhere else to go.

PHS Agencies

Eight agencies compose the PHS. Six of these—the Agency for Health Care Policy and Research (AHCPR), the Centers for Disease Control (CDC), the Food and Drug Administration (FDA), the Health Resources and Services Administration (HRSA), the Indian Health Service (IHS), and the National Institutes of Health (NIH)—afford career opportunities for nurses. In addition, PHS nurses are frequently assigned to challenging medical care and public health positions in the following federal programs: the Federal Bureau of Prisons (BOP), the Health Care Financing Administration (HCFA), the Immigration and Naturalization Service (INS), and the National Oceanic and Atmospheric Administration (NOAA).

Openings for nurses and nurse specialists in some agencies, such as the BOP or INS, are expanding by leaps and bounds. With a primary emphasis on preventive and ambulatory care, the PHS itself does not have any hospital facilities. However, the agencies under PHS do. For example, the NIH, which is the federal government's principal biomedical research agency, has 13 research institutes, 3 research centers, a 478-bed clinical complex, and the National Library of Medicine.

The IHS operates forty-one hospitals of varying sizes, as well as numerous health centers. Within IHS there is thus a demand for nurses in acute care, ambulatory care, clinics, and public health programs. An additional nine hospitals and several clinics are operated under tribal control, and Native Americans have replaced commissioned officers in these settings. The IHS works with over 510 distinct tribes across the country and enjoys cooperative relationships with these tribes. For instance, the twenty-five-bed Acoma-Canconcito-Laguna Hospital in west central New Mexico provides general medical and pediatric care in a traditional Navajo healing setting. When the hospital was being designed, local tribes requested a ritual room. A Native American nurse and architect were instrumental in assisting in the design of the room, which resembles a Navajo hogan and is used by patients and traditional healers. The main door faces east, and in the center of the floor is an open pit, which provides direct access to the bare earth below.

However, difficult challenges confront IHS nurses. For instance, one out of every four Native Americans and Alaskan Natives lives below the poverty line. Further, the risks of illness and premature death from alcoholism, diabetes, tuberculosis, heart disease, accidents, homicide, suicide, pneumonia, and influenza are greater for Native Americans and Alaskan Natives than for the United States population as a whole.

Variety in Nursing

While geopolitical shifts within the United States influence staffing changes within certain agencies, the PHS has a need for not only nurse generalists, but also nurses subspecialtizing in perioperative, obstetrics, pediatrics, critical care, ambulatory care, and public health, as well as advanced practice nurses such as certified nurse midwives (CNMs), certified registered nurse anesthetists (CRNAs), and family nurse practitioners (NPs). Obviously, the roles, responsibilities, and tasks of nurses in the PHS vary depending on the mission of the employing agency. For example, an AHCPR nurse with a master's degree in public health might work with a panel of civilian experts to develop research-based guidelines similar to those recently released for the treatment of pressure ulcers; while an NP for HRSA might be found working in a migrant health center operated by the National Health Service Corps. And yet another NP having seniority within the BOP might serve as the administrator in charge of a Federal Transfer Center operated by this agency.

Unique Aspects of Service

One of the unique challenges of being a commissioned PHS officer is functioning within the directives and requirements of two organizations—that is, the PHS and the agency of assignment. On occasion, this results in "gray areas" and "mixing apples and oranges." For example, nurses in the PHS are officers and, thus, have prescribed uniforms; but some agencies do not require uniforms to be worn in the work setting, others require them to be worn only on certain days, and still others require them to be worn daily.

Unlike the military, the PHS does not have an operational/contingency focus. Rather, in the event of a major conflict, PHS officers may be assigned stateside to replace DoD military personnel who are deployed overseas. However, teams of PHS officers did serve for thirty to sixty days on a voluntary basis during the recent hostilities in both Kuwait and Somalia. PHS officers have also volunteered aboard the hospital ship HOPE, operated by the People-to-People Health Foundation. Staff from various federal agencies may travel overseas on special assignments, working with other nations and international agencies toward solving global health problems. CDC personnel, for instance, traveled to Africa to investigate the AIDS virus and, more recently, the deadly Ebola virus.

FEDERAL CIVIL SERVICE SYSTEM

The federal government is the nation's largest single employer. The civil service system, which is managed by the Office of Personnel Management, has well over two million civilian employees in over one hundred agencies. Civil service nurses can be found working side by side with military and PHS nurses. In addition, positions often are available at other federally operated facilities and institutions. One of the best illustrations of the nurse role in civil service can be found within the Department of Veterans Affairs (VA). The VA, which employs over thirty-seven thousand professional nurses, offers veterans the largest, most comprehensive health care system in the United States, with more than one hundred seventy medical centers nationwide. Furthermore, the elevation of the VA to cabinet status in the mid-1980s has led to an increase in both the quantity and quality of services for veterans. Whereas the Civil Service System as a whole has been heavily impacted by the Base Closure and Realignment Commission (with the 1993 recommendations resulting in nearly fifty thousand civil service jobs being abolished or transferred), the VA has been left relatively unscathed.

Variety in Nursing

Nursing opportunities with the VA include clinical practice, administration, research, and education in ambulatory, acute, and extended care settings. In addition to medical, surgical, and psychiatric units, the VA offers nurses challenging roles in many specialized areas including intensive care, operating room, alcohol/drug treatment, posttraumatic stress disorder, geriatrics, rehabilitation, epilepsy, blind rehabilitation, hemodialysis, organ transplant, and spinal cord injury. The VA also has nursing home care units, day treatment, and hospital-based home care programs to serve the increasing number of elderly veterans.

The VA has assignments available for clinical nurse specialists (CNSs), NPs, infection control nurses, quality assurance nurses, and community health nurses. In addition, because the VA is one of the largest medical research organizations in the country, research is basic to all components of nursing practice. At many VA facilities, in fact, it is not at all uncommon to find doctorally prepared nurses conducting research and providing consultation to other nurses interested in conducting research.

Unique Aspects of Service

The closure of military MTFs could result in increased numbers of veterans who formerly received health care at military facilities obtaining care instead at VA facilities. Some individuals involved in health care reform have even gone so far as to propose that all health care for military retirees be provided by the VA. In one or two places, the VA Medical Center also doubles as the military MTF for nearby military installations, providing health care for active duty personnel as well as retirees (as is the case with Kirtland Air Force Base in Albuquerque, New Mexico) .

Like PHS commissioned nurses, nurses in the VA system do not have an operational/contingency role. However, they may be called on to furnish medical care backup to military hospitals during national emergencies. Also, in the event of a *major* conflict, should a shortage of beds occur in military hospitals, patients could be transferred to VA facilities to make room for "fresh" casualties. During major disasters, the VA also operates command centers to coordinate services through the National Disaster Medical Service.

Because the vast majority of VA medical centers are located in metropolitan areas, many of them have affiliations with both medical and nursing schools. In fact, the VA provides clinical rotations for one out of every three physicians and one out of every four professional nurses in the United States. The VA also provides training for members of various other health care disciplines. Consequently, assisting students in clinical areas and collaborating with faculty can be a major facet of the VA nurse's role.

The Civil Service System uses decentralized hiring, meaning that applications and vacancies are handled directly by each institution. Civil service nurses are covered by a locality pay system (LPS) designed to ensure that nurses' salaries are competitive with those in local labor markets. Thus, salary ranges vary according to facility location. Unlike their uniformed services counterparts, who are salaried workers, VA and civil service nurses do receive shift differentials for evening and night work, as well as premium pay for overtime, on-call, weekend, and holiday duty.

One Nurse's Career Path

Vietnam veteran Joan Furey's seventeen-year career with the VA clearly illustrates the opportunities and roles available to nurses in the VA and civil service. After her discharge from the Army Nurse Corps, she obtained her BSN and MA in Nursing and began working for the VA in Florida. Beginning as a staff nurse, she subsequently worked first as a head nurse and then as a nursing supervisor for several years. Following a year in Maine as Assistant Chief, Nursing Service, she returned to Florida and was assigned as Chief, Nursing Service. From that job, she went to Palo Alto, California, where she was the Associate Director of Education at the VA's National Center for Post Traumatic Stress Disorder Clinical Laboratory and Education. She is currently serving as the first Director of Women Veterans Program Office at the VA headquarters in Washington, DC.

BASIC REQUIREMENTS

Nurses must have several qualifications in order to obtain commissions in the military or PHS. These are listed in Table 15.1, as are the requisites for civil service employment.

Without a doubt, flexibility is the hallmark of a nurse in any one of the four uniformed services. Other critical characteristics include a sense of adventure, commitment, dedication to nursing, a strong sense of caring, creativity, honesty, loyalty, leadership, high energy, solid people skills and common sense. Nurses must also be good team players who are skilled in negotiation, helping others, and communicating professionally with patients and colleagues alike. Certain assignments or agencies may also require special skills. For instance, nurses working in the IHS also must feel comfortable working in settings strongly influenced by the past and be able to demonstrate respect for ancient traditions.

Mobility, or the willingness to move, is another essential trait. Only civil service nurses are not ordinarily subject to involuntary relocation. In the uniformed services, everyone has a choice of assignment location, but officers are subject to assignment wherever they are needed. PHS has an interesting approach to managing assignments. Their nurses must find vacancies for which they qualify, interview for those positions and be selected. This naturally requires networking skills to ferret out openings in desired locations and agencies. On the other hand, they also have the option of remaining in their same jobs and locations. However, doing so may decrease their chances for promotion.

In the armed forces, nurses generally move, or "rotate duty stations," every three to four years. They are offered several options, and are given their first

Table 15.1 Qualifications for Federal Service

Criteria	Air Force	Navy	Army	USPHS	Civil Service
Be a U.S. citizen	yes	yes	yes	yes	yes
BSN or MSN from an NLN-accredited school of nursing	yes	yes	yes	yes	a
Current nursing license valid in the U.S., Guam, or the Virgin Islands[b]	yes	yes	yes	yes	yes
Meet height, weight, and physical requirements	yes	yes	yes	yes	yes
Married or single	either	either	either	either	either
Open to male and female	yes	yes	yes	yes	yes
Age	c	d	e	f	g
Initial obligation	3 yr.	3 yr.	3 yr.	3 yr.	None

[a] State-approved school of nursing
[b] Recent baccalaureate-degree graduates must take the NCLEX-RN exam prior to reporting for active duty and must become licensed within one year.
[c] 18 to 35 years of age(waivers up to 48 years of age)
[d] 31 to 33 years of age(waivers up to 47 years of age)
[e] At least 20 but under 35 years of age (some waivers for prior service)
[f] Under 44 years of age
[g] Basically, no age limit; however, some exceptions may apply.

preferences whenever possible. Overseas assignments have specified "tour lengths" that vary from one to three years. Each branch has established career pathways and senior officers who work closely with each individual officer to ensure assignments and opportunities that will enhance promotion to a higher rank.

Another characteristic required of military nurses is the ability to teach, nurture, and counsel junior personnel, both officer and enlisted. Positive role modeling and mentoring skills are definite assets! In addition, overseas assignments entail the responsibilities of being sensitive toward other cultures and cultural differences, and serving as an ambassador abroad. An issue brought to light on several patient-satisfaction surveys involving a postpartum unit in the Philippines vividly illustrates the importance of cultural awareness and sensitivity. Several caucasian women were distressed that the Filipino women were not taking showers or baths. Unfortunately, the caucasian women were unaware that in the Filipino culture, showering or bathing is taboo for thirty days following delivery. They were equally unaware of the customarily exacting perineal care that their "roommates" were carefully carrying out in the privacy of the bathroom!

Working in any large organization requires the ability to tolerate a certain amount of bureaucratic "red tape." The old days of inflexible, strict routines have all but disappeared in the military and civil service, however. Fortunately, in an era of continuous quality improvement, there is most definitely a place for individuals with vision who are articulate and patient in finding solutions to issues and problems. For example, two navy nurses based in San Diego, California, and having computer/informatics background worked closely with ICU staff and with computer programmers contracted by the navy to design and implement a truly twenty-first-century bedside computer system. "CliniComp" maintains all the data generated by any patient-monitoring system and handles all clinical information about the patient, including manual input such as the nursing care record. The system can calculate drips, rates, and any other pertinent data! Although many regulations govern practice in the military, a nurse who takes initiative can locate great opportunities and resources for innovation. As one renowned navy admiral quipped, "It's often easier to ask forgiveness than to ask permission."

COLLEAGUES

Nurses in the uniformed services work side by side with physicians, pharmacists, dietitians, physical and occupational therapists, social workers, physician's assistants, and the full array of allied health professionals. The professional health care team functions in an atmosphere of mutual respect and cooperation. Physicians value nurses' judgment and often seek their input. Esprit de corps and camaraderie quickly and easily develop among the members of the team. Depending on the location, uniformed staff may be augmented by civil service personnel, or vice versa, as is true of most PHS assignments.

All military hospitals are accredited by the Joint Commission on Accreditation of Healthcare Organizations (JCAHO). Military health care facilities range from small branch clinics to 500-bed, state-of-the-art teaching hospitals comparable to university medical centers and having accredited internship, residency, and fellowship programs. In the larger hospitals with graduate medical education programs, nurses work closely with interns and residents as well as staff physicians.

By and large the majority of ancillary personnel at military MTFs are enlisted personnel, also known as army medics, USAF technicians, or navy hospital corpsmen. Patient-care assignments and administrative paperwork are shared with these staff members, who normally function at the level of licensed vocational nurses (LVNs) or licensed practical nurses (LPNs). Following initial basic training, or "boot camp," these individuals attend advanced training to learn basic nursing skills. In the navy, for instance, this training is fourteen weeks in length, and the bulk of the faculty is composed of Nurse Corps officers. Obviously, one of the primary responsibilities of military nurses in the clinical setting is to assist enlisted personnel in building on the foundation of basic client-care skills. Nurses work very closely with enlisted personnel to ensure that all nursing tasks and procedures are performed safely and correctly. The need for teaching, leadership, and supervisory and delegation skills becomes even more evident in view of the work that these nurses do with these service men and women. Taking the time to carefully and thoroughly orient, supervise, guide, clarify, educate, motivate, and support enlisted personnel results in very functional members of the health care team!

The military health care team provides care to not only active duty personnel and their families, but also retired personnel and their families. The client population spans the spectrum from neonates to the elderly. The health care team and patients represent a cross section typical of American society as a whole. They represent both large and small communities, various backgrounds, and all nationalities and races.

The PHS does not have an enlisted component. Rather, all PHS ancillary personnel are employed through the Federal Civil Service System. The client population served depends on the agency. INS nurses provide care to detained aliens. Nurses assigned to the NOAA provide care to the scientist officers who staff and command NOAA ships and aircraft and to their families. A nurse practicing in the Alaska region of the IHS provides comprehensive care to Alaskan Natives representing seven different tribes, each retaining many of its original customs and beliefs.

Working with the Medicine Man

M any of Anne Gwiazdowski's staff at the IHS Wind River Service Unit in Montana are Native Americans. "I have an MPH (master's in public health) nutritionist, an LPN, and an RN/BSN who are Shoshone; an MPH health educator who is a Lumbee tribal member; two community health outreach workers who are tribal members; and two male public health nurses. The secretarial and clerical staff are also all of Native American heritage." Nurses working in the Navajo area of the Southwest quickly become aware of the special connections between the Navajo people and their traditions. The medicine man or woman functions as doctor, counselor, priest, and historian. He or she works with IHS health professionals in referring patients to medical doctors for the treatment of serious illnesses.

The Patients Are Prisoners

A colleague from graduate school has been a commissioned officer with the PHS for the past six years. Currently assigned to the BOP, he is the Chief Nurse in the Federal Transfer Center located in Oklahoma City, Oklahoma. His staff includes seven contract LPNs, three PHS flight nurses, and one civil service flight nurse. They are responsible for the basic health care of prisoners in a seven-story federal prison and during transit on airlift operations. They work closely with federal marshals in transferring prisoners around the skies of the United States on two Boeing 727 jets, jokingly referred to as "Con Air, where you must be indicted to be invited." A master's degree in nursing, training as a flight nurse, and previous experience as an air force nurse helped him qualify for this position. One of the flight nurses on his staff waited more than one year for a flight nurse vacancy in this particular facility. When the position became available, she accepted her PHS commission. She didn't want to work anywhere else or hold any other position in the PHS.

Nurses in the VA system care for veterans, both male and female. It may be mistakenly assumed that most VA patients are in the geriatric age range. However, even nineteen- or twenty-year-olds who have been medically discharged from the military with service-related injuries or disabilities are eligible for and receive care at VA medical centers. For instance, a young airman who loses a limb in an accident while on duty would initially be cared for in an air force facility and then discharged from the service. At that time, he would be eligible for care through the VA. The same would be true for a service member diagnosed with a chronic illness, such as myasthenia gravis or amyotrophic lateral sclerosis, that precludes him from performing his duties.

GEOGRAPHIC VARIATIONS AND OPPORTUNITIES

Federal service offers wide role diversity depending on location and seniority. Although the vast majority of federal installations are located close to major metropolitan areas, there are also "isolated" facilities and/or assignments where one or maybe two nurses work independently. White House nurse for the president and his family; recruiting officer in Buffalo, New York; nurse anesthesia instructor at the Uniformed Services University of the Health Sciences; and research nurse in Lima, Peru, or Cairo, Egypt, are several examples of potential roles for military nurses.

At a small shipyard in Mississippi there are two civil service occupational nurses. The navy and NOAA have a few, select nursing positions available aboard ship. The INS maintains several one-person clinics similar to its screening center in Puerto Rico. Nurses in such facilities usually practice independently with remote consultation from physicians. All of the uniformed services have flight nurse positions. The bulk of these naturally are found in the air force. Following a highly competitive, six-week course, air force flight nurses have the opportunity to travel all over the world, flying and providing care to patients at 30,000 feet!

There are also headquarters assignments, primarily in the Washington, DC area, where nurses have the opportunity to become involved in long-range planning and policy and decision making. PHS nurses under the HCFA are involved in the administration of Medicare and Medicaid programs. Policy development considers eligibility, coverage, and reimbursement, and addresses whether a person is eligible to have services paid for, whether a certain service should be paid for, and what a service is worth. Military nurses might be found at the Pentagon, working for the surgeon general of their respective branches of service; in the Office of Legislative Affairs, evaluating the impact of pending legislation on the armed forces; serving as congressional fellows; or working in the Office of the Assistant Secretary of Defense for Health Affairs.

One of the greatest opportunities available to military nurses by far is overseas assignment. Between the three services, there are over forty-seven overseas locations, from Germany to Panama, Iceland to Italy, Spain to Puerto Rico, and numerous locations in between. Transportation and moving expenses are paid by the government for all uniformed services nurses and their families. With these expenses paid, experiencing the culture, cuisine, and sights of a foreign country firsthand is a priceless opportunity and benefit. Furthermore, there is no break in or loss of seniority, tenure, or benefits when transferred to a new assignment.

Living abroad is not just an enriching experience, but humbling and sensitizing as well. Nurses who have been assigned overseas return home with a tremendous appreciation for all that we in the United States have, have become accustomed to, and tend to take for granted. For instance, in the Far East, shopping for fresh fruits and vegetables in the local, open-air market is a delightful experience; but, the produce must be rinsed in a bleach solution before it can be consumed. As another example, consider a rural Filipino hospital. Here, the families of hospitalized patients are responsible for providing linens and meals, and even for purchasing IV solutions and medications at the pharmacy in town. These items are then given by the families to the unit nurse for administration.

Many of the smaller overseas hospitals—such as those in Iwakuni, Japan, and Sigonella, Sicily—have a low average daily census. There may only be two wards—one for males and another for females and children. Military nurses in these locations may find themselves functioning more as generalists, caring for pediatric, medical, surgical, and obstetrical patients all on the same shift. Any critically ill or complicated cases are immediately medevaced to the closest MTF or civilian hospital for care. MTFs overseas also have positions for civil service nurses; however, preference is sometimes given to qualified spouses of military personnel.

The PHS also offers enormous geographic diversity. There are opportunities in every state as well as in some United States territories. Under the IHS, for example, most opportunities are in rural areas throughout the California region, except in the highly populated southern part of the state. In the Portland area (which includes Oregon, Washington, and Idaho), all service units are community-based outpatient clinics, and most are within 100 miles of a major city. Nurses working in these units enjoy a great deal of autonomy in practice.

EDUCATIONAL OPPORTUNITIES

Another opportunity afforded by federal service is education. All branches of the military, the PHS, and the VA each offer excellent programs for students in both baccalaureate and master programs. If selected, applicants may receive a monthly stipend, tuition assistance, or reimbursement for school fees and books, or a combination of the three, depending on the service and the educational program.

Student nurses today also have the opportunity to apply for a full Reserve Officer Training Corps (ROTC). Under this program, students receive up to four years of tuition, textbook reimbursement, and monthly stipend. All of these programs are highly competitive, and specifics may change depending on the need for and availability of qualified nurses. There is also a service obligation upon graduation.

Education, particularly in the military, is a priority. Nurses are strongly encouraged to pursue continued personal and professional growth. Opportunities for advanced education leading to higher degrees are available on a competitive basis. For those who qualify, full-time duty under instruction (full time pay and benefits while attending school full time) is available at civilian colleges and universities of the nurse's choice. The nurse must choose an accredited course of study that best meets the needs of the individual and the military. Besides having tuition, fees, and books paid for by the military, nurses continue to receive full pay and benefits while attending school. Of course, there is an obligation of additional active duty service with this program.

Many MFTs are located near large colleges or universities, making it possible for nurses to attend classes during off-duty time. Under the part-time out-service program, nurses can receive tuition reimbursement of 75% for approved courses taken during off-duty hours. In addition, all branches offer advanced or clinical specialty courses. Some of these are a perioperative nursing course, intensive care course, combat casualty care course, air force flight nurse course, and nurse anesthesia course. Besides these in-depth courses, each branch offers one- or two-week leadership and management courses designed to prepare nurses for positions of greater authority and responsibility as they progress in their careers.

An in-depth orientation is provided to all military, PHS, and civil service nurses. Many facilities also have extensive preceptor programs for new graduates. Because most air force hospitals have fewer than fifty beds, the air force offers a twelve-week transition program at its six regional teaching hospitals. During clinical rotations, the new graduate is paired with a preceptor and focuses on learning and improving clinical skills. The IHS has a highly competitive RN intern program, also designed for the new graduate. This program is offered at the Alaska Native Medical Center in Anchorage and the Pine Ridge Indian Hospital in South Dakota. Over a five-month period, nurses rotate to all clinical areas, including the ER and outpatient clinics, to enhance their skills.

All nurses in the federal service are encouraged to participate in professional associations and keep up with the latest nursing practice trends by attending short courses, seminars, and workshops offered by civilian organizations for continuing education credit. In many instances, the government pays the registration fees as well as travel, lodging, and incidental expenses.

OTHER BENEFITS

There are still other advantages and benefits to federal service employment. Compare those listed in Table 15.2 to the benefits typically offered by other careers.

Table 15.2 Benefits Offered by the Uniformed Services and the Civil Service

Uniformed Services	Civil Service
Rank is based on the number of years of education and experience. Eligibility for promotion is based on accumulated experience, length of time in service, or length of time in grade. Officers meeting these criteria, are automatically considered for promotion.	Appointment grade and salary are based on education, experience, and the level of the position to which assigned. Pay is based on the grade of the position. An employee must apply under the merit-promotion plan for a promotion and selection is based on merit.
Automatic longevity pay raises at two, three, and four years, then at every two years, plus cost of living increases.	Longevity and merit pay increases.
In addition to base salary, tax-free allowance for housing and food, and variable housing costs.	
Transportation and moving expenses plus relocation allowance paid by the federal government.	Transportation and moving expenses plus relocation allowance paid by the federal government. *continued*

Table 15.2 Benefits Offered by the Uniformed Services and the Civil Service (continued)

Uniformed Services	Civil Service
Annual vacation of thirty calendar days.	Vacation earned is determined by the years of service: thirteen work days per year for the first three years, twenty work days per year for years 4 through 14, and twenty-six work days per year after fifteen years.
Unlimited sick leave, granted as needed with full pay and allowances.	Thirteen days of sick leave are earned each year, with unlimited carryover.
Free medical and dental care. Free medical care also provided for family members.	Health insurance, with premium payments shared by the federal government.
Retirement pay based on rank and length of service, with no contributions by the individual. Twenty-year retirement option with 40% of base pay, increased to 50% at age 62.	Contributory retirement plan.
Free travel on any space available on military aircraft and discounts on most commercial airlines.	Travel at own expense.
No loss of seniority or benefits associated with relocation.	No loss of seniority or benefits associated with relocation.
Reduced prices for brand-name items at military exchange (department store), commissary (grocery store), beverage store, garden shop, etc.	Civilian stores.
Recreation on base may include Officer's Club, golf course, swimming, bowling, craft and hobby shops, fitness center, movies, etc., all at reduced rates.	At own expense.
If found unfit to perform duties of the grade and rank because of a medical condition, may be retired on disability.	Disability retirement may be granted if employee is totally disabled for useful and efficient service in the position held and has at least five years of credible civilian service.
$200,000 term life insurance policy for only $8.00 per month.	$200,000 term life insurance policy for only $8.00 per month.

RESOURCES FOR FURTHER INFORMATION

For additional information about the U.S. Air Force Nurse Corps, call 1-800-432-USAF or write to:
Air Force Recruiting Service
HQ AFRS/RSOHN
550 D Street West, Suite 1
Randolph Air Force Base, TX 78150-5421

For additional information about the U.S. Army Nurse Corps, call 1-800-USA-ARMY or write to:
Headquarters, U.S. Army Recruiting Command
Fort Knox, KY 40121-2726

For additional information about the U.S. Navy Nurse Corps, call 1-800-USA-NAVY. In Puerto Rico, call 1-800-872-6289. You may also write to:
Nurse Corps Programs Officer
Navy Recruiting Command
4015 Wilson Boulevard
Arlington, VA 22203-1991

For additional information about the Commissioned Corps of the Public Health Service, call 1-800-279-1606 or write to:
Recruitment Branch, BCP
5600 Fisher's Lane, Room 4A07
Rockville, MD 20857

To learn more about Federal Civil Service System positions and vacancies, contact the Federal Job Information Center in your state or the nearest Regional Office of Personnel Management. These offices are located in Philadelphia, Pennsylvania, Atlanta, Georgia, Chicago, Illinois, Dallas, Texas, and San Francisco, California. Telephone numbers are listed in local phone directories under "U.S. Government." If you are located near a military base or a VA medical center, try contacting the associated personnel department for specific telephone numbers.

For more information about VA opportunities, call 1-800-827-1388 or write to:
Department of Veterans Affairs (054E)
810 Vermont Avenue, NW
Washington, DC 20420

SUMMARY

Despite the turmoil and change taking place today in the health care arena, nurses in the armed forces, USPHS, and Federal Civil Service System remain in the spotlight. Challenging and diverse professional opportunities can be found at locations around the globe. For the nurse with a sense of adventure, there is at least one type of assignment that will broaden not only professional skills, but, also, personal horizons.

Chapter Sixteen

Educator Roles

Bette Case

INTRODUCTION

The role of teacher is inherent in the role of nurse. Even nurses who have not yet had the opportunity to gain much experience have certainly had occasion to provide patient education and to present information to classmates. Experienced nurses often precept new staff members or students and provide in-service education. If you have found the teaching component of your practice enjoyable and fulfilling, you may want to explore the opportunities available in education and consider moving your career along an educator path.

Just as changes in society and health care are changing expectations of nursing and careers in nursing, changes in society and health care are also creating new mandates, challenges, and expectations for educators. This chapter explores emerging opportunities for nurses who wish to focus on educating nursing students; practicing nurses, other caregivers, and support staff in health care organizations; patients and their families; and members of the community.

Although a desire to teach may propel you toward an educator role, education encompasses far more than classroom and/or clinical teaching. As one expert suggests, "education brings up a particular box"—that is, teaching (del Bueno, Personal Communication, January 28, 1995). But today, the roles of those responsible for education have broadened considerably and far beyond formal teaching.

THE EDUCATOR ROLE TODAY

Concerns about cost containment and quality in health care have called attention to the effectiveness and efficiency with which educational services are delivered. More than ever before, society, professional organizations, schools, health care organizations, and students hold educators accountable for providing relevant, effective education.

Increasingly, educators must demonstrate the value they add to their organizations. To do so, they must identify how their programs positively impact desired organizational goals and outcomes. Educators must ensure that their activities reflect and further the philosophies and missions of their universities or health care organizations. Educators must carefully consider personal and professional alignment with the philosophies and missions of the organizations within which they work. They cannot succeed when they do not embrace and continually seek ways to further the philosophies, missions and values of their organizations.

No longer can educators remain viable if they function in isolation. Educational programs must reflect community needs and characteristics; such programs must integrate well with the mission of the organization, whether that organization is a university, a hospital corporation, or a health maintenance organization (HMO). Further, educators must collaborate effectively with all other disciplines represented in their organizations.

Society and health care organizations expect educators to produce individuals who have learned the information, skills, and attitudes they need in order to perform safely and effectively.

In the past, some cynics have suggested that for nurses, careers in education were for those who either were physically incapable of practicing nursing or wanted to retire on the job. George Bernard Shaw's infamous quote, "Those who can, do; those who can't, teach," echoes this sentiment. Although effective educators have surely always held themselves to higher standards of professional practice, past circumstances certainly permitted more isolation and less accountability than the present and future environments will tolerate. Today, the education career path is definitely not for the faint of heart.

TRENDS IN SOCIETY, HEALTH CARE, AND EDUCATION

As the twentieth century ends, health care and education in the United States are "corporatizing." Health care agencies and educational institutions are becoming members of larger corporations, merged entities, and regional alliances. As members of larger organizations, they must identify and focus on their contributions to the missions of these larger concerns. To survive and grow, they must ensure that they are doing the "right work" in the context of the bigger picture. They must contribute to fiscal, quality and marketing goals, and, therefore, operate more as businesses than was true in the past.

Trends in health care have created new health care delivery roles and the corresponding need to prepare individuals to perform competently in these roles. Educators are required to prepare more individuals to work in home health care, extended care, and cross-trained roles. Caregivers must learn to function in the managed care environment and as interdisciplinary team members. Postgraduate programs are assisting nursing school graduates in preparing for practice. Self care and care by family and significant others is a growing trend requiring educational support—not only in managing disease, but also in supporting the increasing involvement of men in infant and child care and the increasing complexity of caring for the elderly in their homes.

The explosion of technology and information has special implications for the educator. Besides staying abreast of health care technology and information, educators face the additional challenge of keeping current with regard to new developments in educational technology and information. The information highway, specialized linkages and networks, robotics, computer-assisted learning, and satellite-mediated distance learning all create exciting new possibilities for learning. In addition to using new modalities, educators must address the need to package learning and adjust teaching methods to take advantage of advances in technology and information. Adjusting learning methods means incorporating technology while creating opportunities for adult learners to interact with one another and share experiences.

Societal changes mean that the educator is encountering greater diversity among learners—diversity with regard to not only culture, ethnicity and language (including English-as-a-second-language learners), but also levels of literacy and education, previous and current work experience (including multiple jobs), and a host of other ways whereby adults differ from one another.

Responding to the changes in society, organizations, health care, and education, the educators of tomorrow will venture far from the traditional definition of this role. They will shift away from a controlling and information-giving role and toward a role of facilitating learning and assisting learners to develop strategies that empower them to accept responsibility for lifelong learning. The focus will shift away from providing information and toward practicing strategies for seeking and organizing information, framing and solving problems, and applying principles. These shifts emphasize critical thinking and will require educators to model critical thinking and to reward learners' curiosity and judgment.

Although the educational needs of the future are great, few experts expect the number of educator positions to increase substantially. In fact, the Pew Health Professions Commission advises closing 10% to 20% of the nation's nursing schools as we move into the twenty-first century (Pew Health Professions Commission, 1995).

Nevertheless, the educator of the future will still find opportunities to join the faculty of schools of nursing. RNs will continue to be in demand. However, educational programs will move from an acute care focus to one that better prepares nurses to manage client care in outpatient, community, and home health settings. Educators will also find opportunities to contribute to the education of unlicensed caregivers, including patients and their families. Educators will face the additional challenge of differentiating scope of practice as it relates to the different levels of basic nursing education. For example, how should graduates of diploma, associate degree nursing (ADN), and baccalaureate programs differ in the scopes of their practice and the settings in which they practice? And how should educational programs differ to ensure that these graduates master the competencies specific to their respective practices?

Consistent with the shift in nursing practice toward RNs working through assistive personnel, educators will also work through others: preceptors, trainers whom they train, managers, and learners themselves.

In another departure from tradition, educators will demonstrate efficiency and effectiveness by taking education to the places and times where learners are found. Educators will accomplish some increased access through online and satellite linkages, and through "just-in-time" learning for practicing nurses on the unit or patients and their families in the home. Both technologically mediated and in-person contact will move increasingly toward the places where people live, work, and spend time in professional and service club activities. Educators will continue to expand their concepts of the educational setting, thinking not only of home and community settings, but also of the educational needs of those who give and receive health care and health-related information in space and undersea.

THE EDUCATIONAL PROCESS

Whether learners are nursing students, practicing nurses, hospital staff other than nurses, patients, members of patients' families, or members of the community, the same educational process applies. The educational process has much in common with the nursing process.

Assessing Learning Needs and Resources

Designing educational activities begins with an assessment process. The purpose of the assessment process is to identify those things that learners must learn in order to accomplish specific goals. There are two components to what learners must learn. One component is the information, skills, and/or attitudes necessary for competent performance. The other component relates to the learners themselves, specifically, how much of the information and how many of the skills and attitudes the learners already possess, and how to best facilitate learning with these particular learners.

Depending on the setting, the educator considers different factors when identifying the information, skills, and attitudes that the educational activity or course will address. School of nursing faculty must incorporate certain aspects of the curriculum conceptual framework in planning courses. Staff-development educators must address mandates of the Joint Commission for the Accreditation of Health Care Organizations (JCAHO) and other accrediting bodies. All educators, regardless of setting or learner audience, must ensure that the information, skills, and attitudes they plan to teach reflect current knowledge and standards of care and practice.

Assessing learners varies somewhat according to the educational setting. In some aspects of staff development, continuing education, and community education, educators have greater latitude in designing educational activities, courses, and curricula based on learners' perceived learning needs. In standardized programs, certification programs, and academic degree-granting programs, the curriculum or course is prescribed in advance. Although there is often opportunity to vary methods and time allotments based on the entering capabilities of learners, some parameters are fixed.

In patient and family education, the information, skills, and attitudes to be learned are also specified in advance, but characteristics and previous knowledge of the learners determine the content and teaching methods. Hospitals accredited by the JCAHO must comply with standards related to patient and family education. Patient and family educators also assess their communities and patient populations in order to identify opportunities to place education for maximal effectiveness, such as a nurse specialist in the Southwestern United States who recognizes the tribal council as an appropriate setting to assess and address the health education needs of Native Americans (J. Pelusi, Personal Communication, February 14, 1995).

An additional dimension of assessment involves assessing learning resources. Learning resources include readily available, conventional, printed, educational materials; information in multimedia formats and computer-assisted formats; resource persons; information available on the Internet; and any other source of information or learning experience that can assist learners to satisfy their learning needs. Educators face the challenge of keeping current with regard to available options and creatively tapping into and designing resources within practical constraints.

Establishing Objectives

After making an assessment to determine learning needs, the educator establishes objectives. Objectives are similar to desired outcomes when planning patient care. Objectives specify what the learner will do upon completion of learning—for example, state the five "rights" of medication administration. Objectives drive the educational process; all successive phases of the educational process refer back to the objectives.

Selecting Content, Methods, Time Allotment, and Teacher

Guided by the learning objectives, the educator matches content, learning methods, time allotment, and teacher to the requirements and constraints of the learning situation. This process parallels individualizing a standard patient care plan to ensure effective care of an individual patient.

Implementing and Coordinating Learning Activities

For educators as for practicing nurses, implementing a plan involves both coordination and direct intervention. When implementing and coordinating, educators balance the need to provide an effective, organized structure for learning with the need to provide control, choices, and active involvement to learners. To coordinate effectively, educators need to know the resources available, match resources and needs effectively and efficiently, and continuously communicate with all involved. In nursing education, as in nursing practice, the need to accomplish more through others places increasing emphasis on coordinating skills.

Evaluating Learning

When evaluating learning, the educator refers to the objectives and requires the learner to perform the objectives to demonstrate learning. For example, if the objective states, "List contraindications for TPA (tissue type plasminogen activator) administration postMI," the learner must write or orally recite those contraindications. If the objective states, "Locate findings pertinent to TPA administration in the patient's medical record," the learner must use the medical record to demonstrate learning, rather than merely explaining where to locate the findings in question. Sound, valid evaluation of learning requires specific, measurable objectives.

Besides evaluating the learner's accomplishment of objectives, educators engage in other levels of evaluation. Abruzzese (1992, p. 538) identifies four levels of evaluation: process, content, outcome, and impact. All of these levels contribute to total program evaluation. In process evaluation, learners, educators, and relevant others indicate levels of satisfaction with the educational process, including learning methods, scheduling, and physical facilities and other environmental aspects. Content evaluation uses the objectives to determine whether learners have accomplished the intended learning, as described previously. Outcome evaluation determines whether learners are using the new learning in the practice environment. Impact evaluation measures the contribution of the learning activity to the broader organizational goals related to quality improvement, risk management, job satisfaction, cost effectiveness, and other important indicators of organizational performance. Obviously, the latter levels (i.e., outcome and impact evaluation) are more complicated and costly to plan and perform. Society and organizations, however, will increasingly expect educators to demonstrate accountability by evaluating outcomes and impacts of education.

Feeding Evaluation Results Back into Assessment

Educators use results of all levels of evaluation to plan future programs and practices. In this way, evaluation findings feed back into the assessment process and compose a part of the assessment data that educators analyze to plan future directions and activities.

ADULT LEARNING PRINCIPLES

Educators assist or facilitate their learners in making changes—that is, to what learners know, how they think, and what skills they can perform. Educators also assist learners in developing and appreciating new values, attitudes, feelings, beliefs, and perspectives. Most people experience some difficulty in making changes. Educators make the learning process easier by applying and incorporating principles of adult learning. Principles of adult learning encompass three themes: active involvement, individual differences, and relevance and motivation. The acronym AIR provides a convenient way to remember these themes or overlapping categories of adult learning principles.

Active Involvement

Active involvement means involving learners in all phases of the learning process. The educator looks for opportunities to give learners choices and allow them input.

Within the classroom or clinical learning environment, active involvement means actively engaging learners in the material they must learn. This means moving away from teacher-centered, teacher-controlled methods and toward more learner-centered approaches. Research summarized by Pike (1989) documents increased learning and retention when the learner makes use of more senses. For example, when learners are required to speak or perform, learning and retention increase four or five times over that gained when learners only hear the information. Incorporating the use of additional senses—for example, by adding visual complements to lectures—yields impressive gains. Although time and space constraints sometimes limit the use of highly interactive methods, educators also apply principles of active involvement by doing more asking than telling and designing learning to promote maximal interaction of learners with the material to be learned.

Individual Differences

Adult learners differ from one another in a host of ways. As noted previously, educators are increasingly encountering greater diversity among groups of learners. These differences relate to culture (of both birth and work), experience (life, work, and educational), learning style, personal preferences and approaches, age, development (cognitive, affective, psychomotor, and moral), gender, sexual orientation, talents, interests, presence of disabilities, and roles and responsibilities in family and community. To facilitate effective learning among adults, educators demonstrate respect for these differences. Educators recognize each individual as a unique constellation of differences rather than stereotyping individuals based on characteristics. Educators encourage learners to express their individual differences, particularly experiences. By identifying and incorporating individual differences into the learning process, educators facilitate learners' connecting new information with previous learning.

Relevance and Motivation

Educators realize that adults are interested in learning when gaining new information, attitudes, or skills will enable them to address more effectively meaningful problems and important situations. Educators also realize that they cannot motivate learners, but, instead, must connect with the motivations, needs, and wants that learners bring to the learning situation. Educators sometimes establish the relevance of learning by connecting the material to be learned with problems and concerns viewed as important by learners.

ATTRIBUTES AND QUALIFICATIONS OF THE EFFECTIVE EDUCATOR

Experts in the field emphasize the attitudinal component as being among the qualifications that increase chances for success in the educator role. Certain attitudes toward oneself and one's work fit well with the work of the educator. One of the first attitudes most experts mention is love of learning and commitment to lifelong learning. A sincere interest in learning and helping others learn establishes the context for other educator attitudes and skills.

Sometimes, others fail to appreciate educators' efforts. When this occurs, a sense of security and a strong sense of self can help educators. Learning means changing, and asking someone to change can and often does meet with resistance or anger. Thus, learners sometimes direct negative feelings toward the educator.

Nursing colleagues sometimes misunderstand and question the value of the educator's contributions. Colleagues in nursing and other disciplines occasionally feel that educators are intruding in their realms. Learners, managers, administrators, and others all hold different expectations of educators. The educator's sense of security must extend to confidence in making judgments about priorities and time management. Often, the educator cannot satisfy all stakeholders' expectations.

Because the educator accomplishes much through others and in collaboration with others, feeling secure when working with other experts enhances an educator's effectiveness. To preserve and enhance this sense of security and well-being, it is important that educators learn self-care techniques.

Other important attitudes include sense of humor, high energy, willingness to take risks, creativity, ability to see and openness to a variety of alternatives, and positive attitude and frame of reference. Effective practice as an educator also requires flexibility. Educators juggle many different types of activities: preparing learning materials and tests, teaching in classroom and clinical settings, consulting, advising, collaborating, and working on committees. Particularly in academic faculty roles, educators are also required to engage in research, writing, and other scholarly activities.

Educators balance "going with the flow" and maintaining a sense of direction and purpose. Educators enjoy more freedom and autonomy than nurses who practice in most other roles. Managing freedom and autonomy, however, requires skill in setting priorities and managing time.

Because they usually work in staff rather than line capacities, educators must feel comfortable developing the informal power of influence and expertise rather than wielding formal power. When practicing effectively, educators give power away by assisting others to develop the knowledge, skills, and attitudes that will empower them to function independently and succeed.

An enthusiasm for seeking new information and answers, challenging conventions, and uncovering new approaches fuels the educator's journey toward the future. Traditional educational approaches cannot adequately respond to today's mandates from society and health care. In response to mandates related to fiscal and restructuring initiatives, for example, the educators must find and create faster ways for people to learn, and will reflect critically on their practices to do so. As one noted educator commented, "The more I learn, the more questions I have" (R. Abruzzese, Personal Communication, January 30, 1995).

Educators must acquire expertise in at least two areas: education and one or more dimensions of practice, including both clinical specialties and functional specialties such as administration, systems, or research. To practice credibly, educators must achieve proficiency in the knowledge base, technology, and skills associated with both areas.

Educators must communicate, consult, and plan effectively with learners and other stakeholders. To do so, they must apply interpersonal, assertiveness, and collaboration skills. Educators cannot succeed without respecting and "speaking the languages" of those who represent different interests. Specialized communication skills needed for teaching include listening, coaching, and giving feedback.

To prepare learners for changes in roles and for future practice, educators must develop and revise visions of the future. This requires taking a proactive stance and anticipating and managing change. As mentioned earlier, one recent change requiring special competence on the part of educators is the increasing diversity of student, employee, patient, and community populations.

Experts agree that educator roles require a master's degree. Completing graduate education is one way to model commitment to learning. In addition, graduate education teaches conceptual thinking, or the ability to reframe, rethink, and consider a big picture and many dimensions and components of an idea. Educators interpret, apply, and assist their learners in applying research findings. Graduate education develops the capability to critique, apply, and communicate research findings. With few exceptions, school of nursing faculty positions require a master's degree in nursing.

If not included in the graduate program, the educator must pursue formal education to master skills in educational design and evaluation and to gain knowledge of a variety of approaches to learning and evaluation. Certifications in various clinical and functional specialties also strengthen the educator's credentials.

Experts recommend some self-exploration for those considering careers in education. What does specializing in education mean to you? Why do you want to move toward education? How and where will you pursue your career? Who is your market—not only who you will teach, but who will purchase your services as employer or client? How will you feel about spending less time in direct patient care? How will you feel saying, "I nurse nurses now, not patients" (Karen Kelly, Personal Communication, January 25, 1995). How will you feel about working through others?

DIFFERENCES AMONG EDUCATOR ROLES

Educator roles differ depending on the employing organization (i.e., educational institution or health care agency) and the learner audience (i.e., students, nurses and other health care professionals, patients and their families, or community members). Although this section describes differences among these roles, there are many educators whose practices encompass dual appointments and all of the aforementioned learner audiences. Present trends reflect a move toward more collaboration among specialties, development of collateral skill sets, multiskilling, and otherwise integrating specialties for greater effectiveness and efficiency. The future will hold more opportunities for integrating these dimensions of educational practice in single jobs. For example, an oncology clinical nurse specialist (CNS) might teach university nursing students in classroom and clinical, carry a caseload of patients in a hospital setting, and provide continuing education and staff development on chemotherapy to home health nurses. Carrying a caseload might include providing direct care and patient and family teaching, and practicing interdisciplinary collaboration. This CNS might also work collaboratively with representatives of many disciplines in the hospital setting, addressing quality improvement and policy and procedure concerns, conducting research, and/or providing education in community settings regarding reducing the risk of cancer.

The School of Nursing Faculty Role

Schools of nursing prepare graduates to apply for licensure to practice nursing. The nursing profession has debated for many years over the most appropriate educational preparation for entry into practice. Most nurses entering practice have graduated from a diploma-, associate degree-, or baccalaureate-degree-granting educational program. In 1993, diploma programs, typically hospital based and three years in length, accounted for approximately 12% of United States nursing programs and 10% of the nursing student population (Pew Health Professions Commission, 1993b). In that same year, associate degree programs, typically community college-based and two years in length, accounted for over 50% of the nation's nursing programs and 50% of the nursing student population; baccalaureate programs, usually four years in length and offered by colleges or universities, accounted for just over 33% of the nursing programs and of the nursing student population (Pew Health Professions Commission, 1993b).

Many nurses whose initial educational preparation consisted of diploma or associate programs return to school to complete the bachelor's degree. According to a survey conducted by the American Association of Colleges of Nursing (AACN), RN/BSN completion enrollments are increasing, and graduations increased 6.3% from 1994 to 1995 (Varro, 1996). There are also several graduate programs that prepare individuals who have baccalaureate degrees in other fields to enter nursing practice. The nursing profession continues to explore differentiating practice based on educational level. Some states are planning to create different levels of licensure for graduates of different programs.

In the United States graduate programs in nursing that lead to master's and doctoral degrees have grown in number in recent years. In 1993, 23,000 students were enrolled in 200 master's degree programs, and 2,700 students were enrolled in 53 doctoral programs (Pew Health Professions Commission, 1993b). Graduate programs are enjoying increasing enrollments, while enrollments in entry-level programs are decreasing (Varro, 1996).

Schools of nursing face the challenge of preparing practitioners for the future at a time when turbulent change characterizes the present. As Lindeman (1995) comments, "We must educate for careers in a dynamic system, rather than for jobs in a static system" (p. 535). The coming years will see unprecedented changes in nursing education programs as schools respond to community needs; move away from medical-model, hospital-based learning; identify multiple ways for students to achieve learning outcomes in multiple settings; collaborate more closely with other professionals, community, and business groups; and work toward more meaningful integration of their missions in education, research, and service. Today's leaders in nursing education recognize that schools of nursing cannot survive as isolated, ivory towers. As one dean noted, a number of deans bring entrepreneurial experience to their roles in academic leadership (M. Wake, Personal Communication, February 13, 1995).

Nurses who join nursing faculties in the future will enter different environments than they remember from their student days. Faculty will actively practice nursing, many in community settings. Experts cite excellence in practice as an essential qualification; many, in fact, assign it top priority. Rather than supervising a group of students on a single nursing unit or within a single agency, faculty will supervise students who practice in diverse, physically distant locations and who often have preceptors.

Faculty members often enjoy freedom to work in the library or at home when not conducting scheduled class or clinical sessions, participating in committee work, or holding scheduled office hours. Schools vary in their established scheduling policies, but in general, faculty have more autonomy in setting work schedules than do nurses in most other roles. Although having the authority to schedule time, however, faculty members often feel overwhelmed with the number and variety of activities that they must include in their schedules. Faculty often travel to a number of clinical sites and may each teach and practice in more than one location.

Besides preparing classroom and clinical sessions, teaching, and counseling students, faculty members must also take responsibility for committee, task-force, and other special assignments. Today, many faculty feel challenged in trying to stay current in their clinical fields. In the future, the mandate to engage in more direct practice and develop expertise in more than one specialty will compound this challenge. Academic leaders will have to reorganize programs and faculty roles to permit more direct practice.

In addition to the practice dimension, faculty must factor in time for scholarly activities. These activities include conducting research, publishing in the professional literature, and presenting research findings to and conducting educational sessions for peers and members of other disciplines. Faculty members must meet scholarship expectations in order to receive tenure and promotion in academic rank. Many schools of nursing are examining their requirements for appointment, tenure, and promotion of faculty, and are revising criteria to incorporate excellence in nursing and education practice. Some academic leaders in nursing believe that traditional appointment, tenure, and promotion requirements have forced faculty away from maintaining and enhancing their expertise in practice and teaching. When gathering information about faculty roles and responsibilities in particular schools, it is wise to inquire about appointment, tenure, and promotion criteria.

Some experts predict that within the next twenty years, faculty roles in baccalaureate programs will require a nursing doctorate (G. Donnelly, Personal Communication, Janauary 16, 1995). At present, many nursing faculty have earned doctorates in other fields such as education, psychology, or physiology. Depending on the mission of the university and the track or emphasis of the nursing program, members of a particular faculty may hold doctorates in other fields. In addition to advanced academic preparation, nursing faculty must develop expertise in applying health care and educational technology and in collaborating with other disciplines and representatives of agencies where students practice.

Teaching/learning methods will take advantage of technology and place more responsibility on learners. Faculty, as one nursing leader notes, "will need to learn to love independent learners and not feel threatened by them". She adds, "We have made learners dependent in the past" (Mueller, Personal Communication, January 27, 1995). Students will interact interpersonally in groups as well as interact with computers, the information highway, and various forms of simulation. Faculty will need the skills of expert facilitators, coordinators, and learning-resource experts. As one seasoned nursing leader notes, "faculty will not be paid to teach the book" (V. Farley, Personal Communication, January 25, 1995). Some experts in education believe that the content is merely a vehicle to learn the processes of thinking, critiquing, and applying information.

Experienced educators advise nurses aspiring to faculty positions to look for mentors to assist them in navigating the academic environment as well as in developing skills and expertise.

 ## A New World

Sam finished his master's degree in a pediatric CNS program. As a staff nurse in a children's hospital, he enjoyed working with students and precepting orientees. One of his teachers in the graduate program encouraged him to apply for an instructor position in the maternal-child health nursing department. Sam felt confident that his previous experience and newly acquired knowledge and skills qualified him to take advantage of this opportunity. He had really savored his experiences working with students and precepting orientees. He also thought that the more flexible work schedule of faculty looked pretty attractive compared to the twelve-hour shifts he'd been working. He decided to apply.

To prepare for his interview, Sam studied the school of nursing catalog and requested information about the maternal-child nursing courses from the department chair. He noticed that the concepts stressed in the philosophy, particularly those about self-care principles, were prominent in the objectives of the maternal-child courses.

Sam was thrilled when he got the job. His first year on the faculty expanded his view of the academic world and of nursing. He quickly realized that he was expected to broaden his expertise far beyond his specialty in pediatric oncology. He was glad his specialty had afforded him knowledge and experience with all body systems and all ages of children, because the patients on the general pediatric units where his students had experience represented many different diagnoses and age groups. With the declining inpatient census and the school's plan to increase outpatient and community experiences, Sam needed to broaden his perspective not only within acute care, but also beyond the acute setting.

His oncology experience prepared him well for investigating some potential home health experiences. However, he felt less self assured when the department chair assigned him to visit elementary schools to assess potential for experiences with well children and normal growth and development. Then the department chair announced a plan for pediatric faculty and obstetric faculty to begin learning one another's specialties over the next year!

Sam learned a lot about evaluating students. He took a course in test construction. At first, he struggled with sorting out the differences between standards for student clinical performance and standards for the orientees whom he had precepted.

Sam connected with an experienced pediatric faculty member, Sandy, who agreed to mentor him. Sandy was writing a section of the self-study report required for National League for Nursing (NLN) accreditation. Sam had an interest in writing. In fact, he had taken writing courses and done some freelance writing for *Nursing Spectrum*. So he volunteered to edit some of Sandy's work, and he even wrote some subsections under her guidance. He felt good about contributing while at the same time learning more about the program of the school and the NLN accreditation process.

By the end of his first year, Sam had begun to see academia in a whole new light. He had gotten over the shock of continual challenge to learn something new, and had begun to thrive on the stimulation. He looks forward to the day that Sandy promises him will arrive, when a former student will visit and say, "I'm so glad you demanded as much as you did. Even though I hated it at the time, I was really ready to take care of patients in my first job." Now, Sandy and the department chair are both encouraging him to start thinking about a doctoral program. But Sam isn't sure he's ready for that quite yet!

The Staff Development Specialist

A special feature of the staff development specialist role as compared to other educator roles is the importance of an organizational perspective. The staff development function within an organization directs the educational process toward assisting staff to develop the competencies they need to perform their roles as defined by the organization. Increasingly, educators whose responsibility has been nursing staff development are expanding their scope to include staff of other disciplines and departments and to include organizational development concerns.

In order to take an organizational perspective, the educator needs a broad viewpoint that goes beyond a particular clinical specialty and beyond nursing itself. The educator needs a holistic view of the organization, or, perhaps, of the multihospital system or corporation. To perform effectively and remain viable, staff development educators must earn the respect of other departments, speak the languages of other disciplines and departments, and move skillfully within the system. The educator also must communicate articulately and succinctly.

The needs of organizations increasingly require educators to design, implement, and evaluate training programs for multiskilled workers; to prepare workers for roles in restructured organizations through on-the-job training; and to assist employees at all levels in managing change. In the wake of downsizing and elimination of management positions, organizations are holding employees individually accountable for more aspects of their work lives. Employees, in turn, must learn self-management skills in order to incorporate these new responsibilities. Educators also respond to training needs in the realms of leadership, management, customer service, meeting management, and quality improvement.

Effective staff educators function as internal consultants and collaborate closely with management. Educators often work through others—preceptors or trainers whom they train to deliver unit- or department-based education.

Productivity is a paramount concern in today's cost-conscious environment, requiring educators not only to work through others, but also to demonstrate flexibility in response to rapidly changing needs. In comparison to academic nursing faculty, staff development educators experience a more immediate impact of trends. As one expert puts it, "Our way of being keeps changing" (L. Rodriguez, Personal Communication, January 25, 1995). Organizational and employee needs frequently mandate shortened time frames for education as well as alternatives to conventional classroom learning.

Coming from a nursing background, the staff development educator has the advantage of experience in dealing with many departments and perspectives, as is required within the practice of nursing. By staying in touch with clinical units, where care is delivered, the educator who is also a nurse can gain unique insights into educational needs. The staff development educator balances the need to maintain a nursing identity and an acceptance among nurses against the need to function as a team player outside of nursing. The specialty of the staff development educator is thus education rather than nursing. Staff development educators apply the educational process to organizational needs in support of organizational change, employee competence, quality initiatives, and compliance with requirements of accrediting agencies. The education specialty includes applying research and evaluation techniques in measuring outcomes.

If I Don't Like My Job, I Wait a Minute, and It Changes

Cindy, a former telemetry nurse, joined the nursing education department of a large medical center five years ago. In one of her assignments, she coordinates nursing orientation. She was heavily involved in developing the competency assessment system for new nursing department employees. Although it was a lot of work, she feels satisfied with the results. Her "gut feelings" have proven accurate in the past, and nurse managers often request her feedback. Now she has some objective data to support the impressions she gains during orientation. Using the new system, she assesses and validates the critical thinking, technical, and interpersonal skills of new nursing employees. She then recommends individualized development plans to the orientees and their managers. She also contributed to developing the departmental competency policies, which other departments now use as a model.

In another of Cindy's assignments, she coordinates new-product inservices, often arranging schedules for vendor representatives to provide product inservices on all units and shifts. As a member of the interdisciplinary product evaluation committee, she collects new-product evaluation data from nursing units, compiles it, and shares results with the committee. She then participates in formulating the committee's recommendations.

Cindy also teaches a portion of the preceptor training program. And as chairperson of the clinical ladder committee, Cindy consults with staff nurses to develop unit-based inservices and prepare other projects in support of their applications for promotion in the clinical ladder program.

Last year, the nursing education department expanded its scope. It now serves all hospital employees as the staff education department. As one of its first hospitalwide education projects, the department designed and introduced a program to ensure compliance of all departments with mandatory education requirements. The department, collaborating closely with administration and human resources, created a program for employees of direct care departments, as well as a shorter program for employees of support services departments. At first, the nurse educators struggled to identify essential components pertinent to the needs of all disciplines: nursing, physical and occupational therapy, respiratory therapy, social work, pharmacy, patient transportation, and others. When they had identified objectives and content, Cindy developed some interactive learning activities including a "Safety Shuffle," wherein small, multidisciplinary groups developed and performed skits to illustrate specific elements of important safety information. She also designed a jeopardy game wherein the groups competed as teams to answer questions based on the objectives of the mandatory education program.

Now, in the second year of the program, Cindy has designed a variety of simulations wherein employees identify safety risks and demonstrate their knowledge of safety policies and practices.

Cindy's experiences in the education department have broadened her understanding of both the hospital as a whole and the perspectives of various departments. She feels satisfied in contributing to the bigger picture, and enjoys her access to so many different units and departments.

Although she's learned a lot on the job, Cindy still recognizes her need for further knowledge and skill in education. With the support and encouragement of her boss, she has therefore enrolled in an MSN program. She also participates annually in at least one continuing-education offering related to education and training—sometimes at her own expense.

Cindy feels a certain sense of anticipation every time her telephone rings. Someone might be calling to consult her in relation to any of her diverse assignments. Or, her boss may be calling to advise her of some new organizational change and the role Cindy and her colleagues in the education department will play in the process.

The Continuing Education Specialist

Continuing education specialists may work within hospital or other health care agency education departments, for colleges or universities, or in entrepreneurial continuing education businesses. Educators who focus their practices on continuing education must develop business and marketing skills. Continuing education is broader in scope than addressing the employee-competence needs of a particular employer. Continuing education specialists respond to political, economic, and health care trends when designing and marketing continuing education products. In the past, conferences, courses, and seminars have predominated as formats for continuing education. Today, however, continuing education specialists are complementing their product lines with other formats such as video and audiotapes, computer-based learning, distance learning, and independent study programs.

Effective practice as a continuing education specialist requires interpreting and documenting compliance with continuing education accreditation criteria (e.g., so that the American Nurses Association (ANA) will approve offerings for continuing education contact hours). In order to complete applications for continuing education contact hours and to market programs in a timely fashion, the continuing education specialist must plan far in advance of presenting programs. The successful continuing education specialist not only plans far in advance, but also sets and complies with interim deadlines.

The Patient/Family/Community Educator

Educators who facilitate learning among patients and their families as well as various segments of the community serve a considerably more diverse audience than do educators who work with students, nurses, and health care staff. There are no prerequisite courses or qualifications for patients, patients' families, or community members, other than a need or interest in learning to manage health problems or maintain or enhance health. These learners vary greatly in educational level, life experience, culture, age, motivation, and nearly every other area. The educator thus must translate health care information into meaningful terms and choose methods appropriate to each individual learner's characteristics and circumstances. Effective educators "teach with information, not data . . . and give away to people the power to care for themselves" through the learning process (Byers, Personal Communication, April 5, 1995). As experienced CNSs note, "people aren't motivated to learn what isn't a problem right now . . . " (S. Hall-Johnson, Personal Communication, January 26, 1995). "Most people need a coach [in addition to information] to support lifelong behavioral change" (M. Gulanick, Personal Communication, February 7, 1995).

For nurses, the patient/family educator role—and sometimes the health educator role—is a component of a broader role in practicing nursing with a specified population, as, for example, a CNS, a nurse practitioner (NP), a certified nurse midwife (CNM), a school nurse, or a camp nurse. Selected education courses in continuing education or graduate study can greatly enhance the nurse's effectiveness in broadening a practice role.

Current trends and technologies influence patient, family, and community education. The JCAHO, for example, has established standards for patient and family education. And insurers currently reimburse only for selected and defined aspects of patient education. When patients receive effective patient education, they manage their conditions more proactively, and, therefore, are more likely to avoid the need for costly inpatient care. Both providers and insurers value such cost savings. These facts will help ensure the viability of patient/family education and roles, particularly if reimbursement is extended to additional aspects of patient education.

Shortened lengths of stay for hospitalized patients mean shortened time frames for teaching. In addition, because they are often unable to recover fully prior to discharge, patients often are less physically and emotionally ready to learn while hospitalized. These factors create the needs for new approaches to inhospital patient education and for additional patient education in outpatient and home settings. Wasson and Anderson (1995) describe many examples of such efforts.

The increase in information and information access and management technology has resulted in extensive resources for educators and their audiences alike. Internet services now offer information on health and disease, and teleconferencing, computer bulletin boards, electronic mail, and new CD-ROM developments join older forms of technology to create an impressive array of health care information delivery mechanisms. Such technologies increase the possibilities of providing health care information at accessible sites such as the home, workplace, and community organizations. Matching and applying available technology to educational needs offers an exciting challenge to the creative educator. Specialized educator opportunities include designing formats for education and resource centers such as the Patient Education Resource Centers (PERCs) of Veterans' Administration medical centers (Kathleen Kelly, Personal Communication, February 8, 1995).

Roles in community and health education focus on health maintenance and enhancement. These roles, based in HMOs and various community service settings, are stand alone careers, as contrasted with the patient/family education role, which is incorporated into a nursing practice role. Typically, individuals who practice in these roles have master's degrees in public health education, health education, or public health. A nurse considering one of these positions can expect little emphasis to be placed on disease-oriented education.

SAMPLING EDUCATOR ROLES

Because the educator role is inherent in the role of nurse, you will find many opportunities within nursing to sample education practice. Learn more about the educator role the next time you attend an inservice, continuing education offering, class, or training session. Observe what the educator is doing. Think about the work involved in preparing the learning materials. Ask the educator what a typical week is like. Have lunch with a clinical educator or staff development instructor and ask about their jobs in detail. Talk with faculty members at your school of nursing to gain insight.

For experienced, practicing nurses, precepting offers a chance to practice the educator role. Consciously apply the educational process and adult learning principles while precepting. Doing so will increase your effectiveness with your preceptee as well as allow you to sample the educator role.

Many schools of nursing are increasing adjunct faculty appointments. Adjunct faculty serve as clinical teachers while practicing nursing. If schools affiliate with your hospital or agency for clinical practice, inquire about adjunct appointments. If your employer currently has no academic affiliations, ask your direct supervisor or staff educator whether they have explored this impossibility with regional schools of nursing. Most schools are eager to create new alternatives for student clinical practice.

Get involved in committee work related to education: unit-based inservice committee, education advisory committee, continuing education review panel (if your organization has received accreditation as a continuing education provider), patient education committee, program committees of specialty and other professional organizations. Even committees not carrying the term *education* in their names—such as policy and procedure, quality improvement, and clinical ladder committees—offer opportunities to practice the consultant/educator role. Community service work, such as that associated with PTAs, youth program leadership (like scouts or 4-H), religious training programs, and service clubs, affords opportunities as well.

Volunteer for CPR instructor training, which also addresses principles and practices of classroom teaching. As a certified instructor, you might then be able to assist with CPR recertification of fellow staff members or teach in community-based programs.

Explore the patient education resources of your agency. There may be opportunities to develop materials or provide group instruction. When instructing patients and their families as a component of your current job, consciously apply the educational process and principles of adult learning.

Go to the library and review journals related to educating nurses, staff, and patients. In addition to reading selected articles and inspecting tables of contents, look at the jobs advertised and the reports of news and meetings in order to gain more insight into the field.

If you decide to pursue an educator position, do some networking with persons currently practicing in educator roles. Do not limit yourself only to advertised jobs. Through networking, you may learn of openings before advertisements appear.

Assess your current organization, health care organizations in your community, and your community itself. Identify problems that education and training can solve. Consider political and economic factors. Might there be some opportunities to create a job or service to address the problems you uncover?

SUMMARY

Nurses will continue to find opportunities to practice educator roles. The number of educator positions will not increase significantly, and will decrease within hospitals and as a result of the decreasing number of nursing schools. The educator role has grown beyond the boundaries of classroom and clinical teaching. Depending on the nature of the setting and the learners, the role may also embrace components of nursing practice, organizational development, community assessment and education, business and marketing, research, professional writing, and consultation. Whatever other components a particular role encompasses, educators can expect their roles to require expertise in addition to expertise in education and a particular content area. Many learning needs accompany the accelerated rate of changes in health care today, ensuring a continuing and vital role for educators. Exciting opportunities await nurses who have "fallen in love with learning" (E. Falter, Personal Communication, January 27, 1995), and can view the big picture, flex, and tolerate ambiguity.

REFERENCES

Abruzzese, R. (1992). *Nursing staff development: Strategies for success.* St. Louis, MO: Mosby Yearbook.

Alspach, J. G. (1995). *The educational process in nursing staff development,* St. Louis, MO: Mosby.

American Association of College of Nursing. (1993). *Position statement: Nursing education's agenda for the 21st century.* Washington, DC: Author.

American Health Associates. (1994–1996). *Patient Education Management.* Atlanta, GA: Author.

Avillion, A. (Ed.). (1995). *The core curriculum for nursing staff development.* Pensacola, FL: National Nursing Staff Development Organization.

Campsey, J., Clutten, S., Hotz, M., Jennings, K., & Zaremba, J. (1994). Staff development survey shapes restructure. *Trendlines, 5*(4), 4–5.

Gundlach, A. (1994). Adapting to change: Reconsidering staff development organization, design, and purpose. *Journal of Continuing education in Nursing 25*(3), 120–122.

Kelly, K, (1992). *Nursing staff development: current competence, future focus.* Philadelphia: J. B. Lippincott.

Lindeman, C. (1995). President's message: Nursing's emerging roles. *Nursing and Health Care, 15*(10), 532, 535.

Oerman, M. (1994). Reforming nursing education for future practice. *Journal of Nursing Education, 33,* 215–219.

Pew Health Professions Commission. (1993a). *Contemporary issues in health professions education and workforce reform.* San Francisco: Author.

Pew Health Professions Commission. (1993b). *Health professions education for the future: Schools in service to the nation.* San Francisco: Author.

Pew Health Professions Commission. (1995). *The third report of the Pew Health Professions Commission.* San Francisco: Author.

Pike, R. (1989). *Creative training techniques handbook.* Minneapolis, MN: Lakewood Books.

Puetz, B. (Ed.). (1995). *Getting started in nursing staff development.* Pensacola, FL: National Nursing Staff Development Organization.

Radke, K., & McArt, E. (1993). Perceptions and responsibilities of clinical nurse specialists as educators. *Journal of Nursing Education, 32*(3), 115–120.

Redman, B. (1993). Patient education at 25 years: Where we have been and where we are going. *Journal of Advanced Nursing 18*(5), 725–730.

Rodriguez, L. (1995). *Manual of staff development.* St. Louis, MO: Mosby.

Swansburg, R. (1995). *Nursing staff development: A component of human resource development.* Boston: Jones and Bartlett Publishers.

Tresolini, C. P., & The Pew-Fetzger Task Force. (1994). *Health professions education and relationship-centered care.* San Francisco: Pew Health Professions Commission.

Varro, B. (1996, January 10). BSN enrollment dips as nursing realigns. *Chicago Tribune.*

Wasson, D., & Anderson, M. A. (1995). Hospital-patient education: Current status and future trends. *Journal of Nursing Staff Development, 10*(3), 147–151.

Chapter Seventeen

Taking Off with Your Career

Bette Case

INTRODUCTION

Imagine a launching pad—the launching pad from which you will take off with your career. The preceding chapters have assembled the launching pad from the following components: societal, economic, and health care influences; present and predicted opportunities; and personal and professional experiences, preferences, and strengths. Your unique blend of personal and professional experiences, preferences, and strengths will function as your guiding system, helping you make choices regarding the most promising and satisfying directions for your career.

This chapter concludes the book and finalizes construction of the launching pad by citing additional facts about nursing today and some last minute reminders of strategies and opportunities.

WAYS NURSES ARE WORKING IN THE 1990S

Since 1977, the Division of Nursing of the United States Department of Health and Human Services (DHS) has surveyed national samples of RNs. The division collects data on a variety of characteristics of the RN population in the United States. The most recent results reflect data from the March, 1992 survey (Moses, 1994), which sampled the 2.2 million RNs licensed to practice in the United States at that time. Following are some of the findings that apply most directly to developing your career. Note that trends in the results are as important as are the specific findings.

Selected Demographics

Age. The average age of new graduates in the United States was thirty years. The average age for all RNs was forty-three years, showing a continued rising trend from previous surveys. Only 11% of RNs were under thirty years old.

Gender. The RN population comprised 96% females and 4% males. Although females still formed the overwhelming majority, the ranks of male RNs had increased 97% since 1980—an increase three times greater than the 35% increase in the total RN population.

Ethnic. Only 9% of the total RN population were members of racial/ethnic minorities. Those who live and work in large urban centers or other centers of minority populations may be surprised at the lack of diversity in the nursing profession nationwide. Encouraging and incorporating greater diversity in the future will strengthen the nursing profession and the cultural competence of care.

Marital status. Seventy-two percent of RNs were married; 16.6% were widowed, divorced or separated; and 11% were never married. Many of the nurses who were married and had children were working part-time.

Education. The percentage breakdown of highest academic degrees held by RNs was as follows:

- diploma: 34%
- associate degree: 28%
- baccalaureate degree: 30%
- master's degree: 7.5%
- doctoral degree: 0.05%

Baccalaureate, master's, and doctoral degrees were not necessarily in nursing, especially at the master's and doctoral level. At the master's level, 29% held degrees in fields other than nursing; and at the doctoral level, 62% held degrees in other fields.

Employment Status

The 1992 survey revealed the lowest number of RNs not employed in nursing since the survey began (17%). Of the group not employed in nursing, 26% (100,000 nurses) held nonnursing jobs, a decrease since 1988. Among those holding nonnursing jobs, 44% held health-related jobs, and 6% were seeking nursing jobs.

Of those not employed, only 1.3% were seeking nursing jobs, the lowest number since the survey began. Of those who were seeking nursing positions, most were seeking part-time employment. The majority had been searching for fewer than four weeks, and 23% had been searching less than one week. While it is likely that more may be seeking nursing jobs today, nurses do indeed enjoy strong employability. Of those not employed, most (nearly 75%) were not seeking employment.

Those who were working in nonnursing positions gave as their reasons the following: more convenient hours, more professionally rewarding work, and better salaries. Twenty-three percent believed their nursing skills were outdated, and 18% cited concerns about safety in the health care environment.

Most RNs were employed by the facilities in which they worked. Only 2% were temporary or agency employees (a decrease from the previous survey), and 2% were self employed. Sixty-six percent of RNs were employed in hospitals. Since the time of the survey (between 1993 and 1995), hospitals in the United States have eliminated 44,700 jobs, including a number of nursing jobs (Sullivan, 1995).

Of those employed, 16% held an additional job, compared to 6% of the national workforce who held more than one job in 1995 (Kaye, Butler, & Fisher, 1995). Second jobs are of growing importance in the current environment, not only for supplementing income and serving as fallback positions in case of potential layoff, but also as opportunities to develop additional skills that will add value to primary jobs or to create opportunities for new career paths.

Workweek

Sixty-nine percent of employed RNs typically spent at least 50% of the workweek engaging in direct patient-care—a slight decrease from 1988. With continued restructuring and increasing numbers of unlicensed, assistive personnel, this decrease will continue. The RN role will evolve toward more coordination and management of care. "Nurses can be either proactive or reactive to change, but change is going to happen. RNs of the future are going to be integrators and coordinators of care. We have to learn that it's okay for us to let go of a few patient-care tasks because there's so much more we can do" (Pauly-O'Neill & Andreola, 1995, p. 3).

Restructuring of organizations, increasing emphasis on outpatient services, and other trends will continue to modify the picture of the nursing workweek painted by the 1992 data.

Allocation of time during the workweek differed for those having graduate degrees. Those with master's degrees spent 33% of the workweek in direct patient care, 26% in administration, and 19% in teaching. For doctorally prepared RNs, 35% of the workweek was spent in teaching, 31% in administration, and 13% in research. Research showed a slight decrease since the 1988 survey.

Compensation

The average annual RN salary was $33,898. Those holding more than one job earned an average of $39,674. Those holding only one job earned an average of $32,821. Median weekly income differed between male and female nurses. The median weekly income for male RNs was $709; for female RNs, it was $680.

NEW WORDS, NEW WAYS OF THINKING

A few terms appearing in the current literature provide food for thought and some fuel for career launching.

Career Nursing

Some nurses use the terms *career nursing* and *career nurses* to refer to nurses with advanced academic degrees who work full-time, frequently in administration, teaching, research, or advanced practice. Those who use these terms distinguish career nurses from nurses who have not pursued advanced education and who choose part-time employment in order to participate more actively with their children and in family and community life. This use of the term *career nursing* is unfortunate because it implies that only nurses who are employed full-time in leadership or other more autonomous capacities and have graduate degrees can have nursing careers.

The beauty and excitement of nursing is that there are many ways to develop a career. Nursing careers and career opportunities for nurses proliferate in many more forms than the more limited definition of career nursing suggests. A career is not necessarily a full-time pursuit. In addition, many of the experiences gained in child rearing and community service influence nurses to explore new career paths. New paths do not necessarily require graduate education or full-time involvement.

Job-Morphing

Job-morphing is the practice of rapidly adjusting one's work skills. Picture yourself as an amoebae engulfing and incorporating new skills while constantly changing your shape to fit new, attractive opportunities.

You may job-morph to a new job in your organization, a new organization, self employment, or an entirely new career. In these fast-paced times, getting stuck in a rut is hazardous. "Ruts are secure, but they reinforce weaknesses, as well as strengths. Changing employers might amount to finding the same rut in another organization. Changing careers eliminates the rut" (Kanter, 1995).

Career-Diversity Training

Career-diversity training is another version of multiskilling. One example can be found at the Managed Care College for specialist physicians at Rush-Presbyterian-St. Luke's Medical Center in Chicago, Illinois. The program retools specialty physicians for practice in primary care and in the managed care environment. Physicians, too, are facing new challenges and must look at their careers in new ways. Some medical schools, in fact, are conducting career symposia to assist students in this regard (Schreuder, 1996).

Expect to see more and more opportunities for nurses to retool. Both critical care and long-term care nurses are learning one anothers' skills to practice in subacute care.

Develop your own personalized, self-directed career-diversity training. Or, if you're educationally inclined or thinking of developing a business, you may find a market for career-diversity training programs and consultations.

STRATEGIES FOR SUCCESS

As you embark on your career-development journey, keep in mind the following ten strategies for success.

Discover Problems

When you discover a problem, you discover a potential job. Look for problems to solve in the news you read. The news may have more to offer your career than do the job advertisements. Be ahead of job growth predictions because "the prediction of the week comes too late for the job of the lifetime" (Jackson, 1991, p. 63).

For example, can you identify problems related to the increase in the elderly population? The United States has nine million more people over sixty-five years of age than Canada has people. Sixteen to eighteen million people in the United States are more than eighty-five years old (Curtin, 1995). An Institute of Medicine committee recently recommended that Congress require twenty-four-hour RN coverage in long-term care facilities by the year 2000. Are there services or products you'd like to design and provide to address these needs?

What problems lie in other trends such as the AIDS epidemic, emphasis on wellness, self care, alternative medicine, nutrition, and psychobiotics? Did you ever think about nursing in space? A 1995 conference held in Hampton,

Virginia, and hosted by North Carolina Central University explored the concept of space nurse practitioner.

Begin your search for problems close to home. What is not getting done in your department? Can you turn that need into an assignment that will help secure your job or even lead to a new career direction?

Assume the Role of Engineer of Your Career (Forman, 1995)

Look for work that will satisfy your most important needs, whether those needs be personal or professional. In today's environment, most leadership positions carry "face time" expectations—that is you must be visible and physically present on the job much of the time. This requirement may not suit you if your important needs include spending more time with your children. In fact, some suggest that this factor limits promotion of women to the executive level as much as does the "glass ceiling." Women may choose not to pursue promotions if the requirements of the job conflict with other important needs.

Within an organization, continually look for the "right work" to do. Be sure to direct your efforts toward organizational priorities. To shelter yourself from layoff, ensure that both your performance and your attitude demonstrate commitment.

Always be ready to pursue new opportunities wherever you discover them by, among other things, annually updating of your résumé.

Develop resilience. Be ready to flex in response to changing circumstances. Develop self-sufficiency by preparing to take the next step. Shape your work to showcase your strengths. Most importantly, take care of yourself physically and emotionally so that you can respond to challenges and opportunities.

Generate Jobs That Blend Your Skills and Interests

Jackson (1991) recommends that you list your ten best-developed skills and your ten most attractive interests, and then use these lists to create a matrix similar to the one in Figure 17-1. At each intersection of a skill and

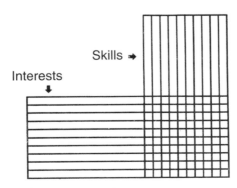

Figure 17.1 Skills and interests matrix

interest—that is, for each combination of skill and interest—invent or recall two or three possible jobs that blend that skill and interest.

Shift Your Paradigm from Loyalty to Professionalism

Neither expect unconditional loyalty from your employer nor offer unconditional loyalty to your employer. Take responsibility for continually growing in your profession and finding the best situation for you to practice.

Learn to Promote Yourself

Prepare factual statements about your contributions to your organization's goals. Be as specific and quantitative as possible. Acknowledging and crediting the work of others strengthens the credibility of your statements and your contributions. Translate your past experiences into contributions to the organization instead of position titles or personal achievements.

Admire a Job

When you find yourself admiring a job, ask yourself, "What do I need to know to do that job?" Career consultant and author Robin Ryan advises to develop two new skills every year (Hansen, 1995). Some admirable jobs are truly one of a kind, such as being a Walt Disney World nurse. One nurse who holds that position today identified her interest four years ago while vacationing at the Disney resort. Although she continued to work in other jobs, she kept her dream alive. Then, twenty-three years into a diverse nursing career that included, among other things, military service, she landed her dream job (Kauffold, 1996).

Peruse Online Resources

Access online bulletin boards and services, such as the America Online Career Center. Study the guides for using online career resources, such as *The Electronic Job Search Revolution* (Kennedy & Morrow, 1994). And look at NurseNet.

Take a Piece of What You Want

To enter the organization or specialty of your dreams, you may need to compromise. It is important, however, not to be seduced by offers that don't fit your career vision. The key is knowing your personal priorities.

Students are wise to work as nurse externs, technicians, unit secretaries or other job positions that they can later cite as evidence of health care experience—especially in organizations where they hope to obtain their first RN positions.

If your career vision is practice in a particular specialty, you may decide to compromise on work location, benefits, salary, or schedule to obtain experience in that specialty. If you continually clarify your, career vision, you will be less likely to let features of lesser importance seduce you.

Investigate Internships—Not for New Grads Only!

Tap local and regional resources to uncover potential internships. Don't wait to see internships advertised. Contact organizations of interest, and ask whether they offer internship programs. If they do not, propose an intern experience based on your career-development goals.

The National Society for Experiential Education in Raleigh, North Carolina, publishes *The National Directory of Internships*. More than one-half of the entries in the 1994/1995 edition sought midcareer professionals as well as college students and recent graduates.

Plan a Winning Interview Follow-up

During any job interview, find out about some of the problems facing the unit or department to which you are applying. After the interview, think about how someone in the position for which you are applying could contribute to solving these problems. Ask yourself what *you* will do to address those problems if you get the job. If you haven't heard from the interviewing organization within one or two weeks of the interview, follow up with a call to the interviewer, hopefully your prospective boss. During this call, describe your ideas for how you will address present priorities.

IF YOU'RE A NEW GRADUATE

"How am I supposed to get experience if no one will hire me without experience?" Many new graduates express frustration because employers are looking for experienced applicants. Employers favor candidates who have demonstrated reliability and performance on the job—especially when skills used in previous employment apply to the position sought.

Look for part-time employment opportunities in hospitals and health care organizations while you're still in school. Don't restrict yourself to nursing assistant or nurse extern positions. Experience as a unit secretary or a patient transporter, or in any number of capacities will prove valuable, especially if you can find employment in the facility where you hope to begin practicing as an RN. Ask the nurse recruiter or employment specialist in the human resources department for suggestions. Although a hospital job may not pay as well as some other part-time work in your community, settling for a lower part-time wage now may prove a wise investment in your future.

Package your past to highlight relevant abilities and accomplishments. Maybe you managed money or resources, or coordinated events as an officer or committee chairperson in a club or other volunteer organization. Although not paid work, accomplishments in such roles translate into job qualifications. Rather than simply listing the office or the purpose of the office, explain the things you *did* in the office. Furthermore, did you finance your own education? Have you cared for children or ill or elderly family members, or coordinated such care arrangements? Employers may find such experiences relevant.

Exhaust the job placement resources of your school. Look beyond the usual placement and counseling services. School of nursing alumni may have information about where alumni are working. You might then contact specific individuals to learn more about opportunities in particular fields or specialties.

IF YOUR JOB HAS BEEN ELIMINATED

Although layoff is certainly a dreadful experience, many who have experienced it say that after the initial shock and numbness, they actually began to feel relief (Powers & Russell, 1993). When the threat of layoff became a reality, energies consumed by anxiety about the threat and feelings about employer disloyalty were freed for more constructive uses.

Most people feel a need to personally regroup immediately after layoff. It is wise to use this time to let reality sink in and to take stock of preferences, strengths, weaknesses, and potential next steps.

After you've regrouped, you have a job: to get a job. Imagine broader possibilities than finding a job that is exactly like the one you just left. You may need to do some homework—through reading, networking, or volunteer work—to educate yourself about new fields and possibilities.

Many people have emerged from the layoff experience to redirect their careers. And many of these individuals say that as unpleasant as layoff was, they might never have looked for or found new and more satisfying paths had they not been laid off.

IF YOU'VE BEEN OUT OF NURSING FOR A WHILE

If you haven't been practicing nursing, you've been doing something else. You've added other experiences to your nursing preparation, such as child rearing, community service, volunteer work, or employment in another field. Whatever you've been doing, make it count to help you reenter nursing. You must package your past to highlight relevant abilities and accomplishments, just as the new graduate does. The good news is that you have much more past to package than does the new graduate.

Think about the skills you've used and the experiences you've gained, and emphasize these in your communications with potential employers. Find out exactly what competencies are required in the jobs in which you are interested. Most employers must specify competencies for all positions in order to satisfy accreditation requirements. Find out what, if any, orientation, education, and training the employer will supply to assist you in gaining the competencies you lack. If the employer supplies none, ask the employer for recommendations regarding where to obtain such assistance. Also, find out whether local community colleges offer refresher or postgraduate courses.

MORE PATHS TO EXPLORE

Following are ten fields of opportunity not discussed in previous chapters. Have you thought of more as you've reflected on your own skills, interests, and preferences?

Subacute Care

The growth in subacute care creates the need for the nurse who wants to develop a hybrid skill set of extended care and critical care nursing skills. Nurses coming from either specialty have succeeded in making this transition. In the subacute care specialty, nurses exercise a great deal of independent problem solving. "What matters most is an attitude—a willingness to provide patient-centered care and to involve the family in virtually every aspect of treatment" (Andreola & Pauly-O'Neill, 1995). The American Subacute Care Nurses Association in North Bay Village, Florida, can supply further information.

OR First Assistant and OR First Assistant, C-Section

Some hospitals have developed training programs to prepare OR nurses for the expanded roles of OR first assistant or OR first assistant, C-section. Check regional continuing education offerings for programs, or contact the Association of Operating Room Nurses (AORN) for further information.

Forensic Nursing

The new and evolving specialty of forensic nursing encompasses providing care to victims of crime, collecting evidence, and providing health care services within the prison system. The International Association of Forensic Nurses (telephone 609-848-8356) can provide further information.

Organizational Restructuring Outcomes Evaluation

Although restructuring of hospital organizations and patient care is sweeping the country, only limited information about the effects of restructuring has been generated. The future will thus see increased emphasis placed on evaluating the effects of restructuring on the quality and safety of patient care and outcomes, and on the quality of patient and caregiver satisfaction. This need for evaluation will result in many opportunities for nurses, whether as assignments within current jobs, ongoing projects in quality management departments, evaluation plan developers, or entrepreneurial consultants in quality and outcome evaluation.

Temporary Services

Most organizations are reducing the ranks of management and exploring ways to reduce operating expenses. Organizations find economies in outsourcing. What services are health care organizations eliminating or curtailing? How could you provide some of these services on a contract basis, either as a single contractor or in collaboration with others?

Family-Friendly Employment Policy Development and Administration

Some organizations are developing policies and practices that allow workers to fulfill parenting and family obligations without sacrificing advancement opportunities at work. Not all businesses are pursuing this course of action, however. Downsizing has placed many workers in the employment pool, and with the resulting increased competition for jobs, companies can locate candidates who are willing to work long hours without accommodations for family responsibilities. Nevertheless, some companies are initiating family-friendly practices. Nurses with an interest in human resource development might offer unique contributions to the human resource departments in such organizations.

Politics

Nurses can contribute much to the political arena. Nurse lobbyists work for nursing and health-related concerns. Nurses have won election to public office. President Clinton appointed a nurse to serve as the first AIDS czar. Because public interest in health issues is running high, political involvement by nurses is timely. Contact your state nurses association for information about political involvement.

Writing

With the increasing interest in self-care and health issues, opportunities abound for nurses to write for the general public, whether in local or regional newspapers, magazines, or newsletters. Contact such publications directly to learn how to submit an article.

Growing numbers of nursing-focused newsletters and newspaper sections create professional writing opportunities. Your regional *Nursing Spectrum* welcomes inquiries from new authors. Editors of nursing journals and book publishing companies are constantly looking for new ideas and new authors. Journals include information for prospective authors in every issue. You will increase your chances of success by proposing your idea to an editor and getting some feedback about developing your idea into an article for a specific journal. When selecting a journal, paying attention to the audience and purpose of the journal will both help you find the most appropriate journal for your article and increase the chances of your work accepted for publication.

One nurse began a company that publishes children's books. Her first book grew out of stories she crafted for her children to teach them about fire safety in their home (Kapinos, 1996).

Writing and publishing do not generally prove financially lucrative, especially initially. At first, your only reward may be seeing your work in print. However, one publication experience tends to lead to others, and certainly creates networking opportunities. If you like to write, investigate opportunities both in popular and professional publications. If you like reporting and public speaking, you might consider preparing yourself for a career as a radio or television health reporter. A full-time career in writing or reporting requires additional education and training.

Environmental Opportunities

In recent years, the environmental protection movement has grown. Governmental agencies and local health departments can provide further information about this growing field. Some college and universities (such as Illinois Institute of Technology, Cornell University, Yale University, and Duke University) have developed environmental management graduate programs, which combine studies in law, engineering, and management.

Entrepreneurship/Intrapreneurship

Chapter 13 focuses on the role of the nurse entrepreneur. The entrepreneurial attitude can be vital to success in today's work world. As corporations have downsized, former corporate employees have developed businesses to perform services for corporations. Interestingly, today women are starting businesses at a rate three times that of men. (Kleiman, 1995). For example, two California nurses created a business to rent breast pumps, provide counseling services, sell maternity and baby products, and offer maternal-child health classes. The business, named Pump Station, also provides services to businesses who want to support and assist their employees who are new mothers (Applegate, 1995). You might develop business ventures to take advantage of opportunities suggested in this book.

If you do not want to develop a business as your major means of support, limited freelance or contract employment in some areas of interest could serve to complement your primary job. Or you might develop a business unit within your current organization. Such business units, called intrapreneurships, can take many forms such as a nurse-run clinic, continuing-education center, or a service offering nontraditional therapies as adjuncts to medical treatments.

Experts advise that to succeed in today's workplace, employees must approach their work with entrepreneurial spirit—that is, they must take responsibility for their contributions to their organizations, manage their own productivity, and continually develop new skills to enhance their value. Maintain an interdependence with your employer. Fully commit to your work, to professional development, and to organizational contribution. At the same time, be alert for and open to other opportunities, other places to apply your skills, and changes in your organization that may signal the need to make a change.

SUMMARY

This chapter cited several additional facts about nursing today and highlighted some important approaches to and aspects of career development. Now, you're ready to take off with your career.

Think of your career as a journey, not a destination. As your journey unfolds, you will explore many routes and courses. If you stay alert for and act on signals of the need to adjust your course, you can find success, joy, and satisfaction. Bon voyage!

REFERENCES

Alderman, L. (1995, July 24). Casting call—Starting out or starting over? Get a line on a new job. *Chicago Tribune.*

Andreola, N. M. & Pauly-O'Neill, S. (1995, February 6). Jumping on the subacute care bandwagon. *Nursing Spectrum Greater Chicago/NE Illinois and NW Indiana Edition, 8*(3).

Applegate, J. (1995, November 1). Nurses turn talents to small businesses. *Chicago Sun Times.*

Brown, M. (1995). *Landing on your feet: An inspirational guide to surviving, coping and prospering from job loss.* New York: McGraw-Hill Ryerson.

Chicago Tribute Staff. (1996, January 19). Presence of RNs recommended for nursing homes. *Chicago Tribune.*

Curtin, L. (1995, October 15). Address to Chicago District, Illinois Nurses Association, Chicago, IL.

Forman, H. (1995, January 23). Tact, craft and ingenuity. *Nursing Spectrum Greater Chicago/NE Illinois and NW Indiana Edition, 8*(2)

Hansen, C. (1995, March 12). Working smart. How to ensure job security? Build career self-reliance. *Chicago Tribune.*

Jackson, T. (1991). *Guerrilla tactics in the new job market.* New York: Bantam Books.

Kanter, R. M. (1995). *World class: Thriving locally in the global economy.* New York: Simon and Schuster.

Kapinos, T. (1996, January 10). Nurses as entrepreneurs. *Chicago Tribune.*

Kauffold, M. D. (1996, January 10). First Person: Nursing in the magic kingdom. *Chicago Tribune.*

Kaye, S., Butler, S., & Fisher, J. (1995, March 13). It doesn't pay much now—But just wait. *US News and World Report.*

Kennedy, J. L., & Morrow, T. J. (1994). *The electronic job search revolution.* New York: Wiley Publishers.

Kleiman, C. (1995, January 19). Women execs say they're aliens in the corporate world. *Chicago Tribune.*

Moses, E. B. (1994). *1992 The registered nurse population.* Washington, DC: U.S. Department of Health and Human Services.

Pauly-O'Neill, S., & Andreola, N. M. (1995, April 3). The restructuring phenomenon: Creative deconstruction in action. *Nursing Spectrum Greater Chicago/NE Illinois and NW Indiana Edition, 8*(8).

Pedersen, L. (1993). *Street smart career guide.* New York: Crown Publishers, Inc.

Peller, M. (1995). *Crisis proof your career: A planning guide for job security and satisfaction in the 90s.* Berkeley, CA: Berkeley Press.

Powers, P., & Russell, D. (1993). *Love your job!* Sebastopol, CA: O'Reilly and Associates, Inc.

Schreuder, C. (1996, January 26). Even medical students have career anxiety now. *Chicago Tribune.*

Sullivan, B. (1995, February 12). Nurses on the front lines as hospitals restructure. *Chicago Tribune.*

Index

Note: Page numbers in **bold type** reference non-text material.

A

AACN (American Association of Colleges of Nursing), 327

AAIN (American Association of Industrial Nurses), 237-38

AANP (American Academy of Nurse Practitioners), 162

AAOHN (American Association of Occupational Health Nurses), 148, 237-38

ABOHN (American Board of Occupational Health Nursing, Inc.), 238

ADA (Americans With Disabilities Act), 245, 246

Adult
learning principles, 323-24
nurse practitioner, 163

Advanced practice nurses, 13-14
acceptance of, 174-75
accreditation of, 174
legal issues concerning, 173-74
reimbursement of, 172-73

resources for, 175

Advocacy/control assessment scale, case management, **254**

African-American women, in the work force, 6

Agency for Health Care Policy and Research (AHCPR), 302

AHCCCS (Arizona Health Care Cost Containment Service), 144-45

AHCPR (Agency for Health Care Policy and Research), 302

AHEHP (Association of Hospital Employee Health Professionals), 238

American Academy of Nurse Practitioners (AANP), 162

American Association of Colleges of Nursing (AACN), 327

American Association of Industrial Nurses (AAIN), 237-38

American Association of Occupational Health Nurses (AAOHN), 148, 237-38

American Board of Occupational Health Nursing, Inc. (ABOHN), 238

American Health Consultants, 239

American Nurses Association (ANA), 238

American Nurses Credentialing Center
(ANCC), 115
Americans With Disabilities Act (ADA),
245, 246
ANA (American Nurses Association), 238
ANCC (American Nurses Credentialing
Center), 115
AOHP (Association of Occupational Health
Professionals), 238-39
Arizona Health Care Cost Containment
Service (AHCCCS), Carondelet's pro-
grams and, 144-45
Assessment, nurse case management and,
154-55
Association of Hospital Employee Health
Professionals (AHEHP), 238
Association of Occupational Health
Professionals (AOHP), 238-39
Attitudes
helpful, 45-47
negative, ignoring, 46
Attorneys, 291
nurse, 295-97
Awareness
career opportunities and, 47
developing, 54-55

B
Berrone, Nan, case management axioms by,
253-54
Bridges, William, on "de-jobbing" trend, 6
Brookfield, Stephen, on mistakes, 53
Bureau of Labor Statistics
health care occupations, 14
on job market growth, 5
Business skills, importance of, 49-50

C
Care
continuity of,
home health care and, 221
promoting, 155
Career
attitudes, helpful, 45-47
change,
awareness and, 47, 54-55
hindrances to, 51-52
motivators, 44-45
preparation for, self-directed, **47-48**
self-confidence and, 53-54
sources of help, 45-51

defined, 37
developing, **36**
myths about, 39-41
nurse,
anesthetists, 168
midwife, 170-71
practitioners, 165-66
nursing, 342
opportunities, 40-41, 78
seizing, 9-16
path, 38-39
myth about, 41
resources for, 24-25
satisfaction, finding greater, 73-75
setbacks, preparing for, 46
sources of help, 45-51
strategies, 17-26
assess yourself, 19-20
increase your value, 18-19
interview preparation, 22-23
interviewing, 69-73
network, 20-21
résumé maximization, 22
search organization, 21-22
success, 343-46
wants/needs and, 41-44
see also Employment; Job
Career management
form, exercise skills application, 78-79
interviewing, 69-73
advanced, 71-73
basic, 69-71
locating information, 61
market assessment and, 60-61
networking and, 61-62
résumé and, 66-69
self-assessment and, 62-65
methods of, 63-65
Career paths
linear, 89-90
linear-nonlinear continuum, 92-97
moving on the, 97
questions concerning, 93-97
nonlinear, 90-92
shift toward, 91-92
Carondelet
Arizona Health Care Cost Containment
Service (AHCCCS) and, 144-45
St. Joseph Hospital, case management at,
136-38, 144-45
St. Mary's, 151

Case management
  advocacy/control assessment scale, **254**
  axioms, 253-54
  beginning of, 241-42
  client/clientele served, **237**
  clinical nurse specialist and, 182-83
  finding/marketing, 156-57
  future of, 256-57
  level actions, **255**
  managed care, 133-34
  models,
    clinical, 136-41
    community, 151-53
    payer-based, 141-42
    program, 143-51
    varied practice, 196
  need for, 253-56
  nurse manager, attributes of, 153-56
  opportunities in, 135
  process of, 135
  professional/certification associations
    for, 239
  relationship with other subspecialties,
    239-42
  resources for, 157-58
Case Management Society of America
  (CMSA), 239
CDC (Centers for Disease Control), 302
Centers for Disease Control (CDC), 302
Certified Employee Health Nurse (COHN),
  239
Certified registered nurse anesthetists
  (CRNAs), 166
Change
  adjusting to, 4
  career, self-directed preparation for, **47-48**
  entrepreneurial nursing/nurses and, 267
  tends indicating, 4-9
Client
  education, clinical nurse specialist and,
    185
  home health care and, 220-21
  honoring choices of, 153-54
Clinical
  care, prevention levels, 249
  case management model, 136-41
  nurse specialist,
    as career choice, 197-99
    as clinician, 181-84
    as consultant, 186-87
    as educator, 184-86

  leadership and, 191
  learning about, 196-97
  as manager, 189-90
  models, varied practice, 196
  overview of, 180-81
  practice models, 191-95
  as researcher, 187-89
  in a staff position, 190-91
Clinicians
  clinical nurse specialist as, 181-84
  decision making model, **252**
  in primary care, 250
  in secondary care, 250
  in tertiary care, 250-52
CM. *See* Case management
CMSA (Case Management Society of
  America (CMSA), 239
CNS. *See* Clinical nurse specialist
COHN (Certified Employee Health
  Nurse), 239
Collaboration, redesigned organizations
  and, 124-25
Communications
  entrepreneurial nursing/nurses and,
    266-67
  importance of, 49
  nurses and, 106-10
  therapeutic, described, 121
Community
  case management model, 151-53
  education,
    clinical nurse specialist as, 185
    home health care and, 229-30
  educator, 334-35
Computerized Patient Record Institute
  (CPRI), 107
Computers
  future of, 109-10
  nurses and, 107
    as programmers, 110-12
  opportunities with, 108-9
    preparation/characteristics of, 109
Consultant
  clinical nurse specialist as, 186-87
  entrepreneurial nursing/nurses, 284-85
  nurse legal, 290-95
    qualifications, 291-92
Continuing-education specialist, 333-34
Cost-consciousness, redesigned organizations and, 125-26
Courage, career and, 45

Cover letter
  résumé, 68-69
  sample, 86
Covey, Stephen
  First Things First, 216
  **The Seven Habits of Highly Effective
    People**, 216, 264
CPRI (Computerized Patient Record
    Institute), 107
Creativity, nonlinear thinking techniques,
    100-103
Creighton, Helen, **Law Every Nurse
    Should Know**, 297
Critical thinking, described, 120-21
CRNAs (Certified registered nurse anes-
    thetists), 166
Cross-diversity training, 343
Cross-training, cost consciousness and, 125
C-section, first assistant, 348
Curriculum vitae (CV)
  cover letter, 68-69
    sample, 86
  job management and, 66-69
  maximizing, 22, 66-68

D

Debtors, importance of, 50
Decision making model, clinicians, **252**
Department of Labor, 245, 247-48
Diagnostic related grouping (DRG), 134
Disability syndrome, 254
  The Diseases of Workmen, 240
Downsizing
  education departments, 260
  experience of, 7
DRG (Diagnostic related grouping), 134

E

Economic trends, 4-9, 318-20
Education
  community,
    clinical nurse specialist and, 285
    home health care and, 229-30
  departments, downsizing of, 260
  management track and, 210-12
  nurse,
    anesthetists, 166-67
    midwife, 169-70
    practitioners, 163-64
  nursing, 39-40
    informatics and, 115-16

process, 320-23
  adult learning principles, 323-24
  establishing objectives, 321
  evaluation of, 322-23
  learning needs/resources assessment,
    320-21
Educator
  attributes/qualifications of, 324-26
  clinical nurse specialist as, 184-86
  role of, 317-38
    continuing-education specialist, 333-34
    differences among, 326-35
    nursing faculty, 327-29
    staff-development specialist, 329-31
EEOC (Equal Employment Opportunity
    Commission), 245, 246-47
Egan, Gerald, on change, 4
EHN. *See* Employee health nurse
The Electronic Job Search Revolution, 345
Employee health nurse
  client/clientele served, **237**
  future of, 256-57
  occupational health nurse compared,
    legal/regulatory responsibilities, 245-48
    roles/responsibilities of, 248-52
    setting/program influences, 242
    special skill requirements, 242-45
  professional/certification associations
    for, 238-39
  relationship with other subspecialties,
    239-42
Employment market,
  assessing, 60-61
  nurse practitioners, 165-66
  see also Career; Job
  nurse
    anesthetists, 168
    midwife, 169-70
  success strategies for, 343-46
  see also Career; Job
  Encyclopedia of Natural Science, 240
Entrepreneurial nursing/nurses, 259-88,
    350-51
  business owners and, 284
  characteristics of, 263
  concerns in, 286-87
  consultants, 284-85
  continuing education and, 283
  defining, 260-63
  as educators, 282-84
  getting started, 268-80

interaction/collaboration, 281-85
private or collaborative practices, 281-82
qualities favoring, 265-68
resource information, 287
staff development educators, 283
student nurses and, 283
working in, 263-68
Environmental opportunities for nurses, 350
Equal Employment Opportunity
Commission (EEOC), 245, 246-47
Ethos, entrepreneurial nursing/nurses and,
267-68
Experience, taking inventory of, 98
Expert witness, witnessing as, 291

F
Family
educator, 334-35
importance of, 50
nurse practitioner, 163
FDA (Food and Drug Administration), 302
Federal civil service system, 299, 304-5
qualifications for, **307**
Feldman, Harriet R., on MBA/MPA pro-
grams, 211-12
First Things First, 216
Flowerdaye, Phillipa, occupational health
nursing and, 240
Food and Drug Administration (FDA), 302
Forensic nurse, 348

G
Gerontological nurse Practitioners, 163
Gladstone Family Nursing Center, 13
Glass ceiling, 5
Goals, satisfying, 3
Grove, Andy, on communicating with
employees, 6

H
HCFA (Health Care Finance
Administration), 134
Health care
challenges facing, 134
occupations, 14
trends in, 7-9, 318-20
Health Care Finance Administration
(HCFA), 134
Health care industry
management, success in, 212-17
management competencies in, 204-9

acquiring, 208-9
new, 207-8
reengineered environment, 206-7
traditional, 205-6
professional growth opportunities, 209
Health Level Seven (HL-7), 107
Health maintenance organizations
(HMO's), 134
Health Resources and Services
Administration (HRSA), 302
Help, sources of, 45-51
Helpful skills, 49-45
HL-7 (Health Level Seven), 107
HMO's (Health maintenance
organizations), 134
Hobbies, taking inventory of, 98-99
Holistic focus, maintaining, 155
Home care nurse, client/clientele
served, **237**
Home health care
agencies,
hospital based, 228-29
private and, 228
proprietary and, 228
public and, 228
community education and, 229-30
environment in, 222
growth of, 220-22
hospital versus, 222-26
assessment/improvisation and, 222-23
autonomy/flexibility and, 225
communication and, 225
documentation and, 225-26
interdisciplinary collaboration and,
224-25
ongoing learning and, 226
technology and, 223-24
work schedule, 223
Home health care (continued)
nurse, clients served, **237**
nursing process, 231-32
nursing roles/variations in, 226-31
agency ownership and, 227-29
agency size and, 226-27
community and, 227
qualifications for, 232-33
Visiting Nurse Association and, 228
Hospital
home health care versus, 222-26
assessment/improvisation and, 222-23
autonomy/flexibility and, 225

communication and, 22
documentation and, 225-26
interdisciplinary collaboration and, 224-25
ongoing learning and, 226
technology and, 223-24
work schedule, 223
liaison nurse/admission planner, 230
HRSA (Health Resources and Services
Administration), 302

I
Industrial health nurse. *See* Occupational
health nurse
Industrial medicine, beginning of, 240
Industrial tends, 4-9
Information
locating, 61
systems,
changing roles in, 106-7
characteristics of, 109
future of, 109-10
nurses as programmers in, 110-12
opportunities in, 108-9
preparations for, 109
Institute for Nurse Executives, 203
on management competencies, 207
Interests, taking inventory of, 98-99
Internet
information and, 107
nursing and, 116-17
Interpersonal skills, importance of, 49
Interviewing
career management, 69-73
advanced, 71-73
basic, 69-71
job, preparing for, 22-23
Intrapreneurship, 350-51
Introduction to Nursing Informatics, 116

J
JCAHO (Joint Commission on
Accreditation of Healthcare
Organizations), 308
Jeremiah Coleman Company, occupational
health nursing and, 240
Job
changing, 40
market assessment, 60-61
growth in, 5
nurse,

anesthetists, 168
midwife, 170-71
practitioners, 165-66
redefining, 10
search, organizing, 21-22
wants/needs and, 41-44
see also Career; Employment
Job change
awareness and, 47, 54-55
help sources, 45-51
hindrances to, 51-52
motivators, 44-45
preparation for, self-directed, **47-48**
self-confidence and, 53-54
Job management
interviewing and, 69-73
advanced, 73-75
basic, 69-71
preparing for, 22-23
locating information, 61
market assessment and, 60-61
networking and, 61-62
résumé and, 66-69
self-assessment and, 62-65
methods of, 63-65
Job shift, 6
Job-morphing, described, 342-43
**Joint Commission for Accreditation of
Health Care Organizations
(JCAHO) Standards for Home
Health Care Accreditation**, 221
Joint Commission on Accreditation of
Healthcare Organizations (JCAHO),
308
Judgment, entrepreneurial nursing/nurses
and, 265-66

K
A Kick in the Seat of the Pants, 102

Kleiman, Carol, on careers, 37

L
Law, 289-98
nurse legal consultant and, 290-95
nurse legal consultants and, qualifications,
291-92
Law Every Nurse Should Know, 297
Lawyers, 291
nurse, 295-97
Layoff experience, 7

Leadership
  clinical nurse specialist and, 191
  in management, 215
  self understanding and, 216-17
Learning
  love of, 46-47
  needs, assessing, 320-21
Lerche, Renee, on women in business, 5-6
Level actions, case management, **255**
Liaison nurse/admission planner, 230
Lienhard School of Nursing, 203
Linear
  career paths, 89-90
  nonlinear continuum,
    finding your place in, 92-97
    questions, 93-97
    moving on the, 97
  see also Nonlinear
Loyola University, Advanced Practice
    Trauma/Critical Care Nursing pro-
    gram, 13

M
Managed care, 133-34
  home health care and, 221
Management
  competencies in, 204-9
    acquiring, 208-9
    new, 207-8
    reengineered environment and, 206-7
    traditional, 205-6
  success in, 212-17
    finding a mentor, 214-15
    leadership and, 215
    mentoring, 214
    self understanding and, 216-17
  track, self-assessment for, 209-12
Manager, clinical nurse specialist as, 189-90
Mans, Rosemary, 6
Marketing, nurse case management, 156-57
MBA/MPA, management and, 211-12
McGarvah, Eleanor, first nurse attorney,
    296
Medical records, 290-91
  reviewing, negligence cases and, 290
Medicare, home health care and, 220
Medicare Conditions of Participation, 221
Medicare Prospective Payment System, 220
Mentoring, 214
Mentors
  finding, 214-15

importance of, 50
Midwife nurse, 169-72
  educational preparation for, 169-70
  employment opportunities/compensation,
    170-71
  personal requirement for, 170
  working relationships of, 170
Military nursing, 300-302
  qualifications for, **307**
Mistakes, as learning opportunities, 53
Models
  case management,
    clinical, 136-41
    community, 151-53
    payer-based, 141-42
    program, 143-51
  clinical nurse specialist, 191-95
  clinicians decision making, **252**
Mommy track, 5
Monitoring, nurse case management and,
    154-55
Motivators, career, 44-45
Moulder, Betty, occupational health nursing
    and, 240
Multiskilling, redesigned organizations and,
    124-25
Myers-Briggs Type Indicator, 64
Myths, career, 39-41

N
National League of Nursing (NLN), 116,
    238
National Organization of Public Health
    Nursing (NOPHN), 237
Needs
  knowing, 41-44
  satisfying, 3
Negative attitudes, ignoring, 46
Negligence cases, medical record review and,
    290
Network, identifying your, 99
Networking
  career and, 20-21
  career management and, 61-62
The New Quick Job-Hunting Map, 64
New England Medical Center, case manage-
    ment at, 136
Newborn, intensive care, case management
    program model and, 144
NLN (National League of Nursing),
    116, 238

Nonlinear
  career paths, 90-92
    shift toward, 91-92
  thinking, 87
    preparing for, 98-100
    techniques, 100-103
  see also Linear
NOPHN (National Organization of Public
    Health Nursing), 237
Nurse
  attorney, 295-97
  career myths about, 39-41
  as case managers, attributes of, 153-56
  as communicators, 106-10
  forensic, 348
  future and, 340-42
  job opportunities, 9-16
    advanced practice preparation and, 13-14
    growth in, 5
    redefining job, 10
    specializing and, 11-13
  managed care and, 133-34
  new graduate, 346-47
  OR first assistant, 348
  as programmers, 110-11
    future of, 112
    preparation/characteristics of, 112
  public perception of, 16-17
  redesigned organizations and, implications
    for, 120-26
  returning, 347-48
  as risk manager, 292-94
  subacute care, 348
  success strategies for, 343-46
  as vendor representatives, 112-14
    future of, 114
    preparation/characteristics of, 114
Nurse anesthetists, 166-69
  educational preparation for, 166-67
  employment opportunities/compensation,
    168
  personal requirements of, 167
  working relationships of, 167-68
Nurse legal consultant, 290-95
  qualifications, 291-92
Nurse midwife, 169-72
  educational preparation of, 169-70
  employment opportunities/compensation,
    170-71
  opportunities for, 170-71
  personal requirements for, 170

working relationships of, 170
Nurse practitioners, 162-66
  educational preparation for, 163-64
  employment opportunities/compensation,
    165-66
  personal requirements for, 164-65
Nurse risk manager, 292-94
  qualifications, 293-94
Nursing
  career opportunities, 40-41, 78
  internet and, 116-17
  military, 300-302
    qualifications for, **307**
  process, home health care, 231-32
  staff education, clinical nurse specialist
    and, 185
  subspecialties, 236
    professional/certification associations,
      236-39
    relationship between, 239-42
  success strategies for, 343-46
  trends in, 7-9, 318-20
Nursing informatics
  changing roles in, 106-7
  defined, 105-6
  educational preparation and, 115-16
  information resources on, 117
  nurses as,
    communicators, 106-10
    programmers, 110-12
    vendor representatives, 112-14
  opportunities in, 114-15

O
Occupational health, case management and,
    148, **148-50**
Occupational health nurse
  beginning of, 240-41
  client/clientele served, **237**
  employee health nurse compared,
    legal/regulatory responsibilities, 245-48
    roles/responsibilities of, 248-52
    setting/program influences, 242
    special skill requirements, 242-45
  future of, 256-57
  professional/certification associations for,
    237-38
  relationship with other subspecialties,
    239-42
Occupational Safety and Health
    Administration (OSHA), 245

OHN. *See* Occupational health nurse
Operating room first assistant, 348
Optimal resource allocation, 126
Organizing skills, importance of, 49
OSHA (Occupational Safety and Health
    Administration), 245
Outcomes, focus on, 123-24

P
Parent educator, 334-35
Parish nurse, client/clientele served, **237**
Patient-care centered redesigned organiza-
    tions, 121-23
Payer
  based case management model, 141-42
  satisfaction, home health care and, 220-21
Pediatric nurse practitioners, 163
Pediatrics, case management program model
    and, 143, **145-47**
Peers, importance of, 50
Perinatal, case management program model
    and, 143, 1**45-47**
Perseverance, career and, 46
Personal life, enhancing, 74-75
Pew Health Professions Commission, on
    educator positions, 319
PHO (Physician hospital organization), 134
Physician hospital organization (PHO), 134
Political sense, importance of, 49
Politics, nurses and, 349
Prenatal programs, high risk, case manage-
    ment program model and, 144
Prevention levels, clinical care, 249
Private agencies, home health care and, 228
Program case management model, 143-51
Programming
  nurses, preparation/characteristics of, 112
  nurses and, 110-12
    future and, 112
    word processing packages and, **111**
Proprietary agencies, home health care and,
    228
Public agencies, home health care and, 228
Public health
  nurse, client/clientele served, **237**
  service, 302-4
Public sector
  benefits in, 313-14
  colleagues in, 308-10
  geographic variations in, 310-12
  nursing opportunities in, 299-316

  federal civil service system, 304-5
  military nursing, 300-302
  public health service, 302-4
  requirements, 306-8
  resource information, 315

Q
Qualitative methodologies, acceptance of,
    188

R
Ramazzini, Bernardino, **The Diseases of
    Workmen**, 240
Recognition, gaining, 55-56
Redesigned organizations
  characteristics/skills needed in, 126-27
  collaboration/teamwork/multiskilling in,
    124-25
  controversy about, 129-30
  cost-consciousness of, 125-26
  economic forces driven, 119
  focus on outcomes by, 123-24
  information resources about, 130-31
  patient-care centered, 121-23
  registered nurses and, implications for,
    120-26
Registered nurses. *See* Nurses
Rehabilitation Act, 246
Researcher, clinical nurse specialist as,
    187-89
Reserve Officer Training Corps (ROTC), 312
Resource allocation, optimal, 126
Resources
  advanced practice nurses, 175
  career development, 24-25
  case management, 157-58
  entrepreneurial nursing, 287
  nursing information, 117
  optimal resource allocation, 126
  public sector nursing, 315
  redesigned organizations, 130-31
Résumé
  career management and, 66-69
  cover letter, 68-69
    sample, 86
  maximizing, 22, 66-68
  sample,
    advanced skills, 83-84
    basic, 81
Risk manager
  nurse, 292-94
    qualifications, 293-94

Risk-taking, career and, 46
RN's, redesigned organizations and, implications for, 120-26
ROTC (Reserve Officer Training Corps), 312

S

Satisfaction, career, 73-75
Scholar, clinical nurse specialist as, 187-89
School nurse, client/clientele served, **237**
Self-assessment
  career management and, 62-65
    methods of, 63-65
  management track competencies, 209-12
Self-confidence and, 53-54
  job search and, 23-24
Self-enhancement, 74-75
Self-management, planning for, 75-76
Self-understanding, management and, 216-17
Setbacks, career, preparing for, 46
The Seven Habits of Highly Effective People, 216, 264
Shortell, Stephen M., on health care management, 209-10
Skills
  helpful, 49-51
  occupational/employee health nurses and, 248-49
Societal trends, 4-9, 318-20
Software, word processing packages, **111**
Specialty practice, **43-44**
St. Joseph Hospital, case management at, 136-38
Staff
  development,
    educators, 283
    specialist, 330-31
  position, clinical nurse specialist in a, 190-91
Stewart, Ada Mayo, occupational health nursing and, 240-41
Subacute care nurse, 348
Success, strategies for, 343-46

T

Team members, linking care, 156
Teamwork, redesigned organizations and, 124-25
Technology, home health care and, 220

Temporary services, nurses and, 349
Therapeutic communication, described, 121
Thinking
  critical, described, 120-21
  nonlinear, 87
    preparing for, 98-100
    techniques, 100-103
Three Boxes of Life and How to Get Out of Them, 64
Time constraints, minimizing, 156
Trends, 4-9, 318-20

U

U.S. Public Health Service (USPHS), 299
Universal health record, 107
USPHS (U.S. Public Health Service), 299

V

Valenti, William, on effective employee health programs, 239
Vendor representatives
  nurses as, 112-14
  future of, 114
  preparation/characteristics of, 114
Vermont Marble Company, occupational health nursing and, 240-41
Vestal, Katherine, on management competencies, 207
Visiting Nurse Association, Home health care and, 228

W

Wants, knowing, 41-44
A Whack on the Side of the Head, 102
What Color Is Your Parachute?, career management and, 63, 64
Where Do I Go From Here With My Life, 64
Women, in the work force, 6
Word processing packages, **111**
Work
  redesigning viewpoints toward, **127-29**
  skills, taking inventory of, 98
  your feelings about, 98
Work force, job growth in, 5
World Wide Web
  information and, 107
  nursing and, 116-17
Writing, nurses and, 349-5

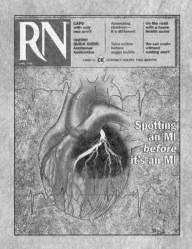
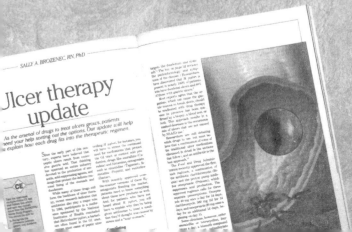